Living *Well* Beyond Breast Cancer

Also by Marisa C. Weiss, M.D.

7 Minutes

Taking Care of Your "Girls"
(co-authored with Isabel Friedman)

Fully Updated Second Edition

Living *Well* Beyond Breast Cancer

A Survivor's Guide for When Treatment Ends and the Rest of Your Life Begins

Marisa C. Weiss, M.D.
Ellen Weiss

THREE RIVERS PRESS · NEW YORK

Published in the United States by Three Rivers Press, an imprint of the Crown Publishing Group, a division of Random House, Inc., New York.
www.crownpublishing.com

Three Rivers Press and the Tugboat design are registered trademarks of Random House, Inc.

Previous editions of this work have been published as *Living Beyond Breast Cancer* by Times Books, a division of Random House, Inc., New York, in 1997, and by Three Rivers Press, an imprint of the Crown Publishing Group, a division of Random House, Inc., New York, in 1998.

Library of Congress Cataloging-in-Publication Data
Weiss, Marisa C.
　[Living beyond breast cancer]
　Living well beyond breast cancer : a survivor's guide for when treatment ends and the rest of your life begins/Marisa C. Weiss, Ellen Weiss.—Fully updated 2nd ed.
　　　p. cm.
　Originally published: Living beyond breast cancer. New York : Times Books, 1997.
　Includes index.
　1. Breast—Cancer—Popular works. 2. Breast—Cancer—Psychological aspects.
　3. Adjustment (Psychology) I. Weiss, Ellen. II. Title.
　RC280.B8W396 2010
　616.99'449—dc22　　　　　　　　2009020648

ISBN 978-0-307-46022-6

Printed in the United States of America

Design by Meryl Sussman Levavi

10 9 8 7 6 5 4 3 2 1

Revised Edition

To Edith and Rosie

Antoinette, Carmen, Kelly, Debbie, Kitty, Ellen, Karen,
and Janelle

Contents

Acknowledgments

We are deeply grateful to the many individuals who infused our book with their extra special blend of expertise, wisdom, spirit, humor, warmth, and compassion. The principal editor of our book, Lindsay Orman, was a pleasure to work with and did an absolutely amazing job. The care and attention and intelligence she brought to her task was beyond anything we could have imagined, or anything other writers we know have experienced. Emily Timberlake guided the book to its launching with thoughtful dedication.

So many voices are heard in this book: the people who shared their stories with us, the patients and their families Marisa has had the privilege of taking care of, and those who have shared our mission. Each person has contributed in a most personal way—eagerly or reluctantly, expansively or cautiously—with honesty and courage and verve—moved by the desire to help others. The book would have fallen flat without the voices of these many good friends. (Most of their names have been changed to protect their privacy.)

We want to acknowledge the diligence, dedication, and unflagging spirit of these many friends—it's impossible to thank them enough. We have also had help from a generous and distinguished group of professionals, and we want to thank them for their invaluable contributions: Zonera Ali, Robert Allen, Jayne Antonowsky, Rachael Brandt, Irene Card, Ned Carp, Carol Cherry, Robin Ciocca, Jan Clark, Martha Denckla, Dianne Dunkelman, Beth DuPree, Brenda Eastham, Barbara Fowble, Kevin Fox, Patricia Ganz, Paul Gilman, Robert Goodman, Generosa Grana, Jennifer Griggs, Barbara Hoffman, Clifford Hudis, Carole Kaplan, Harvey Karp, Rosalind Kleban, Anton Kris, Maria LoTempio, Geralyn Lucas, Cynthia Lufkin, Christina Meyers, Kathy Miller, Lillian Nail, Larry Norton, Kutluk Oktay, Steve Osborne, Edith Perez, Barbara Rabinowitz, Joan Ruderman, Andrea Rugh, Jennifer Sabol, David Sachs,

Romayne Sachs, Andrew Saykin, Mitchell Schnall, Sandra Schnall, Helena Schotland, Leslie Schover, Lynn Schuchter, Joseph Serletti, Gloria Shattil, Lillie Shockney, Robert Smink, Alan Stolier, Margo Weishar, Beverly Whipple, Eric Winer, Anna K. Wolff, and Liza Wu.

We are deeply grateful to our Breastcancer.org friends and Board of Directors: Ray Westphal, Amanda and Conrad Radcliffe, Jenifer and Jeff Westphal, Stevie Lucas, Lisa Kabnick and John McFadden, Peggy and Bruce Earle, Betty Moran, John Chappell, Barbara and Henry Jordan, Marjorie Findlay and Geoffrey Freeman, Sean Rooney, Barbara and Larry Cohen, Jill and Tom Nerney, Noreen Fraser, Patty and Gary Holloway, Aileen and Brian Roberts, Jerry Crowther, Glenn Crowther, Michael Hirschhorn, JoAnn and Joe Thomson, Roz and Chuck Epstein, Sallie and Charlie Grandi, Betty and Phil Harvey, Judy and Michael Mealey, Patty and Brian Holloway, Marge Tabankin, Richard and Maureen Yelovich, Jack Lynch, Elaine Thompson, Sarah Peterson, Erin Dugery, Kathy Schneider, Jessica Laufer, Denise and David Jordan, Sara Vance and Michelle Waddell, Fiona and Lee Yohannon, Lisa Petkun, Eleanor Davis, Shari Foos, Joanne Gillis-Donovan, Richy Glassberg, Sheri Lambert, Christopher Lyons, Jim Monastero, Susan Muck, Nina Montee-Karp, Larry Norton, Debbie and Sam Schwartz, and Hope Wohl. We want to extend a very special thanks to each member of our amazing Breastcancer.org and Lankenau Hospital teams, and to our friends from the Living Beyond Breast Cancer organization.

Always there for support, advice, comfort, care, and feeding, our families patiently endured our neglect and absence as we worked away at this book. Thank you, Elias, Henry, Isabel, and David Friedman, and Leon Weiss—you who waited with such good grace till all this book business was finished and still remembered who we were. Plus a big thanks to our other family champions: Alice, Eve, Nathaniel, Philip, and Stephen Weiss, and Adele Friedman; Aaron, Daniel, Lena and Rob Walker; Cindy Kling; John, Ella and Owen Spencer; Lauren, Sara, and Livia Weiss; Sara Manny, Adam and Ethan Weiss.

And we want to thank each other: for patience and good humor, for holding back and holding on, for drive, energy, and the right word. Close as we are, as mother and daughter, we have a new appreciation for each other's depths and gifts.

Marisa Weiss and Ellen Weiss

Introduction

Living Well Beyond Breast Cancer

Life has thrown you a curve: breast cancer. What do you do with that hit? There is only one you—you are unique, after all—and you have worked so hard to protect your life from the threats and challenges of this disease: subjecting yourself to all manner of tests, procedures, surgery, chemo, radiation, and hormonal therapy, as well as countless medications and then remedies to deal with side effects. You may not have known what was up, down, or coming round the next corner. But here you are: done! It's now time to find your path through recovery to living *well* beyond breast cancer with the best information, solid guidance, new hope, and determination.

Remember, the purpose of all that treatment, all your work, was to give you back your life: joy, fun, comfort, meaning, pleasure, security. And the main reason for writing this book is to help you reclaim, rebuild, and reenergize your life, understanding that you are not alone, as you may have feared.

For sure, you are not alone. In the eleven years since the original publication of this book, the amount of medical information about breast cancer has more than doubled. Almost three million more Americans have joined the ranks of the three million already diagnosed with the disease—and major medical advances have given more and more of these people the chance to live *well* beyond breast cancer.

To make the most of the latest and greatest, you need to be in the know, informed by your link to medical care—your primary care physician. Easier said than done when the average length of a doctor visit has shrunk to seven minutes! So what do you do? Turn to resources available in print, online, wherever.

I wrote this book—together with my mother, Ellen Weiss, a writer and breast cancer survivor—to give you the best medical information and guidance to help you live as long as possible with the best quality of life, and to reassure you that you are not alone. Each page will help you understand the challenges in your path and provide you with many ready-to-use practical solutions to speed your total recovery and reclaim your life.

As a physician specializing in breast cancer for over twenty years, I have had the honor of taking care of thousands of women and men, and their families, facing breast cancer. It wasn't long after I started practicing that I understood the high level of distress that my patients endured on completion of initial treatment. Rather than feeling thrilled to have the breast cancer experience behind them, they were uneasy, often anxious: *What do I do now? Am I really cured? Is it safe for me to get pregnant? Can I take hormones? How do I get rid of extra weight? How do I manage the lingering side effects of treatment? How do I extinguish those horrible hot flashes? How can I stay asleep through the night? What should I tell the man I've just met? How do I deal with the fear of recurrence? What should I be eating, taking, and doing to reduce the risk of recurrence? Does my diagnosis put my daughter at risk?* My patients desperately wanted an intelligent, in-depth, reliable response to their questions as they moved from "I have breast cancer" ahead to "I am leading a normal life."

To provide the best answers to my patients and to countless others beyond the scope of my practice, I started the program Life After Breast Cancer at the University of Pennsylvania twenty-one years ago, then a year later the nonprofit organization Living Beyond Breast Cancer. Both are still thriving today. But to provide a 24/7 resource for medical information for people worldwide, we needed something more. So in 1999, I started the nonprofit organization Breastcancer.org and have worked tirelessly at making it the number one resource in the world for breast health and breast cancer information and the most visited online community for the exchange of personal experience and expertise. I am immensely proud of these absolutely indispensable organizations and all of the wonderful, talented, and dedicated people who run them. Nonetheless, I am most aware of the power and comfort that only comes from a book you can hold in your hand, in the intimacy of time and place.

To provide you with your personal, private, and convenient resource on survivorship, we wrote the first edition of this book, *Living Beyond Breast Cancer*, in 1997. We have been deeply gratified by the many letters and emails we've received telling us how helpful, of the moment, our book has been. And we've been inspired by the demands for a second edition. Thus, we are extremely proud to present our newly titled, fully updated book: *Living Well Beyond Breast Cancer*—our way to help give you countless new opportunities for living a life of health and happiness.

PART ONE

Treatment Over, On with Your Life

CHAPTER ONE

Over, Not Over

I never forget. Cancer has become part of my consciousness, part of my society. With every cancer death, my heart turns over. I'm always amazed at how other people take their lives for granted, as if they'll live forever.

I became assertive, someone I'd never been. I had a new voice. I said whatever I felt, like a cranky old lady. I knew nobody would stop me. I took my husband to an auction, my first post-treatment outing; I bought a few things, and he asked, "What are you going to do with this junk?" I exploded—I just couldn't help myself: "You should be thanking God I'm interested in something again!"

Right after treatment I felt very old, and lost, like I was looking into my grave. I got help, and it took a while, but I came around to feeling reborn, reinvented.

First Things First

I t's over. Treatment, that is. You've survived the initial ordeal. Now what? No one hands you an instruction manual as you go from under treatment to beyond treatment. From Geralyn Lucas' book *Why I Wore Lipstick*:

> I make a list of everything I want to do. Should I quit my job, leave my husband, travel the world? I decide that maybe the most courageous thing I can do is to try to return to my regular

life, with the knowledge that there is nothing regular about it. Since everything has changed, how could we remain the same?

Maybe it's been two weeks, maybe two years, maybe twenty. But no matter how little or how much time has passed, the breast cancer experience is never *completely* over. Active issues, leftover concerns, and reminders can dog you every day or pop up just once in a while.

When it's all over, just when you think you should be celebrating this huge accomplishment, you may feel worse than you did during treatment. How confusing and disorienting. It starts to make sense when you realize that all parts of your life have been touched by the breast cancer experience. It may have taken over your life: bills, taxes, job, vacation, housework, and even children were put on hold.

Now, with the end of treatment, you have to adjust back to normal. But is that really possible? The fact is, life changes after breast cancer treatment. Normal will never look and feel exactly the same. The only thing you can do is to go forward with the rest of your life, one step at a time. You have to find and create your new normal. Many of you speak of how changed you are, almost renewed. This is my hope for each of you as you read my book: a chance to renew your life, one that brings you comfort, meaning, joy, fun, and hope.

Throughout this book, I will help you understand the challenges and identify the solutions to help you live well beyond breast cancer. We'll start by looking at the issues you'll begin facing immediately after treatment.

ℬ Challenges

You can cope with this new life. Countless women have done it and are doing it. When you feel as wobbly inside as a new toddler or as stiff and creaky as a little old lady, draw strength from these other survivors. They understand that your cheery front is covering up the vulnerable, exhausted you. And unlike many others, they appreciate this new you. In time, you will, too.

When chemo is all over, the supportive care is over, too. You're worn down by the accumulated side effects of all your treatments with nearly no pick-me-ups. That's when many of my patients tell me they barely feel as if they're among the living.

Separation Anxiety

After months or more of concentrated attention on you, your illness, and your therapy, you come to that moment when the days mapped out for you by hour and procedure come to an end. Many of my patients felt thrown into an emotional limbo: " 'Come back in three months,' the doctor said. I felt like I was *dumped*, and I was so frightened," Janet recalled.

Your health care team provided emotional support you may not have fully appreciated when so many things were happening to you at once— and at the end of your whirlwind treatment experience, you suddenly miss it. "I felt more scared after treatment was over than I did before it started," said Gena. "During treatment I had peace." The scheduled routine and plan of attack were very comforting, and now they're gone. "When treatment ended, I didn't know what to do with myself," Christy recalled.

With the end of treatment, your family and friends generally conclude the disease is beaten and done with. There's usually a shower of congratulations and celebrations. But you don't feel like yourself. You're still feeling disoriented and conflicted: profound relief and exhilaration mixed with uncertainty and forced enthusiasm. "I dreaded going to my own end-of-treatment party," one woman said. You're expected to feel great and back to normal and ready to get on with your life, but instead you feel lost. Separation anxiety takes on new meaning.

Lingering Concerns

As you move forward, a string of troubling questions can pollute your peace of mind:

- What do I do now?
- Where's my support?
- Can I really get along without my doctors and nurses?
- When do I get to see my doctor again?

- Now that I don't see my doctors every day or every week, how do I get all my questions answered?
- What about that new treatment that I just heard about on TV—does it apply to me?

Flooded with these kinds of questions, you can feel fearful and insecure—making you wonder: *Can I ever handle my life on my own again?*

Cancer Worry

Even if you've been discharged by your doctors, there's likely still that cancer worry in a corner of your mind: "Every time something hurts or I get sick, I think the cancer has come back."

You may also fear that the cancer might grow back because you are no longer doing anything active to keep it away. Annamarie's coping mechanism was ceaseless activity: "I got depressed . . . cancer was still on my mind twenty-four hours a day. I started looking for things I could do, things I still had to decide about, like diet, exercise, tamoxifen, anything I could possibly do to avoid recurrence." You may also worry whether the treatment really worked, whether you're fit to be discharged.

Cancer worry is something you must learn to manage and live with. "Like a whale that moves into your living room" is how one patient described her lingering fears of breast cancer. "Over time, the whale gets smaller, but it never quite goes away completely. A tenant you can't get rid of. Maybe it gets down to the size of a magazine rack. Once in a while you bump into it, and sometimes it swells up into your face again, like when you have a mammogram and they call you back for extra views."

Cancer worry dogs most of the people I take care of—a little or a lot. They carry it with them indefinitely, even as year after year proves them disease-free. Over time, the burden gradually gets processed, loosens its grip, and gets put in its place.

Denial

Quite a number of people shut the door after treatment, saying cancer is over and done with. That may be the only way for them to deal with what's happened. Five, ten, or more years may pass without processing that cancer experience, leaving important issues unresolved and the accompanying fear and anxiety buried deep. They may go on to other things without any difficulty, living their lives without active fear.

Then along the way, something may happen that sets things off:

- A suspicious mammogram
- A bout of arm edema
- Heavy media coverage during Breast Cancer Awareness Month
- A close friend or family member diagnosed with breast cancer
- A daughter reaches her mother's age at diagnosis.
- The recurrence of, or a new, cancer

These events jolt them from the wall of denial where they'd previously sought refuge and into a harsh new reality where buried emotions may erupt with destructive force.

Low Energy Versus High Expectations

You're likely to be bombarded by heavy expectations upon the end of treatment—from yourself and others. Everything you put off till you got your strength back is waiting for you, but you're still dogged by fear and fatigue. You just can't handle it!

The uncertainty of the past, present, and future is still with you, overwhelming and exhausting you. "Not knowing what will be is worse than knowing the worst. It was a living hell." The hardest thing to deal with is this uncertainty—it can consume all your energy.

Even high-energy women are laid low. "I gave up on my superwoman image. It was costing me too much." Some of these formerly high-powered women feel discouraged, useless, and unable to accomplish anything important. "It takes all day to do one thing!" You may be able to do little more than finish up treatment and begin the recovery process.

So there you are, projects waiting, not knowing where to start, still exhausted. And there's your family, waiting for you to take over again, looking for the attention they've been missing all this time. Christy recalled, "I had to act like I could just flip a switch and not be a cancer patient—as if it were possible."

Family members and close friends can only meet some of your needs some of the time. By the time treatment is over, their energy, goodwill, and empathy may bottom out. For Donna's husband, the issue was simple: "I don't want to hear about your illness anymore. Put it away. It's done." "If there are no 'support receptors' in your family, you may not be able to put them there," commented Molly. Support can be as much a part of your cure as anything else; unfortunately, you may need it most when you find it dwindling.

Depression

Is it any wonder that many people become depressed after their main treatment is over? You are most vulnerable to depression at the time of diagnosis and again when your treatment is completed. "I thought I was dealing with everything just fine, but I wasn't. I couldn't. Everything fell in on me. I became clinically depressed shortly after the end of my chemotherapy."

While depression upon diagnosis seems obvious, experiencing depression at the end of treatment is unexpected and counterintuitive. But it's pretty common to be overwhelmed with feelings of helplessness that can peak after treatment is over. It's normal to find yourself angry, sad, and depressed in this period of transition.

There is some good news to help move you through this funk. Time alone solves some things, and there may be some calm after the storm. But you can't just kick back, expecting, waiting, and hoping for things to get better on their own. Don't neglect troubling symptoms. Now is the time to *take care of your whole self.* With this book and through Breastcancer.org, we'll help you find and create small and big opportunities for recovery and renewal.

Telling

Disclosing your breast cancer experience can be hard or easy. Sometimes it just happens. "I didn't want to talk about it, and then this woman I'd just met at a party mentioned her work with breast cancer survivors, and I found myself telling her things I'd never told anyone, years and years after I'd been through with it. Maybe I was just waiting for the right moment, or the right person." Molly was a well-balanced, self-assured woman who surprised herself with the release of this flood of suppressed feelings.

For Sylvie, telling everyone she had breast cancer felt like a responsibility. "I don't think it's good for anybody to be quiet about this disease. Not if we want to find a cure, find the money for research, get women active in the cause." Lily came from a prominent business family in a major city, and telling her story brought her into the public eye on TV and in the newspapers. "I was deluged. All kinds of organizations asked me to speak to their members, and I did. I believe a lot of women went and got mammograms because of my story, as they did with Betty Ford, Happy Rockefeller, and Nancy Reagan."

Some of the women I've worked with are so self-conscious about their illness, they feel almost as though they're wearing a sign and they need to explain: "I stood there in the supermarket, telling this sympathetic checkout clerk my entire history." Others, however, mull over whether or not to share this painful experience with their closest friends. And how do you tell a new boyfriend or lover? (See Chapter 19, on intimacy.)

Others, like Gena, prefer to stay quiet. "I decided not to tell my friends—and my doctor told me not to. This was many years ago. I was very young. I didn't want people clucking over me, feeling sorry for me, being nice to me just because I'd had breast cancer. I kept my mouth shut for twenty years. It was a different time." Betsy would have agreed with Gena. "People ask me, 'How *are* you?' with this woeful eye. Like I'm so brave but really dying. Or they say, 'How good you look!' with real surprise, as though I should look half dead. Or I *do* look half dead and they lie through their teeth and say, 'How great you look!' Who needs all that?" No one really likes a pity party.

Of one thing most of you are sure: you don't want friends telling you sad tales. Annamarie would stop people midbreath and say: "I only listen to stories with happy endings." How can reasonable people be so thoughtless with misplaced reassurance? Maybe they think they must say something but don't quite know what or how. Or maybe they're expressing their own fears. Whatever the reason, these stories about sickness and death that others may want to unload can hurt. Stop them the moment you sense what's coming. Use Annamarie's "happy endings" line. There are plenty of stories with good outcomes for you to hear.

Telling may help others deal with your situation but may do little to help you. You're the one who can end up giving support, often getting the energy sucked out of you to help someone else. Still, most women do tell their friends and co-workers. "I don't like to be with people who don't know," said Florrie. "It makes it so much easier at work. And everyone is so supportive and kind, in many loving ways. Maybe I talk about it too much." Ginnie told her friends but she felt she had to hide it at work because she was worried about keeping her job and her health insurance.

❧ Solutions

Many of you come away from the breast cancer experience with a clearer view of what matters most in life. Cancer has changed your life. And maybe not surprising to you, but surely surprising to people who've never had cancer, is the repeated comment "My life is so much better now," or "We're a much closer family now than we ever were before." That does not include, however, the individuals and families that come apart, unable to manage this crisis. Between these extremes are the people who chug along much like everybody else, dealing with everyday issues and keeping their past health problems on a short leash.

The New You

"I've chucked so much garbage." "I don't suffer fools." "I take risks I never did before." "I take better care of myself." "I'm more assertive." "I don't worry about unimportant details." "I won't let people take advantage of me." "I'm able to make changes I always needed to make." "I stop and look around at new things." "I'm much kinder to myself." "I take nothing for granted." "I don't waste time."

So many people who have been diagnosed with breast cancer have said to me: "I want to find meaning and fulfillment in each day. I want to build memories." Workaholics take time off. Trivial matters are seen for what they are. "I used to get all worked up in traffic; now I'm happy just sitting there." Laughter and merriment are prized; hugging takes on major importance.

Many of you say you no longer put off what you really want to do. "I'm doing things I'd talked about doing for years: I'm going to graduate school, for starters," Vivian told me with pride. Just don't take on too much: "I've been trying so hard to do all the things I enjoy. It's too stressful—it's wearing me out!" Jenny said with irritation. Knowing your priorities will help you save your energy for the things that matter to you most.

Managing Expectations

For self-preservation and self-defense, you have to control and protect yourself from unreasonable expectations. Don't let your family's expectations for you get out of hand. Keep a reality check on work expectations. Even more important, don't expect too much of yourself. Stop comparing yourself to others and judging your performance.

You may know someone who sailed through treatment, went back to work full-time the week after surgery, and seemed to take complete care of her family, job, house, and community obligations. Unlikely—but so what! If that's not you (or most women I know), it's not relevant. Stop measuring yourself against people who may be driving themselves into the ground. Keep your head, and make your family see you as you are and treat you as you need to be treated. Push back on expectations: saying no to a new request or demand often means saying yes to your recovery and renewal. Throughout this book, we'll be giving you solutions for managing expectations and setting reasonable limits.

Fortifying Your New Support Network

There is no reason to go through breast cancer treatment and recovery alone. That kind of isolation without support can itself be life-threatening. Your psychological needs deserve as much attention as your physical needs. You worked extremely hard to get the best treatment possible to protect your body against breast cancer; now it's time to take the best care of your emotional needs and the whole you.

Other people who have experienced breast cancer can provide you with indispensable information and support. You don't need to start from the beginning and explain everything all over again—they understand. Florrie explained: "I decided to go someplace where others knew it wasn't over, where I could tell this complete stranger about my history and feelings, knowing what we share." This shared experience has been the foundation of many beautiful friendships.

For more on building your support network–whether online, by phone, in a group, or though a therapist–see Chapter 2.

Get Answers to Your Questions

You need to acknowledge your fears, rid yourself of uncertainty, and set straight your misconceptions. Start by writing them down, putting your biggest concerns at the top of the list. Assign a go-to person or expert next to each entry. For example, here is just one of many steps you can take to get answers to the following sample questions:

- *Does my diagnosis increase my daughter's risk?*
  ~Talk to your family doctor and make an appointment with a genetics counselor to review your full family history and see if genetic testing would be useful.
- *How do I talk to my daughter about breast health?*
  ~Check out my book *Taking Care of Your "Girls": A Breast Health Guide for Girls, Teens, and In-Betweens* to learn how to get this delicate conversation going and to become knowledgeable about the kind of information she might ask about.
- *What's my risk of recurrence?*
  ~Talk to your oncologist and find out your chances of staying cancer-free and your risk of recurrence. Also ask what additional steps you can take to maximize your chances of doing well.
- *What about that new treatment I heard about on the news—would I benefit from it?*
  ~Breastcancer.org presents research news every day along with a Take-Home Message, making it easy to discuss this with your doctor.

Once you've written out your concerns and ideas for addressing them, follow through to get the information you need. Answering your questions and replacing myths with facts is very therapeutic and will expedite your recovery.

Taking Care of Yourself

Stop and give yourself credit for the hard, hard work you've done to fight for your life.

Now you have to take the time to heal. Push back. Indulge yourself. Give yourself a reward. Treat yourself better. Go on a vacation. "Each year on my anniversary I am in a beautiful place, celebrating life," Jo told me. "If you feel like crying, do it. If you need help, get it. Give yourself time—the biggest gift—for recovery. Don't let anyone make you feel guilty, and don't take on things you're not ready for. It isn't as easy as one might think to put yourself first. Grab what you want and need. I was too brave, always protecting others. Now it's my time."

No normal human being has the time or emotional wherewithal to process the whole breast cancer experience until the major impact of treatment is over. This is one more reason why the end of treatment is such an unexpectedly hard time. "My stress and anxiety became more apparent to me after I finished therapy than when I was going through it," Donna reflected. "I was given this really big test—and I passed. I can wake up and not think first thing about cancer. I can go to work and feel good all day. There is life after cancer! I am who I am; I am not defined by that disease. Breast cancer is behind me."

✄ Moving Forward

It's important to put the recent past in perspective as you focus on a healthy future. "I didn't choose this disease and I wasn't going to let it control me. I had a good life before, and this bad thing wasn't going to change my life for me. I was going to make life good again," Gena said. "You don't want to disappoint yourself; you don't want to let yourself down. So you make yourself come through. That was thirty years ago—and it has been good!"

You did everything you could do to become cancer-free using the best treatments available to you at the time. Moving forward, you will continue to do whatever you can to be healthy. Of course no one is perfect—we can't kick bad habits instantly and completely. But we can set goals and start somewhere.

Form your own conclusions about what your life beyond breast cancer should be, because no one else can supply the answers you need. Many of you want to think of and plan for your future but are afraid to presume that you *have* a future. Don't let fear stop you. *You do have a future*, and you're not daring fate if you think about it and plan what you want to do for yourself, your family, your children, work, vacations, or retirement. You're no different from anyone else on this score, although you may bring a sharper appreciation for the idea of "future." And it's reasonable to hope that your future will mean years and years of a good life.

Remember: your future is built one step at a time. Step one is finding and creating your new normal. How long it takes to get there and what it's going to look like when you get there will reveal itself along the way. Progress isn't always steady, with one day better than the day past. You can take three steps forward, one step back, no step the next day, and then a side step before you make more forward progress again. There is no fixed number for how long it takes to get back to normal. My rule of thumb is that it takes at least as long as the time from diagnosis through the end of treatment.

As long as your overall path is forward, take comfort. Your patience and persistence will pay off. Build momentum whenever you can. Along the way you'll be rewarded as you see glimpses of your old self and piece together a new vision for yourself and your future.

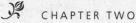

CHAPTER TWO

Support: Building a Network

I found a woman from Johannesburg, South Africa, who is going through the same chemo regimen I went through and we connect two to three times a week on the Breastcancer.org discussion boards. I'm a big help to her and she gives me a lot of positive feedback.

The Breastcancer.org forums have intelligent and savvy women who are really well informed about breast cancer issues. No matter what their educational background, they know what they're talking about when it comes to breast cancer, like how to read a path report and that sort of thing. They can really answer any question that is bothering me.

I needed to go someplace where others knew it wasn't over. It was like going through an invisible wall, with cancer people on one side and everyone else on the other. I didn't need to explain—they understood. That was my support group. They helped me learn to trust my instincts, to take care of myself—nobody else can or will. That's what a support group does.

Getting someone at the other end of the phone was a godsend when I was lower than low, scared by my own shadow, and desperate for a glimmer of hope. That hotline volunteer performed a lifesaving 911 rescue mission for me.

Of all the resources I had, access to my chat room was the best. I could sound off without worrying about consequences, and the practical advice we shared was amazing.

❧ First Things First

Many women believe that the stress in their lives may have caused their breast cancer. While no clear link has been found between stress and cancer risk, stress undeniably pollutes your quality of life. And dealing with breast cancer will definitely increase your stress. The good news is that stress is one of the things you can do something about. Support is *the* big stress reliever.

No matter what the source, support is your safety harness on the breast cancer roller coaster. Don't think you can manage this ride alone; don't even give it a try. It's too dangerous. Stubborn bravery earns you no points. This is not a game; this is no time to play the hero. This is your *life*. Now is the time to reach out for sustenance, to ask for and accept offers of support.

A lifeline of support can come from others like yourself, talking about what's on your mind, what you don't understand, what worries you, what scares you. Expressing all this out loud, in person, by phone or online, to someone else, can be very therapeutic. You need to hear that you are not alone, that other people in the same or similar situation have similar feelings. You also want to take the opportunity to profit from each other's personal wisdom, expertise, and example.

"My doctor said to me, 'You know, I happen to have here a patient that had the same kind of cancer you have, and hers was actually worse. And she talks about this, so I'm free to talk about it. It was spread throughout her body, and that was fifteen years ago and it's been gone since. The drugs these days are very powerful and helpful, and I know she would like to meet you.' I said, 'Wow, then this is not a death sentence!' And she said, 'Oh no, you're going to be fine.' Seeing someone who had been through it all, so happy and healthy, and so many years out, was a defining moment of hope. And that's what I want to do, talking to patients, imparting hope that way."

This chapter will focus on infusions of much-needed support.

❧ Challenges

You may insist on doing everything on your own, and forcefully assert your independence and competency—in an attempt to take back control of your life after feeling so inadequate and disempowered by the whole breast cancer experience.

Running on Empty

Are you finding leaks in your "energy tank" unrelated to the immediate demands of breast cancer treatment and recovery? Think about all the energy it takes to reveal your diagnosis to others, explain your situation, justify (and sometimes defend) your choices, reassure *them* that you'll be okay, and then have to support *them* as they deal with their own emotional reaction. If it were just your children and people in your close support network, fine—but if it also includes co-workers, neighbors, acquaintances, and so on, you may find yourself entirely depleted. Or you might find yourself up against people in denial, pretending everything is okay. They can't get the word *cancer* out of their mouths; to them it's "the Big C," too hard to even think about or imagine. A deep and wide feeling of isolation can envelop you.

The drain on your precious time is also exhausting. Think of all those "time robbers" who talk way too much, dragging out a simple conversation, refusing to get off the phone, calling at the wrong time, failing to recognize the hints and clues that you really, really gotta go. Are you also stuck with people who insist on talking about your health issues during what was supposed to be a relaxing get-together? They are all too much! You find yourself heading the other way, or lying, even hiding, to keep away from them. But as you avoid more people, your isolation deepens; what you really need is more support.

Buried Feelings

Even if you have people within your family or support network to talk to, it may be hard to tell them what scares you. "My family needs my support! I just can't burden them." You may be anxious to protect your family from your own worst fears, to avoid adding to their stress. It's almost as if you have an unspoken agreement to hide your true feelings.

Sadness and fear may have been buried, repressed, denied. "I was afraid that my sadness—especially if I talked about it—would make my cancer come back." It takes considerable emotional energy to keep all that trouble buried—energy better spent someplace else in your life. Stress that isn't released in some way or other can be destructive.

Loss of Confidence

Your energy and ability to connect with other people—including close family and friends—may be severely limited by your feeling fatigued, disconnected, depressed, and anxious, making you too self-conscious, embarrassed, or exhausted to reach out, answer the phone, or write back with an update or even a quick thank-you. The way you think you look might also stop you from connecting to others: nothing seems to fit and you imagine you look awful, your hair is a mess or your wig is out of place.

It's unlikely that people perceive you as you see yourself. But even if all your self-doubts are true, it's still not sufficient reason to hide. Avoiding social interaction, refusing assistance, or not reaching out for help just when you need it most is a big mistake. You need the support that much more—and you're less likely to ask for it. A vicious cycle. More isolation.

Rejecting Support

Unfortunately, only a small percentage of cancer survivors take advantage of support networks. Reaching out for help can be as great a challenge for some people as coping with the concept of cancer, particularly if there are issues to deal with that go beyond the issue of breast cancer. Many are used to being caregivers, not takers. Joining a support group calls for an overhaul of their whole value system and "method of operation."

Some people believe they must work out their problems on their own. It may be a function of denial; they push their anguish out of their mind. "I got it. I had it cut out. I don't want to talk about it again." And they don't, thinking, "If it ain't broke, don't fix it." But many of these same women remain terrified inside, and breaking through this protective barrier—which can be eating away at their lives—may require professional help.

✕ Solutions

The power and appeal of a support resource or network is that the stress and isolation that have become such a burden to you can be alleviated. Connecting with other people who've faced the same or similar challenges can be your greatest source of support—they know what breast cancer is all about, they're familiar with the breast cancer lingo, they feel comfortable talking about the issues, and they know how to get back the energy no one can spare. Just finally acknowledging your fear and telling it to somebody else can diminish that fear and make you feel better. "You can explore ideas that surprise you, stimulate you, and move you to understand yourself as you may never have before."

Stop the Leaks

You need people in your life who can support you right now—not people who need you to support them. Pity-partiers and time robbers only drain your precious energy when you need it most. It's much better to minimize your exposure to time robbers or avoid them entirely, at least for now. Staying away from some people is easier than others. It's particularly difficult if the worst offenders are the people closest to you, like your mother, sister, or mother-in-law—the same people you may also be most dependent on in your everyday life.

Here are some steps you can take to manage personal encounters:

- Only accept obligatory invitations.
- Prearrange to leave social and family events early.
- Don't engage in, escalate, or intensify a difficult conversation, especially if it's one-on-one.

Just because someone says something to you doesn't mean you have to respond to it. Let any thoughtless comment roll out of that stupid mouth and onto the floor and into an imaginary garbage can.

For other types of communication, here are some suggestions:

- Choose mostly forms of communication that you can answer whenever you want: email, voice mail, Facebook, online discussion, or bulletin boards.
- Let emails and voice messages rest for at least a full day before responding (your instant answers will invite too many more of these unwanted emails, guaranteed).
- A note on nice stationery or note card via snail mail—in response to a phone call, email, or letter—works beautifully.
- Keep your responses polite, nice, simple, and short.
- Do not provide extra information and other hooks that will give anyone a reason to delve in deeper or trigger a whole new unwanted conversation.
- Politely set expectations and limits (only happy stories).
- Learn nice but firm ways to say "no, thanks" (e.g., "Thanks so much—but sorry, that doesn't work for me right now").
- Avoid promises or new commitments.

Later on, you can reevaluate your approach—but only after you've made your way through the jungle of treatment and recovery.

Build Alliances

Shaping people's perception of you is always a challenge—particularly during and after breast cancer, when you might feel like you're being watched or judged. You can influence how you are perceived. You may need to do a little caucusing with the people of influence in your life. Establish alliances with people who are in the know and are pleased to follow your wishes and ground rules; let a few of them know what's on your mind, what you plan to do, and how you want people to respond to you. Then ask for their help in getting the rest of the people in your life to follow along.

Tap into Support Networks

A support network will help you restore the confidence that the diagnosis of cancer may have shattered, reclaim the control of your life that cancer has stolen from you, and draw you into a community of understanding people with whom you can quickly and fully connect. Together you can share good and bad news, exchange practical advice, make each other laugh, and work on your recovery and renewal. If you're an information junkie, searching out everything and anything about fighting cancer and staying healthy, support networks can be a great educational resource. (But you must still vet all information for yourself.)

Support comes in many different forms: support groups, online forums (including chat rooms, discussion boards, and bulletin boards), and telephone hotlines. You can pick more than one from the menu of options, and later change your lineup and mix of resources as new needs and preferences emerge. It's easy to be flexible with your choice of options, as support networks and groups are free to you—a compelling factor after the cumulative expense of this illness.

Online Support

Online forums can do much of what face-to-face support networks did for people in the past. With the widespread availability of the Internet, people dealing with a burning question or serious health challenge have learned to make the support come to them, rather than have to travel out to get support.

The ability to communicate across vast distances—at any time of the day or night, according to your evolving needs and convenience—and to find comfort and support as well as knowledge, clarity, and confidence when you need them is a unique advantage of the Internet. It's hands down the fastest and easiest way to connect with other women who share your concerns. In the beginning you have your own screen name, which becomes your "official" online identity. But then over time, community members may choose to get to know each other further, share real names and contact information, and sometimes meet offline. Friendships—perhaps as groups or clubs—may develop.

Many online communities have a moderator, who oversees, guides, nurtures, and manages the various questions, activities, and dynamics. The moderator (there can be more than one) helps facilitate positive interactions between the people utilizing the forums; at times she may intervene, resolve disputes, and establish calm if things heat up or boil over.

Once you sign up within a particular website's online community, you can participate at different times and in many different ways:

- **Right away**
  You can connect at the same time with other people (live, "real-time," or synchronous communication) primarily in a chat room. You have a conversation by typing online, similar to what you would have with voices by phone conference call.
- **Now or later**
  You can connect to other people at the same or different times (asynchronous communication) through discussion boards, blogs, journaling, photo exchange, and bulletin boards. In each of these forums, you post your comment and others respond to it at their convenience. Sometimes you might jump into an ongoing conversation by posting a comment, and get included in a lively discussion. Or you can visit the forums, read the posts, and observe the dynamics without any direct participation.

You have countless online options for support at your fingertips. Breastcancer.org has the largest and most active online community of chat rooms and discussion boards on nearly every subject relating to breast cancer, operating twenty-four hours a day, seven days a week, and is thus a great place to find and connect with someone who matches your unique situation—whether in your local community or at a distance. It's a safe and nurturing place to get practical information and real support.

You have to poke around and find the forum and format that serves you best. While the huge menu can be overwhelming, flipping around from your home computer is certainly a lot easier than checking out a long list of face-to-face support meetings. Plus, you're never stuck in any online forum; you can drop in and out of the forums whenever you want.

These are some of the most popular online options for support:

DISCUSSION BOARDS. Discussion boards contain conversations started by the online community, conversations that get recorded and accessed whenever a particular member gets online. Advice is shared and problems are worked out together. "These people understand me, more than in the real world!" one Breastcancer.org participant commented.

Breastcancer.org's more than seventy discussion boards contain about two hundred thousand different conversations. Here are a few examples of topics they cover: Just Diagnosed, Waiting for Test Results, Help Me Get Through Treatment, Fitness and Getting Back into Shape, Humor and Games. Visitors are welcome to join any of them. Take your time looking for discussions most aligned with your interests and style of communication.

CHAT ROOMS. In chat rooms, everyone talks by typing in real time. There can be a few or many people in the chat room, who jump in and out of the conversation. The depth of conversations tends to be light, because the conversation flows so fast and topics shift very quickly. There is more opportunity for slower and deeper discussion when only a few people are in the chat rooms during off hours.

YOUR PERSONAL NETWORK. You can also utilize an online community to organize your own network of family and friends—particularly useful when you need help with day-to-day tasks such as: providing a ride home from a test or doctor appointment, cooking a meal for your family, or watching the kids when you're in a pinch. In a typical scenario, one of your close friends or family members would facilitate scheduling of to-do list items. A system that spells out actionable to-do items takes the burden off you to ask people for needed help and instead allows people in your network to select tasks that best fit their schedules and talents. Breastcancer.org and Caringbridge.org offer this service.

PERSONAL BLOGS AND JOURNALING. A blog is like an online open diary where you can explain your diagnosis and treatments and share anything else you'd like with family and friends. Keeping a blog can help relieve the burden of explaining things over and over. It can also provide an easy way to share the facts of breast cancer with loved ones, as the basis for what you've done, what you're doing, and what you're planning to do. You can save a ton of time and energy by communicating this way.

Another big bonus to writing a blog or keeping a journal is the satisfaction, self-awareness, and emotional relief that can come from writing down your thoughts and expressing your feelings. A word of caution, though: when you're experiencing a rapid flow of intense new feelings, it can be very difficult and emotional. Go slow to avoid feeling overwhelmed. You may also want to journal more privately. (Some of the women I take care of have an offline journaling group that's facilitated by a writer and guided by a psychologist.)

ONLINE PHOTO ALBUM OR SCRAPBOOK. Sharing photographs, milestones, and memorabilia is a great way to show support and be supported. You may want to put up photographs or other images to highlight a reunion, vacation, or another special occasion to go along with your online posts. For example, Breastcancer.org community members often organize offline get-togethers and then share photos after the event.

Offline Support Groups

A face-to-face support group is a natural way to get support if you like to talk and listen, to share your feelings, process your thoughts, tell your stories, and help solve some of your and other people's problems. "People who care about you won't let you off the hook. They urge courage and honesty—but they do it with great kindness and affection. It can be magic, what goes on in a group." They really want you to think about yourself and devote more attention to what's happening in your life. "It's time you came first." The social network of a breast cancer support group can help you overcome some of your fear of cancer, reestablish control over your life, and connect you to an understanding community of individuals.

Support groups may be organized by your personal situation: breast cancer stage (newly diagnosed, dealing with recurrence or advanced disease), treatment status (under or over treatment), or hospital affiliation. Some groups may be based on a theme, emphasizing a personal interest or concern, such as "How to Eat Organic" or "How to Talk to Your Children." It can be topical, pragmatic, or spiritual, focused, or wide-ranging. Or group members may have nothing else in common with each other besides this one thing, cancer.

Besides word of mouth, the most likely way to find a support group is through your treatment center or a local nonprofit organization such as the Wellness Community, Gilda's Club, or SHARE. Some women organize support groups on their own if there are no existing local options available.

Group meetings are usually scheduled once a week or once or twice a month for a one- or two-hour session, usually on a weekday evening. Sometimes groups allow an open-door policy, allowing you to attend only the meetings that interest you or fit your schedule, but some groups require that you attend most of the sessions in a series. There is no perfect-sized group, although many people have strong opinions about what works best. Basically, you want to have enough people to keep the conversation fresh, interesting, varied, and energetic without sacrificing a sense of trust and familiarity.

Participation in a support group can be a powerful experience, and only a trained facilitator can contain that power and deflect and channel it for the benefit of all present. The facilitator is usually a therapist or social worker who helps:

- Guide the progress of the group
- Keep the focus on the goals, spirit, and purpose of the group
- Make sure that everyone has a chance to participate and no one is allowed to take over or be put on the spot

The facilitator should be attentive, aware, authentic, knowledgeable, caring, practical—and able to create a therapeutic, tolerant, nonjudgmental, broad-minded environment so people can open up and share—and trust that their feelings, thoughts, and privacy will be respected. Occasionally, the facilitator must step in to handle challenging situations. When buried feelings finally start to come out, they may be disturbing to the person expressing them, as well as to the other people listening. Individual counseling may be recommended for people who are struggling or troubled. If conflicts emerge, the facilitator may need to enforce community rules to keep the group dynamics rolling smoothly and maintain positive interchange between group members.

Still, support groups don't work for everyone. "I couldn't sit there and listen to all those painful stories. I had enough to do just taking care of myself; I couldn't deal with other women's complaints, as justified as they might be. I felt I was doing better than they were, and they were dragging me down."

Individual Counseling

Millions of people with and without breast cancer benefit from one-on-one support with a mental health professional, which might include medication. The therapist could be a psychologist, psychiatrist, social worker, member of the clergy, or other empathetic individual. For your physical battle against breast cancer, you had a radiologist (to read the mammogram and other tests), a pathologist (to analyze the breast and cancer tissue), a surgeon, a radiation oncologist, and a medical oncologist. But most likely you've had no professional help for your emotional concerns. It's probably time you got it. If you decide that individual counseling would be helpful to you, ask your doctor or other members of a current support group or online community for recommendations.

Self-Help Groups and Other Options

You might seek support from a nontraditional peer-led support group network, like a coffee klatch, a book club, or a self-help group. These often have more participants than a typical support group, plus an easy come-and-go arrangement. "It's another level of friendship. We deal with loneliness, isolation, fear—many of the issues I explored in the hospital-sponsored support group I was part of for a year. While it provides emotional support, nobody 'spills her guts' here. We tend to keep a little distance. We bring in speakers and focus more on education than unloading."

Help for Partners and Families

There are also support groups for partners or spouses who are dealing with the stress of their loved one's breast cancer situation. Some centers offer support groups specifically for children. Partners often are in real need of ventilating the concerns and tension that they are unable or reluctant to express at home to the person who is actually suffering from breast cancer. Hospitals or wellness centers are generally the organizers of these groups, having a large pool to draw upon. Lesbian partners may have a harder time adjusting to this type of support group, because most participants are men, even though many of the issues are shared. Specialized chat rooms and discussion boards are also available for partners of people dealing with breast cancer.

Selecting the Best Source of Support for You

Experts say that a take-charge person tends to recover faster and do better in the long run than someone who feels like a victim, stuck in disaster and unable to take constructive action. A support group is one important way to take action and propel yourself forward—with others, not alone. But not everybody should join a support group; not everybody is ready for a support group; not everybody needs a support group. There are people who get all the support they need from their existing networks of family and friends

> **SUPPORT GROUPS ARE NOT FOR EVERYONE**
>
> A support group may not be for you if you:
>
> - Tend to be impatient
> - Prefer to talk much more than listen
> - Dislike group process
> - Are uncomfortable dealing publicly with difficult subject matter (like talk of recurrence)

and online forums. And there are others who might benefit much more from one-on-one therapy.

Time-Sensitive Needs

Timing is important, too, in terms of what kind of support you want and need and when you're ready for it. For example, it might be too soon to join a support group when you've just been hit with a diagnosis. Instead, you may first jump online to connect with others in the same boat—perhaps in Breastcancer.org's "Understanding Your Pathology Report" or the "Help, Just Diagnosed" discussion boards; or the Young Survivors Coalition's discussion boards for young women with young children. Or you might call Living Beyond Breast Cancer's help line (888-753-5222) or the Breast Cancer Network of Strength's hotline (800-221-2141). But some time later—three to six months, a year, or maybe more—you may find yourself ready to look for personal exploration and renewal in the form of a support group. "It was a year till I had the energy for a support group," Mary explained.

Group Disconnect

Mismatches can stress rather than support you. Sylvia went to one support meeting. "Breast cancer amplifies everything. There were too many of other people's issues and feelings I wasn't prepared to deal with." Nancy left her support session in tears: "Everyone there had someone at home for them. I had no one—no husband, no lover, and my mother had just passed away. There should be a group for someone who has nobody." If you find yourself in what seems to be an inappropriate group, you'll have to decide if it's worth it to you to continue. For example, if you have noninvasive breast cancer (which doesn't spread to lymph nodes or other parts of the body) and you share a group with women undergoing tons of chemotherapy for dealing with advanced breast cancer, you may leave the group's session worried and convinced that you need to hurry up and get your own chemo. The reverse is also true: if you're dealing with metastatic breast cancer, it's hard to empathize with women who've been diagnosed with early-stage disease. It's almost always worth the extra energy to leave and find a more suitable group if you're in such a mismatched situation. If you find yourself in a support group or network that's unsuited to your needs, try switching before giving up altogether. You do have other options.

Your doctor, nurse, or hospital may be able to come up with suggestions and ideas for establishing a support group or help network. Your support group facilitator can also help place you in the most suitable group for your needs. And don't overlook your church, synagogue, or mosque as a source of support: your spiritual leader may be willing to organize a support group to meet your needs, as well as offer you immediate individual support and comfort.

❧ Moving Forward

Life is a series of millions of moments. If the moment you're in now is stealing your moxie, rocking your confidence, draining

GROUP BURNOUT

Challenges

Support groups can experience burnout—particularly if they have been in existence for a long time. Reasons for burnout include:

- Flagging energy
- Loss of interest
- Distress due to deaths in the group
- Departure of an admired facilitator
- Rehashing the same issues as new people join the group
- Irritating group members
- Angry group members
- Poor organization (e.g., sessions canceled without notice)

Solutions

The facilitator can:

- Reassess the group's purpose and goals
- Talk with other members to see if their needs are being met
- Reconfigure the group
  - ~ A new group may emerge with another focus.
  - ~ The same group may be revitalized.
  - ~ Individual members may shape up or ship out.
- Make a commitment to start and end the sessions on time; keep an up-to-date schedule online
- Help you find another source of support

Help is out there, and no one should be shy about looking for a caring connection, in person or online. You owe it to yourself to find support that works for you.

your energy, or pulling you down, remember that the moment will pass. You can ready yourself for your next moment, feel your strength—even if it's just little by little. Now is the time for you to make your support a top priority. Doing so will facilitate your recovery. Channel your energy into the thoughts and actions that will lift you up and propel you forward. Don't overthink it; just try one type of support network or connection at a time, then later you can add another one or two into the mix. But you may have to open your mind to new possibilities outside your current comfort zone. Jump in and give it a chance over a few weeks before making any judgments or final decisions. The return on your investment will come: the precious support, comfort, new knowledge, and confidence you need to fortify and rebuild your future.

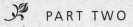

PART TWO

Additional Care Beyond Treatment

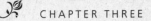

CHAPTER THREE

You and Your Doctors: Continuing Care

The surgeon was in and out of the consultation room in less than five minutes. How was I supposed to trust him with a five-hour surgery to remove and rebuild my breast?

I waited so long to see the doctor, I completely forgot what I was going to say.

My doctor said very little at first, but then I warmed him up with a joke and a few compliments. Now I can tell him anything.

I had a very good, calming doctor; she listened thoughtfully to whatever I asked her. I trusted her to tell me everything. She explained it all in detail, and gave me the statistics with a positive spin. She cared about me. She's still a great source of support. I need to trust my doctor completely. If you don't have that, you don't have the full value of medical care you're entitled to.

❧ First Things First

Y ou and your doctors have come through an exhausting, demanding, emotional, intimate, and frightening experience. You probably feel older and wiser, and, I hope, still confident in your doctors.

When you were given that diagnosis of breast cancer, overnight you became dependent on a team of health care professionals responsible for your life. You had to choose doctors you could trust, or your choices may have been limited by your health care plan. You had to become an expert on a subject you may have known little about, and to make critical choices you may have felt unprepared to make.

Now that treatment is nearing completion, or is over, you may want to reassess, reaffirm, reshape, or reconsider your relationship with your medical team:

- Have you been satisfied with your care, or do you want more?
- Are these the people you want to take care of you in the future?
- Do you feel like making a change in your team?

Ongoing Care

You're not about to be abandoned, if that's one of your fears. After your cancer treatment has concluded, you will be scheduled for regular visits with the physicians who have participated in your cancer care. While reassuring, all this scheduling may once again be overwhelming—so many appointments when you're already so tired. And with all the piles, tasks, and obligations that have been waiting for your return to health, you may find yourself hard-pressed to fit in so many follow-up visits to doctors.

But it is important to continue your care. At this point, your doctors will:

- Monitor any unresolved side effects of your treatments
- Evaluate your response to treatment
- Ease your physical adjustment back to a full life
- Assess your overall health status
- Watch for signs and symptoms of possible recurrence
- Focus on cancer prevention and the promotion of your health and sense of wellness

The importance of your relationship with your doctors has not diminished.

✖ Challenges

Now that the breast cancer diagnosis and treatment crisis is past and you are taking steps to maximize your future health, make sure you're getting what you need from your doctor. Maybe you can make changes to improve an existing relationship, or maybe you should start afresh.

Lopsided Relationship

There's an intrinsic imbalance, a lopsidedness, to the patient-doctor relationship no matter how wonderful the doctor, no matter how fine the communication. And that's intimidating. Bottom line: you have much more at stake than your doctor. It's your life on the line. You've been dealing with a threat to your health, whereas your doctor is presumably well.

There are many other inherent imbalances to the relationship—and that's no one's fault. Your doctor is the expert and may have more access to your medical information than you do, as well as a deeper understanding of its significance and medical terminology. Tests are an example: your doctor usually gets results before you do, and you may need help to understand what the test results mean. Another lopsided part of the relationship is the time, anxiety, and expectations leading up to an appointment. Compare your preparation to see the doctor with your doctor's preparation to see you. When did you make your appointment for your visit to your doctor? Weeks or months in advance? It's their schedule, not yours. During the appointment, your doctors touch you, you don't touch them. You reveal important private information about yourself; they reveal only their names and office phone numbers. And you're paying the tab.

Self-Image

What's the state of your self-image, and how does it get mixed up in the relationship with your doctor? How do you feel about yourself? "Of course your doctor likes seeing you," said one woman to her good-looking friend. "You're attractive and young. I'm neither. I sometimes think it must be a drag to have to take care of a lumpy old bag like me." You should not feel any less well treated or respected than any other patient. Your doctors should care about you whether you are young, old, thin, fat, beautiful, or otherwise. Most doctors see past the superficial to where their focus needs to be.

Still, many try too hard to please their doctors, to present themselves as attractive, appealing, and clever. One woman, determined to make an indelible impression on her surgeon—so he'd remember her forever and always look forward to seeing her—took a Magic Marker and drew a "smiley face" on her chest, with the mastectomy scar as a smiling mouth.

Some people, used to VIP treatment, make the big mistake of pushing past and over receptionists and nurses to play favor directly with the doctors. This approach belittles the very people who run the doctors' schedule, obtain each patient's medical records and test results, and coordinate the care of their patients; behaving in this thoughtless way will likely result in negative consequences.

Uncomfortable Feelings

You may grow particularly fond of your doctor and show your gratitude with letters or gifts. It's also not uncommon to develop a crush on your doctor. "My doctor was a little too handsome for my comfort back when I started with him; he was an active part of my fantasy life. Then over the years he put on weight, lost some hair, got a little puffy; it came as a relief to me. I feel a lot more comfortable with him now."

Anger can also get mixed into the relationship. Anger that is generated from your cancer diagnosis, treatment, frustration, and long waits has to express itself somewhere, sometime: *Why me? What did I do wrong? Why is this taking so damn long?* Sometimes it lashes out against the doctor or his staff. A trivial incident, a thoughtless remark, or an extended wait may trigger an explosion. Unfortunately, not everyone is as forgiving as you might need them to be. Getting beyond the moment and back to a caring patient-doctor relationship can be a challenge. If anger gets in the way of treatment or care, you need to look into it and work through it in some constructive way. Or perhaps start fresh with a new doctor.

Complaints

When a relationship is complex and important—and when so much is at stake—things can easily go wrong. Feelings can be misinterpreted; oversights can trigger trouble.

While the multidisciplinary cancer center team with combined follow-up is a great concept with much to recommend it, you may also discover its potential disadvantage: the fragmentation of your medical care. "One doctor examines my uterus and does a Pap smear. Another does my radiation. Another does my blood work; another, my arthritis; another, diabetes; another, my eyes; another, chemo. I'm all over the place! Who sees me as a whole person and puts all these pieces together?"

In this next section, I'm going to share a whole pile of difficult situations that women have shared with me. Then later on, I'll provide a whole bunch of tried-and-true solutions.

False Reassurance or Wrong Information

What upsets people most about their doctors? Being given a misdiagnosis. Being told they're going to be fine, and then the tests come back: cancer. It happens. "I told him my symptoms, more than once. He missed the diagnosis. I know my body; I knew something was wrong, even when he said there wasn't. When they finally did a biopsy, he told me the frozen section looked good, go to work. Three nights later I'm eating dinner, the phone rings: my doctor. 'It's malignant.' And I'm in total shock. You mustn't let anyone tell you it's nothing till they absolutely know it's nothing."

The shock of bad news after good expectations (for example, from a premature upbeat prognosis) can be devastating. "I can't take any more optimistic predictions. They were all wrong. First they said that because the lump was perfectly round, there was only a very remote possibility of cancer. When it turned out to be cancer, they said it was so small there was virtually no significant risk of lymph node involvement—and then there were eight out of fifteen nodes with

SEPARATING THE MESSAGE FROM THE MESSENGER

Sharing bad news and difficult information during uncertain times automatically makes the relationship with your doctor complicated. The message "You have breast cancer" is devastating; the messenger, usually a physician, tries to present the information with all the sensitivity and support possible, which can sometimes be unrealistically reassuring.

Doctors want the best for you, but they are human. The preliminary view looks okay, and they really think they "got it all," and they want to pass on good news. You desperately need reassurance—and you may even ask or beg for it. But then, over the next few days, the pathologist who provides the biopsy results may find cancer cells. Given the statistics—80 percent of breast biopsy results show no cancer—doctors are generally not far off in their optimism and with their reassurance. But if you are part of that other 20 percent, that optimism is misleading. Remember: it's a very delicate and difficult balancing act for your doctors, figuring how to be reassuring without giving unrealistic expectations.

disease. Why bother with optimism for a few days of supposed peace of mind when they don't know what's really there? I failed each of their predictions and, on top of everything else, I had the peculiar feeling I'd disappointed both my doctors and myself. I was ready to come apart."

Arrogance and Condescension

Besides mistakes in diagnosis, women resent arrogance and condescension. "My doctor thought I just wanted attention—and there I was so sick I ended up in the hospital again," Catherine said, bitter about her doctor's indifference to her reported symptoms. June still bristles over the reception she got from a new doctor: "I went to this specialist—he didn't even look at me when he asked, 'Who do you know who got you this appointment with me?' What an egotistical jackass!"

"I had this list of questions I'd been writing down about what was bothering me. 'You don't need to know all that stuff,' my doctor told me. He didn't welcome any questions. I was left with all my worries and he made me feel like a dunce." "He never told me what to expect." "He took it for granted I didn't want or need to know anything. I was never included in making decisions regarding my care. Being a patient became synonymous with losing all control of my life."

Sophie's doctor was unbearably condescending and never picked up on her discontent—and it was too difficult for her to share her feelings. She finally gave up. "It was hard to make the break; it took me months, but I had to find someone more attuned to what I needed, to what worried me."

Push came to shove for the husband of one patient. "My wife didn't want chemo, and I agreed with her. And this pompous 'high-class' specialist says to me, 'Don't you love your wife?' I couldn't believe it! 'You haven't even looked at her report!' I told him. He hadn't. And when I mentioned going to the university hospital, he sneered, 'They don't know what the hell they're doing.' I couldn't wait to get out of that office, let alone get my wife out of his care."

Disrespect and Insensitivity

Another major complaint: insensitivity. "I'd be sitting there with my husband, and my doctor would be talking to *him*, like I was invisible. 'Do I exist?' I wondered. And later, I'm lying there almost naked while he unwraps the bandages five days after the mastectomy—in a roomful of students, all of them in their clothes, me more than naked. I call that cruel and unusual punishment. I was so young. I got so old after that. I have rights. Now I speak up—that's what my voice is for."

Justine's father was a prominent physician, but at forty-five, Justine was in charge of her own life. She left the doctor who'd been her primary physician when he told her he was planning to call her father and discuss her health with him. "It was such a clear violation of my right to privacy! My father was eighty years old; I was trying to protect him. I switched doctors immediately."

"I don't like it when my doctor walks into the examination room, I'm there half naked, and he brings along another doctor, maybe a parade of doctors, who stand there gawking. It's not fair. It's humiliating and embarrassing. I hate it. He wouldn't treat his wife like that!"

Negative Vibes

Linda had another reason for switching doctors. "I couldn't get past his attitude. He was so pessimistic. You go to a doctor, feeling bad—and he makes you feel worse! Then he kept repeating it. Believe me, there's only one time you need to tell a patient a negative diagnosis. No one wants to hear it over and over. I'll be seeing my doctor the rest of my life; I deserve more. My new doctor told me I was going to have one lousy year, and then I'd get better. And that's what happened—six years ago."

If the relationship between you and your doctor is not going well, both sides of the equation may have lost confidence, interest, goodwill, respect, and willingness to make it work. Once anger and bitterness creep in, the disconnect can be too toxic for you and the doctor to manage.

"If you don't like your doctor, there's a good chance your doctor doesn't like you," says Dr. Larry Norton, from Memorial Sloan-Kettering Cancer Center, "and that's a good reason for changing doctors." It may be impossible to figure out who started it—and it may no longer matter. If you've hit a dead end and neither you nor your doctor is able to turn things around, it's time to move on.

Long Waits

The inevitable waits can further complicate your relationship with your doctor. "Waiting is a hot-button issue. They should be able to schedule better than they do. Are we so unimportant?" You may have started with your doctor some years ago, and now you find there's a lot less time allowed for you than back then. The practice has enlarged, and the waits have lengthened.

Unfortunately, a physician's schedule is predictably unpredictable. Almost every day there are crises, beyond even the extra space in the day doctors do allow: a woman with a new diagnosis of breast cancer needs to talk about it ASAP, another patient must make her final decision about chemo and has to review the pros and cons again, a third is anxious because she's waiting for mammography results complicated by unexplained extra views (did the radiologist order more X-rays because he or she suspected a problem?). You don't want your doctor to rush through important things for you or anyone else. But when the wait becomes the backdrop for all of your accumulated stress, frustration, and anxiety, being reasonable may be an unreasonable expectation.

Interruptions

You finally get in to see your doctor—and then your precious seven minutes (the average face-to-face time during your doctor visit) is interrupted. It may seem rude; there you are in the middle of your talk time with your doctor when the phone rings, your conversation stops, and your doctor's attention is transferred to someone on the other end of the line. Ideally, only the most pressing calls get through: a patient who is having a problem on the radiation table or in the recovery room, or a return call from a doctor your doctor's been trying to reach for days to clarify a patient's therapy. Try to remember that one day it could be your call that interrupts someone else or your important questions that throw off the appointment schedule for patients after you.

✣ Solutions

Most people take more time and care checking out a car they want to buy than they do with the physician who will look after their health. You now have an important opportunity to modify and fortify your health care team and then reaffirm and reinforce the relationships that are working well for you. But before you go out and shed noncontributing members from your team and finalize your "top picks," it's essential for you to take some time to figure out what you're looking for in a doctor.

Finding the Right Doctor for You

Professional Qualifications

You need to pick a doctor who has the necessary medical expertise, experience, and judgment in the areas where you need it. Here are some of the medical qualifications that you should know about any new doctor:

- What medical school did he/she attend?
- At what hospital did he/she complete his/her residency and specialty training?
- Is he/she board certified in his/her field of medicine?
- How many years has he/she been in practice?
- What hospital does he/she admit patients to?
- How did you hear about this doctor?
- Does your primary doctor recommend this new doctor?
- How old is he/she?

You want someone young enough to be around for as long as you are, yet someone with enough experience to manage any complex issues your cancer care requires.

Personal Qualities

Besides these important qualifications, it's often the personal qualities that seem to matter most to the women I speak to.

Over the ten years of delivering my performance *7 Minutes! How to Get the Most From Your Doctor Visit* to people worldwide (now available in book form at www.Breastcancer.org), I have collected all kinds of feedback and ideas regarding the things people look for when choosing a doctor.

TRUST. You need to believe that your doctor is putting your interests first, above his/her own self-interests as well as the pressures from hospital, practice, or financial interests. You also need to know that he/she will pay close attention to the important details in your medical chart and take the time necessary to answer your questions and address your concerns.

DISCLOSURE. You need to trust your doctor to tell you the truth—the whole truth, even the hard-to-hear stuff. Said one woman, "Could you trust a doctor who avoids serious subjects?" Some patients worry that their doctor may be withholding information, that there may be collusion to keep a bad diagnosis hidden, or that their doctor may not be doing everything possible to help them because it's expensive and the added cost may reduce their income.

Your doctors will take their cue from you, but it always helps to be direct with your preferences. Be sure to let your doctor know your limits. That way you'll get as much or as little information as you want.

LISTENS, TAKES YOU SERIOUSLY, SHOWS RESPECT. "The best thing about my doctor? He *listens*." Over and over that's what women truly appreciate. "He takes the time to listen." "She listens to what I say." Listening is essential in a good doctor-patient relationship; a doctor who listens shows that he or she respects you.

You are entitled to a doctor who treats you with respect and dignity. You need to be part of the process so that you can maintain control of your life.

Sometimes doctors can forget to give you the consideration and respect you're entitled to. I took one of my children to a doctor last year, and we were sitting in the examination room together when a substitute doctor walked in studying the chart and immediately proceeded to ask questions. (No introduction.) Then he started examining my child without a friendly word to either of us. No eye contact, not even a smile or a nod, much less a greeting. So I interrupted him, introduced my child and myself, and asked him his name, and finally he realized that he had overlooked an important first step. By correcting the situation and releasing my anger in an assertive (but nonconfrontational way), I set a positive example for my child, and we were both able to relax and get what we needed from that important visit.

UPBEAT AND CARING. People want to feel cared for and hopeful—even when times are tough. "My doctor said, 'You didn't cause this disease; no one knows what caused it.' I finally didn't feel guilty." Concern for you as an individual is essential: "He asks about my husband, about my farm animals, things like that." An optimistic outlook can be so therapeutic: "I loved his positive attitude. He transmitted the belief that I would live a long life. His attitude and his body language said: *You will prevail.*" "My doctor communicated his optimism to me. He was always cheerful." "My surgeon was always upbeat: 'We can handle this.' That 'we' is so important. The better the sense of teamwork, the greater my sense of well-being." When you leave your doctor's office, no matter how good or bad your outlook, you should always be helped to feel a little better.

GOOD CHEMISTRY. You want to like your doctor—but you don't really have to love him or her. You also want to have a good feeling about how the relationship works.

It's all about chemistry: the way it feels, a shared attitude toward risk, treatment, and timing when questions arise. Is this the point to hold back treatment, the moment for testing, or the time to try something new?

Look for a doctor whose style of decision making is most like your own. Communicate your preferences to the members on your team, particularly to your referring physician, who connects you to the specialists

PACKAGE DEAL: THE HOSPITAL AFFILIATION

You'll be choosing a hospital affiliation when you choose your new doctor, who only has privileges in specified hospitals in the area. The hospital you decide on may be determined by the treatment you'll require or by medical insurance regulations, as well as by your doctor's affiliation. Because you're starting fresh, you should think through what kind of hospital you prefer.

- Do you want a community hospital close to home, with a readily accessible cancer center staffed by physicians trained in university hospitals, practicing alone or in a small group without a large team of medical students and residents-in-training?
- Would you rather go to a large university hospital teaching center with claims of state-of-the-art equipment, new treatments, and access to a wide number of research protocols?

In a way, you can do both: you might choose a community cancer center with a university hospital affiliation for breast surgery, radiation, and chemotherapy, and the main university hospital center for more complex procedures, access to clinical trials, and intermittent advice and guidance (such as my practice environment at Lankenau Hospital).

you see off and on and helps you select who's best for you based on your needs and inclinations.

Do you want a doctor who'll act as a partner in your care, or do you prefer the old-fashioned model of the doctor as authority figure? Some women prefer the traditional old-fashioned relationship with a white-haired male physician; others want a same-sex physician of similar age for the ease of communication and camaraderie they feel they should have in a modern patient-doctor relationship.

"One was the best in his field, but simply too cold and business-like for me. I need someone I can turn to for support and encouragement, as well as good medical care." Gena went to a number of doctors before she found the right fit.

ACCESS. "She's always available for questions—I wanted a doctor who didn't have one foot out the door." "She is never too busy to answer my questions. I felt I could really talk to her." "He answered all my questions, directly and honestly, didn't pull any punches." "He always returned my phone calls—and explained everything."

FEELING THE LOVE. One of the things that I look for in a doctor is if he or she loves being a doctor. Such a doctor is more likely to continue improving his or her skills and enjoy taking care of me, and inspire a high level of morale and patient care from his/her staff. A doctor who enjoys being a doctor will also be excited by new medical advances, not threatened by them.

Choosing Your Doctors

To select your doctor, follow your instincts; listen to your inner voice to guide you to the best decision. And keep listening, even after you make your choice—your intuitive sense may be more helpful than you think. You make this decision with the hope that it will work out well, but your decision is not permanent or irreversible. If you've switched doctors, it's possible to switch again, or even to go back to your original doctor.

> **VET YOUR DOCTOR**
>
> In addition to any questions of your own, this list will help you evaluate your choices:
>
> - Is he or she well trained, with expertise in the area that concerns you?
> - Is communication good?
> - Do you get a sense of warmth and respect?
> - Is there any note of condescension or sexism?
> - Is he or she willing to provide you with full information about your condition and related health issues?
> - Is the office clean and cheerful?
> - Is the examining room comfortable and adequate?
> - Is the staff helpful, forthcoming, and competent?

Who Sees You, How Often, and Why

Once you've reaffirmed your relationship with your doctor or selected a new one, it's time to establish a routine for long-term care. You may have been caught up in your cancer care to the exclusion of your other health needs. When were you last at the dentist? Gynecologist? Eye doctor? All of you should be reassessed and paid attention to now, with a holistic perspective that takes into account the big picture of your medical care.

Changing Needs

It's important to keep in mind how your needs may have changed: your gynecologic needs may have changed because of hormonal therapy (see Chapter 7), natural or chemotherapy-induced menopause (see Chapter 14), or treatment side effects that may have sexual repercussions (see Chapter 19). Your general medical care should resume with attention to physical fitness, stress reduction, nutrition, and weight control; minimizing the risks of heart disease, diabetes, high blood pressure, and osteoporosis; and monitoring your risk of uterine, ovarian, or colon cancer. This is also a good time to work on kicking bad habits such as smoking, excess alcohol consumption, or recreational drugs.

Pick a Team Leader and Coordinator

As you wind through treatment and healing, it's important to have *one* doctor who exercises a holistic approach to your care, keeping track of your physical, emotional, and social needs. This doctor talks to your specialists and makes certain that everything necessary for your care is arranged and scheduled, and happens. If you run into any problems as you go along, this doctor can run interference for you.

Although your cancer care doctor may take the main role in your overall care while you're undergoing cancer therapy, the best person to oversee this holistic approach to your medical care before, during, and after treatment is your primary care physician. (If you are in an HMO, your primary care doctor is the gatekeeper of your care and may be managing more of your medical services than if you are in a non-HMO plan.) She or he is used to covering that big picture for you, to being your advocate with other doctors and with your medical insurance company. Your relationship was probably established prior to your cancer diagnosis, and seeing each other during treatment reinforces the prospect of your return to the routine of a normal life after treatment's over.

Prepare for Your Doctor Visit

Doing your homework ahead of time increases the chance of getting what you need and want out of your doctor visit. Writing out questions and concerns helps to organize your thoughts and ease your mind.

Before a visit you should also minimize distractions and unnecessary sources of stress: pick out what you're going to wear, make sure the kids are covered, check that there's enough gas in the car, and allow enough time in case of traffic or parking hassles.

Know What You Want Going into the Visit

We're all different, and your doctor can't presume to know how you want to handle your medical affairs and what questions and concerns you may have unless you communicate them. Some of my patients tell me they've read everything there is on the subject of breast cancer, and they are active and informed about decisions in their care. Others rely mostly on me for up-to-date information and the choices available to them. In any one day, I may see thirty people with altogether different styles of handling information and making decisions.

CHECKLIST: WHAT TO BRING TO YOUR DOCTOR VISIT

- ✓ Health insurance card
- ✓ Photo identification
- ✓ Social Security number
- ✓ Credit card or checkbook
- ✓ Completed forms you were sent ahead of time
- ✓ Copies of relevant documents
- ✓ Pathology slides
- ✓ List of questions
- ✓ Pen and paper
- ✓ Referrals required by your insurance company
- ✓ Something to eat and drink
- ✓ Charged cell phone
- ✓ Backup phone numbers in case you get stuck

Organize Your List of Questions and Concerns

Prepare a list of what you think is important to discuss: a symptom (don't hide any), questions, concerns, your child's troubling comment, time off for a family wedding. *No question or concern is trivial or stupid.* If something is on your mind, put it on your list. Some questions may scare you. Putting them in writing may help you defuse their fearfulness. "When I wrote out the things I was worried about, they seemed a little less frightening."

Organize your questions in order of their importance, so that you address the most pressing issues first. Ideally you'll get to all the questions on your list, but if you have to postpone some questions, let them be the least important.

Have your list of questions in hand so you can ask them with ease; write them out in large, clear print on a single piece of paper, so you can read your notes without fumbling or missing a question that's important to you. Avoid scribbling on bits of paper—you won't be able to read your own handwriting. If you give up on asking, you won't get answers.

Describe Your Symptoms

Report a careful description of each of your symptoms, using the guidelines below:

- What symptom(s) do you have?
- What does it feel like?
- Where is the symptom located?
- When did it start?
- What were you doing at the time?
- Have you ever had it before?
- Has your symptom changed?
- How long does it last?
- Is it better or worse or the same?
- What makes it better?
- What makes it go away?
- Does it happen at any particular time?
- Are there other signs that go along with the symptom?
- What medications are you taking, any new ones?
- Have you used any new products recently?

Make things as easy as possible. You may feel nervous, anxious, and under pressure—especially if you're preoccupied with a specific question or concern, like what's in your test results or a new pain in an odd spot. Everything you planned to ask about just goes out of your head, so be sure to have it on paper, in your hand. All of the effort you put into your homework will pay off big time at the doctor's office.

It is helpful to bring someone along with you to your appointment—a close family member or friend—who can help you listen, understand, and remember all that your doctor has to tell you in a short space of time.

MANAGING THE WAITS

So, other than taking a whole day off from work, or rearranging your child's entire carpool schedule, what do you do about the waiting?

You can try booking your appointment first thing in the morning, just after lunch, or at the very end of the day, when appointments tend to go on time. Your doctor's appointment secretary can help you pick the best time for the most streamlined visit. Arriving early for your appointment helps only if there's been a cancellation or if they're running ahead of schedule. If all appointments are filled or they're running late, coming early may only add additional time to your waiting, especially to your perception of waiting a very long time. It may help to call the doctor's office before you leave home, to find out if appointments are running late and by how much.

If you have appointments with two doctors (or a doctor and a test arrangement) on the same day, let the first doctor's secretary or nurse know about the other commitment so, if possible, you can be moved through without delay and on to your next appointment. Or if you're running late, call your next appointment to let them know of your delay.

If you feel you have waited unduly long, it is possible they have forgotten about you. Go up to the receptionist and be sure they know you're there and that you're on their schedule. Check back occasionally to be sure you are not forgotten. If you have been waiting an unavoidably long time, your doctor or his staff should do what they can to recognize your inconvenience.

For these inevitable waits, I always bring work, knitting, a good book, and/or stationery to catch up on all the letters I've been meaning to write. (This way I don't feel I'm wasting my time flipping through old magazines or fretting about what I could be doing instead of being stuck in a crowded waiting room.) A friend who's addicted to National Public Radio always brings a small portable radio with headphones. You might also want to bring a snack and something to drink in case of long delays.

If you are annoyed with frequent delays or lack of attention, you may decide it's a serious enough situation to warrant switching doctors. But continuity of care is essential, so if you find the level of care and communication to be good, don't let waiting be the sole criterion for making a change. Tell your doctor about your frustration. There may be ways to make things better.

KEEPING IT CLEAN

When I go to my doctor, I'm not there to swap germs. A doctor's examination room is a busy place, and a doctor's hands go unmentionable places. I get especially bothered by seeing my doctor fingering his nose, mouth, or mustache, then reaching over to shake my hand or examine me. That's why it's important for me to see my doctor wash his/her hands in front of me. The office, the table paper, the gowns, the doorknobs, and the nurse's and the doctor's hands had better be clean.

You may not give much thought to this issue, but your doctors should and usually do. I keep my nails short, and I start off the physical examination of my patients by washing my hands in front of them, or letting them know that they've just been washed. This fuss about hand washing, besides being a health measure, is a way of letting patients know they are important and a way to help set the scene before we get on to what we're both there for. If your doctor doesn't wash his/her hands before touching you, then you can quickly say, "One of the things that I really appreciate about you is that you *always* wash your hands before you examine me!"

At the Doctor's Office

Greetings

The first time or anytime, whenever you meet with a doctor, you should expect eye contact, a greeting, and an introduction to anyone in attendance with your doctor. It helps to assert your individuality when you greet your doctor to stand up, eye to eye, hand extended to shake his or hers. If you're in a hospital bed, you can still reach out for a handshake and establish eye contact.

If your doctor wants to invite students or residents to observe, he or she should first ask whether it's okay with you. You should feel able to say no if you find that having an audience is uncomfortable. In turn, you should introduce anyone who has accompanied you, indicating that person's relationship to you. Just as doctors occasionally forget to introduce themselves, patients sometimes forget to identify the person or people they're with. In my own practice, my nurse who does the initial evaluation always makes sure to find out everyone's name and relationship to the patient so I know who everyone is. Then, when I do come in, I introduce myself first to my patient, and then to everyone else.

If you're not comfortable with how you and your doctor address each other, it's never too late to discuss it. I suggest taking your cue from your doctor on how he or she wants to be addressed, or just ask what he or she prefers, and say what you prefer to be called. Remember, you have the privilege of being addressed the way you wish.

Sharing Information

After the greeting, it's time to discuss the purpose of your visit and raise any concerns. It's very important to let your doctor know what kind of information he/she may discuss in front of the people you've brought with you. Patient privacy laws (HIPAA) are very strict, and your doctor would rather withhold information than spill it. To avoid getting only partial information, tell your doctor up front about what kind of information you feel comfortable sharing.

In my practice, if I'm unsure I check with my patients privately about what they find acceptable to discuss in front of the person they're with, even if that person is a husband or partner. With important, delicate matters—sex, for instance—I can't assume that they will want to discuss it with anyone, including their partner or me.

That said, never hesitate to ask your doctor a question for fear that it may be awkward. Getting your questions answered will leave you able to concentrate on the agenda of the day—on what your doctor has to ask you and tell you.

When I meet a new patient, I make a point of letting her know I've prepared for our meeting. "Even though we haven't met before today," I might say, "I feel I know you a little: I've talked with your other doctors, I've read your medical records, and I've studied

GUIDELINES FOR FAMILY/FRIENDS WHO COME WITH YOU

- Always let the patient or doctor speak first.
- Do not talk over or interrupt the patient or doctor.
- Wait for your cue to join in.
- Ask permission to speak up.
- Use names when speaking about each other.
- Bring pen and paper, and possibly a tape recorder (always get your doctor's permission before recording his or her voice).
- Be patient.
- Give the patient privacy during the physical exam, unless you have an understanding otherwise.
- Stay on topic (don't drift over to your personal health concerns).
- Turn off cell phones.

FOR GAY WOMEN

Lesbian patients may have an extra burden in their struggle with cancer care: their doctors may find themselves uncomfortable and particularly awkward in dealing with their patient's partner. The medical community is generally conservative, but personal beliefs should in no way diminish the quality of care your doctor is committed to giving you. You may want to let your doctor know you are gay and to introduce your partner to your medical team, especially if she is your primary caregiver. If you have decided to keep your family in the dark about your personal life, you may be even more grateful for the backup support of your physician, so it's worth the effort of bringing your doctor and your partner together as part of your health care ensemble.

your radiology and pathology reports." Then I tell something about myself, information every patient has a right to know about her doctor: my background, my qualifications, my special interest in breast cancer, and how my office and practice operate—an implicit way of expressing respect for my patient, redressing some of the imbalance I spoke of earlier. We move on from there.

Asking Your Questions

Don't ask your questions in the middle of your physical exam. Few people can do two things well simultaneously. On the other hand, you can't wait until your doctor's hand is on the doorknob. The best plan is to tell your doctor right off—when your visit begins—that you have a list of prepared questions, so enough time can be allotted to answering them. Bring up your major concerns first, to get the most important answers and to ease your anxiety as soon as possible. Don't forget to stop and actually listen to your doctor's answers between questions. (When you're nervous the tendency is to keep talking.) Always thank your doctor for each answer before moving on to the next.

You may feel time is running out as you go down your list of questions, or maybe you have too many questions for the length of your appointment. Be direct: "I know time is running short, but I still have questions. Do you have more time now? Should I make another appointment? Arrange a phone call? How about email? Are there other doctors or nurses to whom I might direct my questions?" Don't let unresolved issues gnaw away at you.

Ask your doctor if there are any important questions you haven't brought up, or if there's more you should know or think about that you haven't been aware of. Your doctor's role as a communicator is to explain complex concepts in understandable words and images and to give you access to information such as test results, new medications, or new protocols on the horizon.

Don't ever let yourself fall into a mind-set where you are afraid to ask questions because you anticipate a brush-off or rejection from an overloaded, harried, or arrogant physician. (Patients don't want to be labeled a pain in the neck.) At the heart of this issue is the fact that patients are generally not encouraged to ask questions. Remember: you are paying for your doctor's services and are entitled to have your concerns addressed. This is *your* life on the line, after all.

There may also be questions you don't want answers to. Not everyone wants to know everything about this disease; some in particular don't want to know about their prognosis, especially if it's grim. In fact, very few of my patients ever ask. Respect your own limits regarding information, but at the same time, don't live with secret fears that are most likely worse than reality.

Being Heard

You may not have specific questions that need to be answered. You may just need a doctor to listen to the concerns you've been turning over in your head and give you some kind of feedback. As you talk with your doctor, you realize it's the listening that matters. A doctor who listens is providing the ultimate in care: empathy, support, understanding. That listening may be the "answer" you've been looking for. When you assert yourself with questions and collect information important to your health, you take an active role in your health care—which is really the only way to give yourself that vital sense of control and to stay as healthy as possible. It also makes it easier for your doctor to take care of you.

Expect to stumble over some awkward subjects. For example, it's a good thing to discuss how your sex life may have been profoundly affected by your breast cancer experience. Most women want to talk about it but won't bring it up unless asked. (In a survey of breast cancer survivors we found that most women wanted to discuss sexuality with their health care giver—doctor, nurse, social worker—but few do.

Health care givers were more likely to discuss sexuality with women having few, if any, problems. Least likely to ask for help were women suffering the most significant problems with sexuality.) But don't be surprised if your doctor doesn't ask personal questions. Doctors are not generally trained in this sensitive area of care. Also, they may not have the answers you need, or they may be without the insight and experience required to come up with practical suggestions.

There should be someone on your team who can handle these issues for you: the nurse, your primary care physician, your gynecologist, the hospital social worker, or the support group facilitator or therapist. Ask your doctor to direct you to people who can address your concerns if she's uncomfortable or unable to address them herself.

Doctors may also customize their questions to their patients. Three women who shared the same gynecologist were talking about their gynecologic exams and the questions they were asked. The first woman said, "So then he asked me whether I had any concerns or questions about my sex life." "He's never asked *me*." "He's never asked me, either. Why you, not us?" After they talked it over together, they decided it was because the first woman was the most outgoing and stylish of the three.

Before You Go Out the Door

Before you leave your doctor's office, take a moment to ask yourself these questions: *Did my doctor listen to me? Did he or she answer all my questions? Did I understand what I was told?* If not, let your doctor know.

Remember, it's a privilege for doctors to take care of you. And it's a privilege for you to have the care of good physicians. When you're happy with your doctor and your care, let your doctor know that, too. Positive feedback will enhance the quality of your relationship and your future health care. As we've said before: your relationship with your doctor is of utmost importance.

After You Leave the Doctor's Office

When Should You Call?

How do you decide, after treatment is over, when it's important or simply okay to call your doctor with a question or concern? You should always report any new, persistent, or possibly progressive symptoms such as fever, arm swelling, back pain, headaches, stress, or continuing weight gain. Ask those nagging questions that trouble your peace of mind. Although you may be seeing much less of your doctors than in the recent past, they are there for you when you feel you need them.

Getting Medication Prescriptions Refilled

Perhaps you're calling because you need a prescription filled or refilled. It's best to have the doctor who originally prescribed the medication renew the prescription for you. Patients often think any one of their doctors can renew a prescription for them. But a prescription is given for very specific reasons, with awareness of other medications you may be taking, and only the doctor who originally prescribed the medication for you should order your refill.

RX REFILL: BE PREPARED

When you call your doctor for a prescription refill:

- Have your most recently filled prescription bottle right in front of you, ready to read off the medication's name, amount given, and other information.
- Provide the name and phone number of the pharmacy you want your doctor's office to call to fill your prescription. Know the pharmacy's hours, so that if you reach your doctor in the early morning, evening, or on a weekend, you are not asking him or her to call after it has closed.
- Ask if a generic version of the medication is acceptable.
- Make sure the medication is affordable, through insurance or other resources. If you get to the pharmacy and can't afford to pick up the prescription, you're without medicine, and you may feel humiliated.
- Know your other medications. Even if you are a longtime, well-known patient of your doctor's, don't expect him or her to recall your specific allergies or current medications.
- Remind your doctor about any medication restrictions, including allergies.
- Ask about drug-to-drug reactions whenever you experience new symptoms and when you've been prescribed a new medication.

Supplying this information will help you get the best care possible.

Facilitate Team Communication

You can't assume good communication among your doctors; your primary care doctor may be uninformed of your current status. You can and should take a personal role in this communication process. Make sure that each of your doctors calls and/or sends progress reports to the others, and also make sure that radiology and pathology reports are sent to every one of your doctors. Call or send a note to keep your primary care doctor personally informed of your progress. Sharing communications with your medical team is greatly facilitated by electronic medical records, and it's good if your team employs them.

Coordinate Your Follow-up Appointments

It's important for you to ask your team of cancer care doctors to help coordinate their follow-up schedules so you can make sure the full year is covered and also establish some kind of control over your time. Continuing care from this team will command the most attention in your health picture for the first five to ten years after treatment ends, when the risk of recurrence and lingering side effects remains highest.

APPOINTMENTS IN SEQUENCE. Any doctor who participated actively in your cancer care should continue to see you for routine checkups; that may include a surgeon, a medical oncologist (if chemotherapy or tamoxifen was part of your care), and a radiation oncologist (if you had radiation). Most doctors see you one month after their particular treatment is finished, then every three or four months thereafter, either by themselves or by another member of the cancer center team. So your surgeon will see you one month after surgery, your medical oncologist one month after chemo, and your radiation oncologist one month after radiation is completed. After that, for example, you might see your surgeon in January, your medical oncologist in April, and your radiation oncologist in July; that pattern then repeats. By alternating doctors in this way, you can minimize your visits to doctors' offices. This rotation system works, however, only if communication among your doctors is cooperative and coordinated. It's important for one of your doctors to take charge of your regular follow-up tests so they don't get missed.

FREQUENCY OF VISITS. Your doctors will want to see you more frequently depending on:

- How serious your cancer diagnosis is
- The treatment you have received
- Ongoing therapies you're on
- Lingering side effects you're experiencing
- Active concerns you have

Some doctors may need to see you every three to four months, independent of other team doctors' schedules, to:

- Watch over ongoing therapy
- Keep a close check on a physical finding
- Monitor side effects

Other doctors may stop scheduled follow-ups and become part of your reserve unit once the treatments they delivered—as well as their side effects—are over, resolved, or stabilized. These doctors then see you on an as-needed basis, staying involved through test reports and letters from other doctors providing your active care until an issue presents that requires them to reactivate their direct care. I have been in practice for over twenty years, and many of my patients have graduated from active to as-needed follow-up. Once I go into their reserve unit, I might not see them for two years, but then see them twice the following year—all depending on how I can be most helpful. As medicine becomes more specialized, major cancer centers are developing follow-up specialists, "survivorists," who specialize in the primary care of people who've survived cancer.

Second Opinions

No doctor knows everything, and one doctor can't take the best care of *all* your needs—not in today's world. Given these normal and expected limitations, at times your doctor or you may need to call another doctor in for help or confirmation. No one should feel threatened if you feel you need more information before making a crucial decision.

A second opinion is a chance for a fresh new perspective on your care—giving you more information so you can get the best care possible. It's when you or your physician decides to seek advice from a medical professional beyond your immediate health care team to evaluate, confirm, or disagree with the current diagnosis and treatment plan, or suggest an alternative diagnosis and/or treatment approach.

Fear of Alienating Your Main Doctor

Some people are concerned they'd be perceived as disloyal if they ask for a second opinion, but it's not so. Your relationship with your doctor is not a commitment like marriage—a second opinion is not like having an affair. Having said that, expressing your appreciation of your existing relationship with your doctor can ease any awkwardness and make him/her still feel valued.

Conflicting Opinions

It's not uncommon to have a couple of different opinions without a clear consensus. "My doctor told me I should have both breasts removed. I didn't feel I needed my breasts, and I didn't think it would make a difference to my husband. I was ready to go ahead, but my husband said, 'Let's just get a second opinion.' I told this new doctor I didn't need my breasts. 'Look' he said, 'you're still a relatively young woman, and a double mastectomy is a complex and serious operation. I don't think it's called for in your situation. I recommend lumpectomy and radiation.' I went with his treatment after we talked it over, and I've never regretted it." There can be several correct ways of interpreting a medical problem. (It's not as though you're a car and there's just one way to fix you.)

Resolving Conflicting Opinions

There is always enough time to get the extra information you need—even a third opinion if that's what's called for. (Some women get more than that.) Linda got three differing opinions—and she became absolutely confused. "I thought they'd all agree, but they didn't. I found that very disturbing. I felt the doctors should have spoken to each other about my care and created a solid front. Each said what he felt was best, but it was left to me to sort through the advice and tie it all up."

The final word on a treatment decision is yours. If you are beyond your initial therapy, you may be deciding whether you should start hormonal therapy, whether to go ahead with the reconstruction you originally were unsure about, or how you can boost your immune system. To that end, you need all the information and expert advice you can collect, even if it's confusing at first. Online resources, including Breastcancer.org, can also help you collect information from a patient's perspective, hearing how other people have dealt with similar issues.

MAKING DECISIONS WITH INCOMPLETE INFORMATION

We all know that medicine is an inexact science, and sometimes a decision must be made based on insufficient data, without clear-cut answers. So how do you work with your doctors to settle on a course of action? How do you decide what's best for you based on the information available? Should you start taking a new medication three years after you've finished your main treatment for breast cancer? What is the healthiest diet for your needs? Should you proceed with genetic testing?

Your best possible decision will be guided by your managing doctor's best medical judgment, your knowledge of your body, and your personal needs and wishes. Your primary care physician can be especially helpful here, with the greatest commitment to you and the least investment in your specialists' presentations. She or he can facilitate discussion among consultants with differing opinions, suggest questions you should ask, and give you a perspective on choices, values, and long-term considerations.

Listen to all information, gather all points of view (including those from family members closest to you), and think about each one carefully. Then find someone with whom to bounce around ideas. Make up a balance sheet of various topics: hormonal therapy, for instance. Have one column listing which benefits from hormonal therapy may apply to you, and another column stating which side effects might apply to you. Circle the factors that matter most. Finally, get back to your managing physician with your information and hammer out the details of your treatment decision together.

Changing Your Team

You spend so much emotional energy investing yourself in your relationship with your doctor. It's difficult to wrench away and find somebody new. But it makes sense to make a switch when you've identified a meaningful problem that won't go away, if you need to address new priorities, or when you're moving to a new location or insurance plan.

No matter what the reason for switching doctors, it's important for you to take control and establish a good doctor-patient relationship with

CHANGING DOCTORS FOR NONPERSONAL REASONS

New Medical Insurance Coverage

Are you being forced to change physicians because your doctor is no longer a member of your insurance plan, or because you've just changed insurance companies and your doctor is not part of your new health plan—reasons that have nothing to do with the competence of, or your relationship with, your present physician? You may adore your doctor, but her bills won't be covered if your insurance has dropped her from its list or she was never on it.

Whether the doctor you want appears on your list depends on many factors, including the time required to identify, recruit, and sign up particular doctors and the time and facilities needed to complete necessary paperwork (which includes the financial conditions of contracts, for example). Doctors often participate in multiple plans, and popular doctors may find themselves besieged by multiple companies at any time. It can take them a lot of time and effort to sort out the details of joining one insurance company plan over another, which further limits their availability to patients. Or in order to control the size of an already too busy practice, or to avoid an insurance plan known for extra paperwork and hassles, a doctor may decide not to participate. Or maybe your doctor is a member but the hospital in which he/she works doesn't participate. It can be a deal breaker if your doctor is covered but the treatment or procedure isn't (surgery, radiation, chemotherapy).

Moving Away

Sometimes a switch is necessary because you or your doctor is moving out of town. A few people manage to keep their doctors, even when they move away; they have too much at stake and care too much for a doctor they trust, so they travel to their doctors a couple of times a year. But even if such an arrangement works for you, don't neglect the need to have someone close to where you now live to take care of you. At the very least, you should have a primary care physician close at hand for ordinary and emergency health care needs.

If you are moving away, ask your current team if they know anyone in the area you're heading to. Medical specialists share a small world: doctors know each other from training, through the literature, from medical conferences, and from the media. And if they don't know anyone personally, there's always the medical grapevine they can turn to. There's also the directory that each specialty publishes, which lists doctors by location and provides information about training and experience. You can check them out further yourself on Google.

If you're using a physician referral service for the name of a doctor, don't expect unbiased information; the service may be one based at a particular hospital or one that includes only doctors who pay to be listed. Ask your friends and trusted neighbors for the names of doctors they recommend, especially if they also have experienced breast cancer. Remember, however, that many such recommendations are made on the basis of bedside manner rather than clinical expertise.

If possible, check out a doctor with other medical professionals who work near or with her or him but have no vested interest in a recommendation: hospital nurses, interns, or residents. Google can give you all kinds of information about his/her professional activities to back up recommendations: papers written, TV appearances, and speaking engagements, as well as accolades and controversies.

your new doctor. But don't be surprised at how hard it may be for you to make this switch—even if that relationship is clearly not working. (You have a personal investment in this important connection; it's difficult when it ends.) In the midst of the switch, don't waste personal energy explaining your decisions or telling off the doctor you're switching away from. Keep your focus: first work on making the new relationship a good one.

✌ Moving Forward

After three years, your risk of recurrence continues to decrease and lingering side effects of treatment usually have subsided or at least

TRANSFERRING RECORDS

Once you've established a relationship with a new doctor, arrange to have your full medical records delivered to the new office:

- Printed materials can be mailed or faxed. Some doctors also do email or utilize an electronic record system
- Written permission is required to transfer records and allow your new doctor to get access to them.
- Call ahead to the radiology and pathology departments to have your radiographic studies (in a film jacket or burned onto a CD) and pathology slides ready, and set a time to collect them.
- You or a family member (with your signed release) should pick up the studies yourselves and bring them to your new physician; you don't want them getting lost in the mail.

stabilized. The frequency of your office visits can be cut back to every four to six months.

As more years go by, the risk of recurrence diminishes further. After five years, you'll probably need only twice-yearly follow-ups. After eight to ten years, checkups once a year will probably do. The risk of recurrence is so low after ten years that many oncologists recommend having your primary care physician conduct your checkups. For quite a number of women, in fact, their primary care physician has handled most if not all follow-up care since their treatment was completed.

You can tailor your follow-up schedule to your needs, the recommendations of your health care team, and your convenience. I have patients who don't want to graduate to longer intervals between appointments because they want the reassurance of continued close supervision. Other patients have to be convinced that they need to see *any* doctor on such a regular, frequent basis. Most patients find comfort and encouragement in these steady visits (allowing, of course, for the anxiety that comes before each visit).

As medical insurance companies establish new regulations to streamline cost, your visits to specialists may be restricted. To protect your access to your cancer care physicians, you and your primary care physician may need to act with persistence to have these follow-up visits paid for.

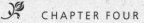

CHAPTER FOUR

You and Other Health Care Professionals: Allied Care Team

The therapist who administered my radiation was the most wonder-ful person in the world. She tried to tell me at least one joke each time I saw her. But one time when I was feeling blue, she told me I needed to cry—and she cried along with me.

The first person I came in contact with at the cancer center was the receptionist. I must have talked to her fifteen times on the phone. I didn't like her at first: she was tough, humorless, and demanding—insisting that I fetch all my records and films from three different hos-pitals; otherwise the doctor wouldn't see me. But then I realized that all this hard work was for my own good. When I finally met her in person, I thanked her—a little reluctantly. Bingo: big smile! From that day on she was my advocate for anything I needed.

I was a grouch, but the nurses were gentle, soft-spoken, and very kind to me—and they were always ready to listen.

After surgery, I couldn't get my arm up above my shoulder. The phys-ical therapist worked with me week after week, for nearly three months. Now I can do almost everything I used to except when it comes to styling my hair. I have to go to the beauty parlor for that. Not too bad.

I loved the gentleness and open-mindedness of my yoga teacher. Each week she helped get another creaky part of my body moving and grooving again.

My social worker was outstanding. I don't think I could have managed my treatment if she hadn't helped arrange the day-to-day details for me.

❧ First Things First

You've probably already met or worked with a number of the members of your health care team other than your doctor: secretaries, receptionists, nurses, physician's assistants, radiation therapists, complementary medicine practitioners, genetic counselors, social workers, nutritionists, physical therapists, psychologists, chaplains, and more. They can be as much of an ally, a lifeline, and a resource for you as your physician. Working with them effectively—and particularly ensuring that communication lines stay open so your overall care is coordinated with each and every team member—will improve your outlook and welfare significantly as you move past treatment to recovery and renewal.

❧ Challenges

You will experience unrealistic expectations, unnecessary frustration, and incomplete care if you assume that all of your care will come directly from your doctors. Determining who else on your health care team can and will look after your best interests, and learning how to coordinate their separate and complementary roles, can be an ongoing challenge. If your team is all perfectly coordinated, great. But if it isn't or if new needs emerge, you will need to manage the coordination and communication.

Of course you want everyone to like you and enjoy taking care of you, and you don't want to alienate *anyone* who is in a position to help you. What a bind! I tell my patients I want to know if anything falls short of their expectations. I've listened to many accounts of difficult interactions and assumed an active role in working things out in such situations. Most problems can be fixed, and confidence restored between patient and caregiver. Typically the problem results from some misunderstanding or miscommunication or from unrealistic expectations. Communication between team members may be absent, insufficient, strained—even hostile. Your doctor, an office manager, or a hospital/patient facilitator or ombudsman can be brought on board to help defuse or correct the problem.

Given the state of health care economics, the setting in which care is delivered can feel sterile, impersonal, and degrading, making you feel disrespected, insignificant, or dismissed. When so much is at stake, it's hard *not* to take this situation personally and get upset.

Let's start by taking a look at the role each of these nonphysician members of your health care team plays. Then we'll move into how to solve any issues with them as you move past treatment to the rest of your life.

Secretaries and Receptionists

Secretaries and receptionists are the front line of professionals, your primary connection to your doctors, nurses, and technologists. Their role is critical to the skillful delivery of your care and support. These are just some of the things that they can do for you:

- Take, deliver, and respond to phone and email messages
- Gather medical records and test reports for each visit
- Transcribe and send communications between all of the health care professionals on your team
- Coordinate procedures, tests, and visits
- Facilitate treatment
- Make sure your file is complete before you arrive for your appointment

- Spend time tracking down your radiology studies and pathology slides
- Call your next obligation if your appointment runs late
- Obtain precertification (preapproval, often called "precert") from the medical insurance company for coverage of your tests, procedures, and treatments
- Do the paperwork and billing
- Check the referral process from your primary care doctor to your specialists
- Facilitate prescription refills

Besides all of these important roles, secretaries and receptionists squeeze you in when you need to be seen in an emergency and do what they can to smooth your passage through treatment and beyond. You want them on your side, as an advocate, when you're in a tight spot.

Nurses

Nurses are indispensable to your recovery and follow-up care. "My oncology nurse always made me laugh, made me feel so good I didn't mind the treatment; I felt I was being taken care of by a good friend." Oncology nurses have a very effective and powerful professional organization, the Oncology Nursing Society, which helps nurses who specialize in the care of cancer patients grow professionally, facilitate the best care for their patients, and embrace new medical advances.

Your oncology nurse can be the most accessible and attentive member of your health care team, helping you:

- Evaluate new signs or symptoms
- Get answers to your questions and concerns
- Communicate with your physicians
- Navigate the system
- Solve problems and overcome challenges
- Access your port for flushes, blood work, and IVs
- Deliver ongoing medicine therapy, such as chemotherapy

• Facilitate other forms of ongoing therapy and your follow-up
  care

Nurse practitioners are trained to take on the role of primary caregivers, able to manage many medical and surgical concerns, working
along with, or independent of, your doctor.

Visiting nurses can provide a full range of in-home services, much
of which maybe covered by insurance. LPNs (licensed practical nurses)
and nurse's aides are trained to provide important supportive services to
the nursing team on your behalf.

Physician Assistants

Physician assistants (PAs) are trained as an adjunct to the doctor, not
as an independent practitioner, as are nurse practitioners. They may
assist the physician with a broad range of medical procedures; they also
provide a wide range of primary services on their own. Some receive
certification after two-year programs; others may have been paramedics
or nurses who have gone on to further training in this specialty.

Depending on their particular background, expertise, and experience, these are just some of the things that PAs may be able to do to take
care of you:

• Gather your medical records and radiographic studies
• Record your medical history
• Perform your physical examination
• Evaluate any new signs or symptoms
• Collect or conduct special tests
• Arrange prescription refills
• Facilitate communication with your doctor

A PA can help make the process of getting your care feel effortless
and efficient, allowing for more quality time with your doctor. In addition, the PA is one more important person on your team who cares
about you, and who may be the one most available to help you when
you're seized with a burning question and can't reach your doctor.

Radiation Therapists

Radiation therapy, for your initial treatment as well as for any ongoing treatment, takes place five days a week for weeks, and it's the radiation therapists who:

- Work closely with your doctor during the initial planning session (called simulation), mapping out the areas to be treated
- Give you your daily radiation treatments to the designated areas
- Facilitate the management of any radiation side effects with your radiation nurse and doctor

Radiation therapists see you often, get to know you, and provide a daily dose of support and reassurance.

If your radiation therapist doesn't think you're feeling or looking well, or you know you're not feeling right but you're not scheduled to see your doctor, your therapist will let your doctor know that you're feeling somewhat off so you can be evaluated then and there. You may really miss this personal connection and support when your treatment finally stops and this caregiver is no longer part of your daily life.

Social Workers

Social workers handle the complex logistics of situations you might otherwise find overwhelming, making your health care delivery as accessible and manageable as possible. They work within the hospital or in an outside setting for in-home services, such as postsurgery care and hospice. They have the skills and resources to:

- Help arrange insurance coverage and discounts for home-care nursing as well as medications, nutritional supplements, wigs, etc.
- Arrange transportation to and from hospitals or doctors' offices
- Coordinate free services and resources, community services, and hospice
- Help settle bills and arrange for supplemental medical financing

Social workers may also provide important support and counseling services. They may be able to:

- Organize and lead support groups
- Provide individual counseling for you or for members of your family, to relieve the stress and pressures that have built up because of this illness

Unfortunately, health care cutbacks may have compromised or even curtailed your access to a social worker, especially for follow-up assistance. You may have to press the hospital administration to come up with a solution to work for you. Be persistent; it's the squeaky wheel that gets attention.

Physical Therapists

Physical therapists can provide you with essential care after breast and underarm lymph node surgery, to help you:

- Recover your arm's range of motion and flexibility
- Reintroduce exercise
- Regain and increase strength
- Reduce and manage pain
- Lower the risk of arm edema and manage the condition, if present (see Chapter 10)

You may need to start working with a physical therapist sooner rather than later if you're unable to raise your arms high enough to start your prescribed course of breast radiation therapy or to wash or brush your hair.

Significant progress can be made in a few weeks of treatment that may involve stretches, exercises, massage, a custom-fit elastic sleeve, or specialized wrapped bandages.

SELECTING A NUTRITIONIST

When you find a nutritionist who interests you:

- Investigate his or her qualifications (training in the area of your concern).
- Ask about his/her approach to your care and how it will be integrated with your conventional therapy.
- Ask how much it will cost.
- Find out how results will be assessed and when.
- Beware of the nutritionist who makes grandiose claims, promising results for an endless list of diseases or enormous benefits for exactly your kind of cancer.
- Be cautious if he or she constantly criticizes conventional medicine or insists that you pursue nutritional therapies to the exclusion of other treatments.
- Avoid high-cost therapies that come from a bottle instead of the vegetable stand.
- Don't become a slave to a complicated, time-consuming, costly, and rigid nutritional regimen that steals your pleasure from eating.
- Be sure to inform your conventional doctor of what your new diet is all about.

Nutritionists

It's important to understand what you want from a nutritionist. Traditional nutritionists, within the hospital and medical practice setting, help people establish a balanced healthy diet and manage their weight. Most of their expertise is with people dealing with chronic conditions for which diet and weight control are cornerstones of treatment, such as diabetes, cholesterol issues, heart disease, and inflammatory bowel disease. Most of the same principles apply to people focused on their recovery and renewal after breast cancer treatment.

If you are seeking cutting-edge advice about the potential anti-cancer benefits of specific foods, vitamins, and supplements, you will most likely have to seek a nutritionist within a progressive, innovative, open-minded cancer center with a strong commitment to cancer prevention and risk reduction, or outside the traditional medical setting.

Finding a reputable and effective nutritionist who will meet your expectations and help you fulfill your goals is no easy task, particularly since it's not routine practice for breast cancer patients to see a nutritionist (even though it should be). Ask for suggestions from your doctor, your nurse, and other patients, as well as local breast cancer and wellness organizations. Be careful: while traditional medications are carefully regulated, alternative medicines and supplements do not benefit from the same kind of regulatory supervision (see Chapter 17 for more information).

Psychologists

Dealing with breast cancer requires adjustment to new physical and emotional situations and new ways of looking at your life. A support group can help you deal with this issue (see Chapter 2), but sometimes you need more than group help; individual counseling may be more what you need right now.

Psychologists work with psychiatrists (physicians with advanced training in mental health and disease) to give and manage medications for anxiety, depression, and other emotional conditions. Neurophyschologists often take the lead on helping you manage "chemo-brain" or mind-fog signs and symptoms (see Chapter 13).

Health insurance coverage for psychotherapy may be minimal or complete, depending on your plan. In general, crisis care plus follow-up sessions are more likely to be covered than nonurgent (but still very important) treatment to address the impact of the breast cancer experience on your life.

Complementary Medicine Practitioners

You may already be an alternative or complementary medicine devotee, but most people—although curious—have not had much to do with complementary medicine beyond vitamins from the corner drugstore or supplements that looked intriguing in the natural food section of their local food market.

Your interest in complementary medicine might take center stage once your conventional medicine treatment is over. Complementary medicine practitioners typically are healers and restorers; they generally spend more time listening and talking to you than your conventional medical team members. Meditation, massage, and anxiety relief feel a whole lot better than someone coming at you with an IV needle and chemotherapy, even if the conventional treatments actually do more to make you cancer-free. Whether you merely sample complementary medical care or jump in completely, it is vital that you keep your conventional medical doctors informed about what you are doing so there are no overlapping concerns and so your overall care can be coordinated.

Spiritual Leaders

Many religious people who have breast cancer seriously question their faith in God at some point: "How could God have let this happen to me?" And they are angry that their body has betrayed them, allowing cancer cells to destroy their well-being and threaten their family's welfare. "Is there a spiritual meaning to all this?" they might ask. "Was this some kind of test from God?"

Your own spiritual leader may help you navigate these complex concerns and get answers to your pressing questions. But you may also get invaluable help from a hospital chaplain as you work to reconcile conflicting feelings and gain better insight and perspective on these spiritual questions. Most hospitals have a chaplain on staff who is trained to be nondenominational—able to work with people of all religions, and who qualifies in a broad sense as a health care provider. The chaplain traditionally visits patients within the hospital who are in particular need of spiritual counseling.

As outpatient care supplants inpatient service, some chaplains have expanded their role to circulating through the emergency room and checking with patients who come and go within twenty-four hours.

❧ Solutions

Achieving harmonious teamwork is a major accomplishment but not always possible. Each team member is like a spoke in a bicycle wheel—you can feel a wobble if one isn't pulling its weight. But when everything is aligned and coordinated, you really feel taken care of. This section will help you identify opportunities to improve your team dynamics so you can feel respected and get the best care possible.

Connecting with the Front Office

When you connect with your care provider's office, first ask the name of the person to whom you are speaking. Greet that person by name and find out politely her/his position in the department. You might say, "Mary, I'd appreciate your helping me as I try to get to know how Dr. Jones' office works. Can you tell me what your role is on the team?" Knowing each person's role on the team helps you know to whom you should direct any particular question, request, or concern. Make sure to thank anyone and everyone who has been helpful to you.

Even if you're calling the office regarding a private matter, be sure to provide some information about the purpose of your call. When your care provider or doctor gets a blank phone message with only your return phone number, he/she is unable to prepare for the callback— and is possibly uneasy not knowing the nature of your call. The result is more likely to be a delay in the callback rather than a way to expedite it. A blank message also makes the receptionist look bad to the care provider or doctor—even if it was your choice to withhold information— since she is expected to obtain complete and specific messages.

Mutual Respect

"Overwhelmed and upset about my situation, I lost control and wigged out at the nurse. My words hit her like a tsunami. I felt terrible, but it was too late to take everything back. Later I apologized."

Double standards are unacceptable. Expect to be treated with respect, and treat every member of your health care team with respect. The receptionists, nurses, and therapists communicate directly with your other health care providers all day long. Your doctor will find out immediately if you are less than truthful, forthcoming, kind, or otherwise to the receptionist staff. If, for example, you call and say you're a "close friend" of the doctor and you must get in right away, you can bet your doctor will be asked to verify this claim. If it's not true, they'll see you as a pushy, manipulative patient. If you are nasty or belittling to a receptionist, this will be communicated like lightning to other members of the staff. Of course you deserve every benefit of the doubt (we all can have a bad day), but everyone benefits when patient and staff get along well.

Dealing with Your Concerns

If you are unsatisfied or upset about the way you've been treated by a member of your doctor's team, it's important to let your doctor know. Before reporting the incident, write down a clear account of what happened, noting:

- Name of the specific team member(s) involved
- Day and time
- Where it occurred: by phone, by email, in the office
- Details of the encounter: what went wrong and what went right (try to find both, if present)
- Series of events, including what happened just before and after the incident.

It's critical to separate the facts from your emotional reaction to what happened. Start with the facts. Later you can express how the episode or encounter made you feel.

If you are prepared to speak up yourself, do so: "When you spoke to me so sharply just now, it really upset me. I'm not used to being spoken to that way." You may be nervous speaking up, but you'll feel good about yourself afterward. If you don't feel comfortable handling the problem directly, speak to your physician, the head nurse, or the hospital's patient ombudsman or patient-relations person.

Every hospital or office practice has some way of responding to patients' complaints and resolving conflicts; a patient-relations representative (ombudsman) will help you get attention, better care, a switch in your caregiver, or maybe simply an apology.

If the problem is with another member of your team—say, a nutritionist or therapist—you always have the option of choosing another person who provides that service and with whom you'll be more compatible and better able to get along.

Most of my patients tell me only good things about the other members of my team. "The radiation therapists always listen." "That nurse brought me flowers and she hardly knew me!" A smile and a warm thank-you are always appreciated and can make someone's day brighter and better.

Positive Reinforcement Strengthens Relationships

When people are particularly helpful or kind to you, it means so much when you do something thoughtful to acknowledge what they have done. It doesn't have to be much, just something that says thank you in a personal and meaningful way, such as bringing bagels, muffins, or fruit now and then when you come in for treatment or a follow-up visit. More significant is a word or a note to a superior—the head nurse, the head radiation therapist, or, even better, the president of the hospital. Letters count big time: they can increase a worker's job satisfaction and might even help with a raise or promotion. It's a special way for you to say thank you. When you put your thank-you on paper it goes into the person's career file.

Establishing and keeping up a good relationship with your health care provider and her office personnel can make everything go more smoothly. It can speed up and smooth out many of the things you have to do:

- Get a convenient appointment
- Have your calls returned in a timely manner
- Facilitate referrals to other doctors
- Expedite approvals and precertifications for tests
- Get paperwork filled out for work, disability, and other benefits
- Have prescriptions called in to your prescription provider

❧ Moving Forword

You're all on the same team, not on competing teams. Each member of your health care team adds an important new dimension, which can greatly enhance your overall care and sense of well-being. For more practical tips on how to get the information you're seeking about your care, check out Chapter 3 on the relationship you have with your doctors.

CHAPTER FIVE

Tests: Peer, Poke, Prod

I wasn't looking for surprises or trouble; I just wanted to keep watch over my health, have the routine mammogram my doctor told me to get. Something worried somebody, because I had to have more pictures, then come back for a biopsy. I thought that would be like a needle stick—but it was a real operation. I should have been warned about that, but I can't really complain. What they took out was benign, and I'm okay.

My cancer didn't show on the mammogram. Only the MRI found it. Why can't I skip the mammogram and just get MRIs in the future?

I freak out every time I get my mammogram. With each year it got worse, not better, so I had to figure something out. Now I go with a friend and arrange to always have the same radiology technician and radiologist at the mammo center—and they give me my results before I leave.

I had both breasts off so I'd never have to have another mammogram.

I don't understand why my doctor won't order repeat tests of the rest of my body to check for recurrence. They were all over me to get my mammogram every year, but for some reason they don't seem to care about the rest of me.

First Things First

Your body is an absolutely fascinating organism, made of and operated by an incredibly complex network of parallel, cascading, and interconnected functions, which are affected by an infinite number of internal and external influences. Tests are a window into what's happening inside your body and can measure:

- What something looks like (e.g., a mammogram to examine your breasts)
- How something is functioning (e.g., a blood test to check liver enzymes)
- What something is made of (e.g., a microscope to check the type of cancer cells)
- How much something produces (e.g., a blood test to check the bone marrow's production of immune cells)

Tests can look at something as large as your liver (by ultrasound, CAT scan, or MRI) and something as small as a tiny part of one gene (BRCA1 or BRCA2 gene mutation testing).

Tests attempt to unlock these mysteries:

- How the breast cancer got started (the HER2 gene)
- What's making it grow (hormone receptors)
- How far it's spread (for example, a bone scan to see if there is abnormal activity in the bone)
- Has it responded to treatment (blood test for cancer markers)

We can use tests to identify people at high risk for cancer who are ready to take steps to reduce their risk (genetic testing). The most common use of breast tests, however, is for early detection of breast cancer for all women over forty and for younger women at increased risk.

For people just diagnosed with breast cancer, testing helps determine the stage (pathology reports on cancer tissue), nature of the disease (Oncotype DX or another type of microarray analysis), and response to treatment (MRI). And for people who've had cancer, tests help with early detection of any possible new cancers in the same or other breast (mammography, MRI). Depending on your risk of recurrence and the need to assess response to ongoing treatment, your doctor might order various tests (blood markers, bone scans, PET/CAT scan).

Tests can also measure:

- Shifts in your body's internal environment (hormone levels to assess fertility or to document early menopause)
- Lingering side effects of treatment (neuropsychological testing for mind fog, aka "chemo brain")
- Ongoing treatment effects (DEXA scan to measure bone density in women taking an aromatase inhibitor)

Working with your doctor, you can choose the best tests at the right time to efficiently and accurately answer a question, assess a situation, monitor your health, and maximize your quality of life moving forward.

⚘ Challenges

Tests can be nerve-racking and a nuisance, but as you know, they are an indispensable part of your diagnostic evaluation and continuing care. The breast cancer experience itself is a major test of you and everyone and everything in your life. How you are feeling and functioning is often the first sign that you're doing well or that something is not right.

Feelings of Failure

Tests can produce performance anxiety—making you feel like a success or failure, and dragging up miserable old memories of final exams at school. But you can't study for a medical test—the results are generally beyond your control. About the only tests you must prepare for are a colonoscopy (with bowel prep) and a blood sugar test (by fasting).

Sometimes you may feel that tests have failed you—for example, your mammogram failed to find the breast cancer early, despite your diligence in going for one every year. This may make you skeptical of all these tests and possibly angry that we have nothing better with which to detect the presence of cancer. Having to accept the limitations of a test that you entrust with your life doesn't feel good.

Result Reports: Clear or Confusing

Tests can create uncertainty, anxiety, or confusion. Some tests have precise objective numerical results generated by a laboratory machine; other tests depend on a trained person's subjective interpretation that's reported in a kind of medical mumbo jumbo.

Because tests don't always deliver clear answers, you may wonder if your result is really correct or as good as it possibly can be. Perhaps you've already received two different interpretations from two different pathologists on the same piece of tissue—how confusing.

Sometimes one test leads to more tests. For example, if you get a bone scan, you're just about guaranteed to have "a little this and a little that" in your back area—signs of aging-related arthritis—and the radiologist says, "Probably arthritis; rule out cancer." Their reports are extra cautious and they tend to order additional studies before issuing a precise interpretation of the findings.

Other times a test reveals something unexpected. You can be very upset (for example, if the pathology report shows lymph node involvement after you were reassured that your lymph nodes felt normal) or relieved (if your lymph nodes felt abnormal but turned out to be clear).

Anxiety Waiting for Test Results

Waiting for test results is haunting—most people tend to imagine the worst. Getting your test results sooner than later helps lessen the uncertainty and eases your worries, even if the news is grim.

Understanding your test results is yet another challenge. So many of the results are expressed in highly technical language (borderline HER2 overexpression by immunohistochemistry) or complicated medical terms (intratumoral lymphatic and vascular invasion). I'll give you plain-speak explanations throughout the book, but for any words that still puzzle you, go to Breastcancer.org.

✣ Solutions

The good news is that we have a broad range of highly sophisticated and useful tests that are ready for you to take advantage of immediately. Old-fashioned tests have been greatly refined—for example, digital mammography is a big improvement over film mammography; combining the complementary roles of PET and CAT scans provides more sensitivity (picking up an abnormality when it's very small) and spatial resolution (seeing it clearly). Advances in technology and genetic and protein research are promising many new breakthroughs on the horizon.

Another reason to feel hopeful: treatment advances are finally starting to keep pace with the ability of tests to characterize targets within the cancer. For example, when I first started to practice medicine, we were able to test cancer for the HER2 oncogene, present in aggressive cancers, but we didn't have a treatment that could do anything significant to fight it. Can you imagine what that was like? We'd have to tell a patient that she had an aggressive form of breast cancer but that we were nearly powerless, without a treatment that could change her odds to a good outcome. Now we have Herceptin (trastuzumab), plus many other medicines on its heels, including Tykerb (lapatinib).

Advances in testing will make possible future success with personalized medicine. The improved ability to gather full inside intelligence to characterize each person's unique cancer will lead to a custom-designed, targeted treatment approach that will maximize benefits and avoid or minimize side effects. And, of course, one day we hope that the power of testing can help identify individuals at significant risk and keep them from ever hearing the words "You have cancer."

Tests to Guide Your Care

There is a test for every step along the way, from wellness to diagnosis through treatment and beyond. In this section, I will describe the "beyond" tests that are specifically used during your follow-up care, including the tests listed below.

Breast tests
- Breast self-exam
- Breast exam by doctor or nurse
- Mammography
- Ultrasound

- Magnetic resonance imaging (MRI)
- Tracer-uptake studies
- Digital tomosynthesis
- Thermography

Body tests
- Blood tests
- Chest X-rays
- Bone scans
- Computed axial tomography (CAT) scans
- Positron emission tomography (PET) scans
- DEXA scan
- Biopsy

No one test is perfect, but when we combine several complementary tests and correlate their findings together with your personal story and physical findings, you get the greatest benefit.

Breast Self-Exam

If you don't love the idea of examining your own breasts, you're not alone. All women worry that they don't know when to do it, how to do it, and what to look and feel for. *Everything* feels like a lump, and it's hard to know what's normal and what's not. But learning the right technique and getting in the habit of performing regular breast checks can make a difference. With practice, you'll become familiar with the "neighborhoods" of your breasts and what's normal *for you.* Then it's easier to recognize a change or something new that you don't remember feeling before. Picking the right time of the month can make a difference if you haven't gone through menopause yet; examine yourself just after your menstrual period is over, when your breast tissue has settled down from the high hormone levels leading up to your period.

There is more than one effective way to examine your own breasts. The most important thing is to look over and feel through all of both breasts: from top to bottom, side to side, and front to back.

The first part of the exam is where you do a careful inspection. Stand in front of a mirror and look carefully over both breasts in two positions:

with your hands on your hips, then with your hands above your head. Notice the shapes of your breasts in both positions. Check the skin for color changes, rashes, pimples, and spots, and look for any changes in shape and size, dimples, indentations, bulges, and unevenness.

The next step is to feel throughout each breast in two positions: sitting or standing, and lying down. You can do this part of the self-exam in your bed, or just the sitting or standing up part in the bathtub or shower—wherever you feel most comfortable. The shower or bath has a built-in advantage because the water and soap make your fingers slide over your breasts more easily. Plus it's a quick add-on to the washing you're already in the middle of. (Some women find that using baby powder on their skin makes breast self-examination much easier outside the shower.)

Feel the front to the back of each breast by slightly increasing the amount of pressure you apply. Use a light touch tó feel the breast tissue closest to the surface of your skin, a firm touch for the middle section of breast tissue, and a bit more pressure to feel the deepest breast tissue.

There are two patterns of examination you can use. It's important to use one pattern to examine both breasts completely during each examination.

• Move your fingers horizontally up and down your breast, as if you're mowing a lawn.
• Move your fingers around in a spiral direction, starting from the nipple and circling out toward the edge of your breast.

As long as you cover your breasts entirely, both methods—up and down or spiral—work equally well. Look and feel for anything that stands out from or feels different than the rest of your breast tissue. Remember the *Sesame Street* TV show's lesson: "One of these things is not like the other." When you're examining your breasts, one area might feel like a mountain range, another area might feel like a rocky road, another region like a sandy beach, a bunch of grapes, or a bag of marbles. In each neighborhood, see if you can feel something that's different from the other parts. For example, if you feel a rock on the sandy beach or a peanut in a bowl of oatmeal and it does not go away, let your doctor know. It's probably perfectly normal, but it's still best to check it out.

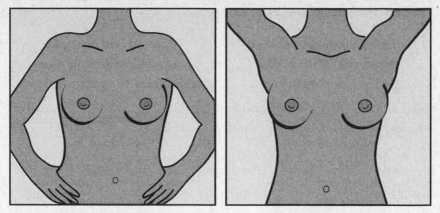

Inspect your breasts carefully, with arms down, then arms up, in front of a well-lit mirror. Check for any change is color, size, and contour.

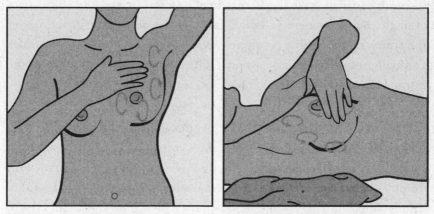

Feel your breasts with the pads of your first three fingers using a circular motion. Apply a light to firm touch as you feel from the front to the back of your breast.

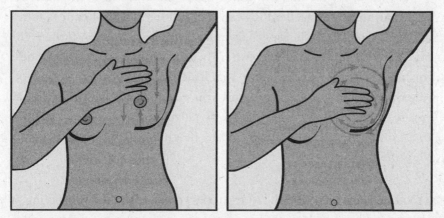

There are two ways to examine your breasts. Start on the side, and then move up and down as you make your way across your breast. Or you can start in the middle and move in a circular fashion, out to the edge.

Your Doctor's Exam

Getting a breast exam by your doctor is an important part of your regular evaluation. It is done in the same systematic way that you would do it. If your doctor feels anything unusual, ask her to point it out to you so you can follow it on your own between visits.

Breast Exam Changes After Breast Cancer Treatment

AFTER LUMPECTOMY AND RADIATION. If you have had radiation therapy, you may find that your whole breast is firmer. In addition, the area where the cancer was, where surgery and boost radiation were focused, can have scar tissue that may be even firmer and difficult to evaluate. Some women, however, can feel the absence of tissue under the scar (corresponding to where tissue was removed). As the firmness gradually resolves, don't be surprised if you're able to feel more of the normal lumps and bumps that have been there all along.

AFTER MASTECTOMY WITHOUT RECONSTRUCTION. If you have had mastectomy without reconstruction, concentrate your examination on the skin, soft tissues of the chest, and the scar. You need to apply only minimal pressure on the skin and soft tissues. In addition, it's helpful to simply slide your fingers up and down over the whole chest wall area to detect small bumps or irregularities of the skin.

If your breast is removed, your ribs are much closer to the skin surface than they used to be. Ribs can feel just like a breast cancer lump and scare you to death, especially at a point several inches to the right and left of your breastbone, where cartilage meets your rib bones, forming a heaped-up junction that can become tender. The good news is that ribs don't move, and you can figure out whether what you're feeling is bone or soft tissue by moving the soft tissue back and forth over the hard, fixed rib. (Also, neighboring ribs can be easily identified.)

AFTER MASTECTOMY WITH RECONSTRUCTION. Reconstructing a breast after mastectomy results in other problems for self-examination. Hard, irregular lumps can occur with transplanted tissue, usually near its outer edge, close to the incision. These lumps are "fat necrosis"—fat that didn't survive the transfer process, shrank into a ball, and hardened. They pose no threat but can drive you crazy until you can prove that they are not something worse.

If you had a silicone or saline implant or tissue expander placed after mastectomy, your body may make a scar tissue capsule around the implant that can make it feel hard and unnatural. If you received chemotherapy treatment through a venous port (usually located a few inches beneath the collarbone), this will feel like a big button under the skin.

> **WHAT RECURRENCE FEELS AND LOOKS LIKE AFTER MASTECTOMY**
>
> Recurrent cancer can occur as a discrete lump, a pale or reddish nodule just below the skin surface, a swelling, a persistent and progressive red rash, or a dimpling of the skin (the lump is beneath the surface, pulling the skin down). A rash or lump near the surface can develop into an open sore.
>
> Keep in touch with your body—literally—and you'll learn to make sense of the different things you feel or see.

Report Changes to Your Doctor

If you feel or see something that concerns you in between your routine doctor visits, don't wait; make a special appointment to get it checked out. Your doctor (gynecologist, internist, or family practitioner) can usually handle most issues, although you may prefer a dermatologist (skin doctor) to deal with breakouts, rashes, spots, or unwanted hair. Your regular doctor may send you to a breast specialist if she or he thinks the breast concern at hand should be looked at further.

To keep a closer watch on any area of concern, your doctor will probably schedule another breast exam in a few weeks or months, depending on your situation. Sometimes a breast test may be recommended on one or both sides to check out a breast lump that you or your doctor may have seen or felt.

Mammography

Mammography, a picture of the breast, is the only proven screening tool in women age forty and older that can detect breast cancer early, improving the chance of surviving breast cancer by about 35 percent. Mammography itself does not prevent breast cancer, but it does save lives by finding breast cancer as early as possible, when it's in its more curable form. The National Cancer Institute, the American Cancer Society, and the American College of Radiology (ACR) recommend annual mammograms for women starting at age forty, but starting younger for women at increased risk (a strong family history of breast cancer, a known breast cancer gene in the family, a personal history of breast cancer or other biopsy results showing precancer changes, or a history of radiation exposure as a young woman).

After breast cancer treatment, some doctors recommend that you have a mammogram every six months, until the effects of treatment have settled and your results have stabilized. At the least, you'll need a mammogram once a year.

Mammography is very effective for evaluating a change you notice in your breast—a lump, thickening, or palpable mass in the breast. Its value is improved when its results are correlated with prior mammograms and other methods of early detection, including your own breast self-examination and your doctor/nurse practitioner's breast examination, and sometimes ultrasound and MRI.

About 40 percent of breast cancers are found by mammography alone, about 35 percent are palpable lumps also seen on mammography, and about 25 percent are found by physical examination alone (not seen on mammography). Most of the lumps found by touch are found by the women themselves or by their partners. Breast cancers found on mammography alone tend to be smaller and to have a more favorable prognosis than cancers found by physical examination.

HOW MAMMOGRAPHY IS DONE. Since this book is for people who've already had breast cancer, I'll spare you the details about how mammogram images are obtained—an experience you never forget. But as unpleasant as getting a mammogram might be, it is still essential to your ongoing health care if you still have breasts.

Once you've had breast cancer, your mammogram is considered a diagnostic study rather than just a regular screening test. Extra attention is needed to make sure you get the most complete and careful mammogram possible. The mammography technician should mark both ends of your surgical scar on your breast by taping tiny metal balls (also called "BBs") to the skin, which show up on the image and indicate where treatment-induced scar tissue lies. Your scar helps define the surgical bed where the breast cancer used to be—the site with the highest risk of recurrence. If you are having a mammogram to evaluate a palpable abnormality, the technologist will place a BB over the abnormality in order to direct the radiologist to the area of concern.

FILM OR DIGITAL. Mammography is an X-ray picture of the breast. Digital mammography technique is identical to film mammography, except that instead of recording the image of the breast on film, the image is recorded directly into a computer (just like taking a photograph with a camera, the image can be recorded on film, as with an old-fashioned camera, or it can be recorded on a computer, as with a digital camera). It takes an instant to produce a digital image of the breast, and about five minutes to develop an image on film. Once a digital image is registered within the computer, it can be quickly checked to see if the whole breast got into the picture and if there is an area of concern. The computer can then zoom in and get a closer look at a particular area of concern to check it out further, such as an irregular lump, a region of thick tissue, or a group of calcifications. To get a closer look with film mammography requires taking additional images—and if you've already left the facility, you have to come back in for those extra pictures. There's less need to be called back for additional views with digital mammography.

High-quality film mammography can be just as good as digital mammography, but digital is better at imaging women age fifty and younger, women with dense breasts, and women with breast enlargement implants (not implants after mastectomy). Digital is more expensive and less available than film mammography, but that extra cost is usually covered by health insurance, and over time, more centers will have this new technology.

Of course, any quality of mammogram is better than no mammogram. Even if mammography failed to find your breast cancer in the past, that doesn't mean it can't find an early stage of breast cancer in the future—and possibly save your life.

MAMMOGRAM INTERPRETATION AND REPORTING. Mammograms can be read as soon as the images are available, assuming there's a radiologist present. If you are getting a diagnostic type of mammogram (because you've had breast cancer, are at high risk for it, or have had prior breast surgery), then the images are reviewed while you wait. This is to make sure the entire breast has been pictured and that anything unusual or suspicious can be further pictured or evaluated—likely sparing you from having to return at a later time for more pictures. Further evaluation of a potential abnormality can be done with zoomed-in digital views, magnified film mammogram images, or ultrasound.

Some centers have two radiologists read each study separately, one after the other, to reduce the possibility of missing an abnormality. This improves the accuracy of the interpretation, picking up 10 to 15 percent more cancers than only one reading. You can always request that your report be read by two radiologists, although it's unlikely that your mammogram will be double-read while you wait; the second reading is generally done at a later time, just before the official report is written. Film images can be read by a radiologist, together with a computer-aided detection (CAD) program. The radiologist first does her interpretation, then the CAD points out any other areas of potential concern, which the radiologist can evaluate further.

Computerized images can be burned onto a CD to get a second opinion from another radiologist. If two hospitals are electronically connected and share the necessary software, your images can be transmitted electronically to a radiologist at another location (or anywhere in the world) for interpretation. This is a better and cheaper way to transport images than to mail original mammo films, which can be lost in transit (radiologists prefer to review original films because the images are much clearer).

CHOOSING YOUR MAMMOGRAPHY CENTER. Getting the best-quality mammogram and interpretation is critical. You should only get your mammogram at a center that is accredited by the American College of Radiology (ACR), meaning it meets the ACR guidelines of standards for the doctors who read the films, as well as for the technicians, reports, mammography machines, and even film-developing materials.

Mammography can be performed in a mobile unit, in a freestanding center, or in a traditional hospital setting. The quality of mammography equipment generally depends more on its age and capabilities than on where it is located. To pick a center, call the National Cancer Institute

(800-4-CANCER) or the American College of Radiology (800-227-5463) for the nearest certified mammography provider.

I advise that you seek out a center with an on-site radiologist, if at all possible, because of the adequacy and accuracy of the study, attention to scars, and faster test results—especially for women who have

- A personal or family history of breast cancer
- A persistent change in the breast, like a lump, thickening, or inverted nipple
- A previous breast biopsy

MAMMOGRAPHY AFTER RECONSTRUCTION. Mammography has no role after mastectomy and implant reconstruction (the breast is no longer present, and the remaining tissues at risk—the skin around the implant and the chest wall tissues behind the implant—are completely blocked by the implant which appears as a large, bright white object). Most doctors also believe that mammography after mastectomy and tissue reconstruction is not clinically useful, because essentially no breast tissue is present and the main tissues at risk are at the surface (the skin). There are special circumstances, however, when mammography may be helpful:

- If you are at high risk for local recurrence and you feel a worrisome change in the way your breast looks and feels

HUH? FAT NECROSIS?

Fat necrosis is when some fat tissue doesn't survive after surgery. It is most common after mastectomy and tissue transfer reconstruction; occasionally it happens after partial breast removal (without reconstruction). The dead fat cells then scar down, forming a lump that usually contains calcifications that can show up on a mammogram. An MRI can also be helpful in showing a lump without blood flow (whereas cancer has increased blood flow). Areas of fat necrosis stay the same or get smaller over time, whereas cancer tends to get bigger over time. Doctors can usually distinguish the two without a problem. But in a woman at high risk of local recurrence having trouble figuring out which lumps are the same or getting smaller or bigger, it's helpful to have an imaging test to sort things out and provide reassurance.

• If you have big lumps in the reconstructed breast that your doctor
says is fat necrosis and it's very hard for you to keep track of them
and figure out if they are changing or if there is a new lump

In each of those circumstances, ultrasound would likely be the first
choice before mammography. And while your doctor might recommend
a fancier test next, such as MRI scans, I have seen several recurrent breast
cancers detected with mammography in women who have had tissue
reconstruction. Mammograms are cheaper and easier to get—and they
are probably better at tracking fat-necrosis-related calcifications and distinguishing those benign findings from cancer changes. In addition,
many of you may have limited access to MRI because of its high cost,
because of health insurance restrictions or absence of insurance, or
because you live somewhere that doesn't have this technology.

Occasionally, a woman who has had a very large lumpectomy may be
left with significant distortion of the breast. After cancer therapy is over,
she may choose to have the missing area reconstructed with transplanted
tissue. Mammographic interpretation after this type of combined treatment can be quite tricky. Fat necrosis can occur, producing groups of calcifications. But once a baseline mammogram has been established and
treatment effects have "cooled," mammograms in this situation usually
become easier to interpret.

GETTING YOUR MAMMOGRAM RESULTS

Each center has its own policy regarding how it reports mammography results,
good news or not. Some tell you all results on the spot; other centers will not
reveal any information directly to you, no matter how much you insist.

It may be possible to get the results of your mammogram right away at a
center that has a radiologist present to review your study. If your test is negative (that is, it shows no abnormality), you're given the information and you
go home. If your films are suspect, however, you may or may not be informed
at the time; you might just be told you'll be hearing from your physician. (But
you may already suspect something because of the extra views you've been
called back for.)

In general, the best person to give you your mammography results is your
regular doctor or the one who recently examined your breasts and ordered

the study. This doctor has an ongoing relationship with you and knows you best. Some radiologists regularly perform both the mammogram and the physical exam, in which case an immediate reading of your study is appropriate. Many women want an instant interpretation of their mammogram by the reading radiologist even if there is no physical examination associated with it. They don't want to wait till their physical exams can be assessed or their referring physician notified, but it can be very awkward for one doctor to tell another doctor's patient any news, particularly bad news.

If you have come in for a mammogram without a doctor's referral, the delivery of test results can be more complicated. One experienced radiologist regularly has this dilemma: "If a woman has no referring physician, it may be hard to reach her after she leaves. I may be the only doctor at hand who can tell her the results and recommend further evaluation. She has a right to the information and she does need to know it."

If you are the kind of person who must have results quickly to prevent anxiety, choose a high-quality center that will accommodate your wishes to immediately communicate your results. Unless your mammography center has an explicit policy to the contrary, as long as there is a radiologist on-site who can read your mammogram, your demand for immediate results can usually be met.

Regardless of who orders the mammogram, who does it, and who reads it, some immediate feedback is needed if you are called back for extra views. Ask to speak to the radiologist who will be reading your mammogram so you aren't left to go home feeling puzzled and anxious. Whatever the test you have, make sure that all of your doctors and nurse practitioners are sent a copy of the report. When you sign in for the test, write their names on the top of your study request form, and note that each one is to receive a copy of the report to follow.

Ultrasound

Ultrasound is a diagnostic tool that produces high-frequency sound waves that travel through the breast and are transformed into images appearing on a monitor.

Ultrasound can detect many breast abnormalities, determining size, shape, consistency, and location. It is complementary to mammography—not a substitute for it—allowing further interpretation of what was first seen on mammography, to determine if the lesion is solid (such as a benign fibroadenoma or cancer) or fluid filled (such as a benign cyst), but it cannot determine whether a solid lump is cancerous or not. Nor can it detect calcifications—a helpful indication of early forms of cancer that can be seen by standard mammography.

Ultrasound is usually the first method of radiographic evaluation for a woman under thirty with a palpable breast lump. (Mammograms are difficult to interpret in younger women because younger women's breasts tend to be glandular rather than fatty, and gland tissue appears densely white on X-ray, much like a cancerous tumor.) Most breast lumps in young women are benign cysts or clumps of normal glandular tissue.

If a biopsy is ordered for an abnormality that's not palpable, ultrasound can be used to guide biopsy needles precisely to suspicious spots in the breast, without radiation exposure.

Magnetic Resonance Imaging (MRI)

Magnetic resonance imaging (MRI) is a powerful, sensitive (and expensive) diagnostic tool that uses magnetic fields, not radiation, to

---

MRI'S SENSITIVITY: GOOD AND BAD

MRI's greatest strength and weakness is its sensitivity. It is unlikely to miss an abnormality in the breast, but it risks overreacting to something that's nothing (a false alarm or false positive) that can lead to extra tests, procedures, trauma, and costs. This fault is officially called "limited specificity." MRI's sensitivity and specificity, however, can be improved by:

- Using a contrast agent. MRI can examine both how the abnormality looks and how it behaves (by how it takes up the contrast agent given through an IV during the procedure).
- Having an experienced radiologist interpret your MRI. There's a learning curve for every new radiology technique. The risk of false positives drops significantly once a radiologist has had a few years of experience with a new complex test.
- Getting repeated MRIs over time. There is also a learning curve for every new radiology technique as it's applied to each individual. The risk of a false positive MRI decreases once a radiologist gets to know your breasts better and compares any new MRI to your past MRI studies.

• Scheduling your MRI consistently at the best time of your menstrual cycle. Your breast tissue gets excited by the mix of high hormone levels leading up to your period (that's what can make your breasts enlarge and become tender). Once your period starts, your breasts settle back down. The best time to get an MRI is around day fourteen out of a twenty-eight-day menstrual cycle (day one is the first day of your period).

These steps can help MRI compensate for its weaknesses and build on its strengths—making it superior to other imaging techniques under certain circumstances, and delivering what matters most: invaluable information to guide you and your doctors to your optimal care.

create images of the body. It's not used as a screening test, like mammography, because of its high cost and hypersensitivity.

HOW MRI IS DONE. For a breast MRI, you lie facedown, with your breasts falling into two wells. A magnetic field is pulsed on and off around the part of the body under study. When it is on, the molecules inside the cells get excited and start spinning; when it is off, the molecules relax, giving off a special signal that is received by an amplifier and then translated into an image. (You don't feel the spinning or relaxing.) The area to be studied can be better distinguished from normal surrounding tissues by injecting a contrast agent such as gadolinium. While the image information is collected, the machine—which looks like a doughnut-shaped round tube—makes a thumping sound, and confinement within the tube can be claustrophobic for some people. (Some facilities have an open MRI machine to avoid this problem.)

An MRI study takes about forty-five minutes to an hour, depending on how much area has to be imaged and if both noncontrast and contrast images are taken. Remaining nearly motionless through much of this time is very difficult for some people, aside from the noise and claustrophobia issues. Get comfortable and relax if at all possible.

People who have had an aneurysm clipped with a magnetic metal or have a pacemaker in place cannot have an MRI because the MRI's magnetic field can dislodge these metal devices. And people with tattoos made with metal-based ink can experience burning pain in the area of the tattoo during the MRI scan.

BEST USES FOR BREAST MRI. MRI's main use is in women at high risk of breast cancer, who have a:

- Recent or prior history of breast cancer
- Strong family history of breast cancer
- Known breast cancer gene abnormality
- Prior history of Hodgkin's disease and treated as a young woman with radiation

In such women, MRI follow-up has proved better than mammography and ultrasound at finding the earliest signs of invasive breast cancer when it's most likely to be curable.

MRI can also be useful in the evaluation of women with an area of serious concern identified by other studies who have:

- A palpable mass not visible with ultrasound or mammography
- A lesion that's barely visible (by mammography) in a very dense glandular breast, and which is difficult to analyze by any other imaging method

MRI is also helpful at the time of initial staging in a person just diagnosed with breast cancer who presents with:

- A strong family history of breast cancer or a known breast cancer gene abnormality, to see if there is any other breast cancer in the same or other breast
- More than one palpable area in one breast to see if there is more than one site of disease
- Breast cancer in the underarm (axillary) lymph nodes without a breast abnormality detectable by physical exam, mammography, or ultrasound (mastectomy is typically recommended in such a situation, but if MRI can find the site of origin within the breast, it can help make it possible to do lumpectomy and radiation instead of mastectomy)

- A large breast cancer or a cancer in the very back of the breast, where more information is needed about the relationship between the cancer and the chest wall (muscles and rib cage) in order to know if the cancer is without chest wall invasion and is removable by surgery, or with chest wall invasion and not removable at this particular time

During and after treatment, breast MRI can help

- Assess response to treatment (for example, chemotherapy done before surgery to shrink down a breast cancer)
- Evaluate a significant change in a lumpectomy scar
- Sort out various lumps in a tissue-reconstructed breast in a woman who is at high risk of recurrence
- Detect leakage from a silicone-filled breast implant (silicone gel has its own characteristic appearance on MRI, easily distinguished from surrounding normal breast and chest wall tissues)

As powerful as MRI is, it cannot replace mammography (which is still the only proven screening test that can reduce the risk of dying of breast cancer by about 35 percent). Mammography is the best at finding grouped small calcifications, which are the warning signs for ductal carcinoma in situ, a curable, noninvasive breast cancer. MRI is less able to detect these calcifications.

Tracer-Uptake Breast Imaging Studies

Most breast tests show what the breast tissues *look* like; tracer-uptake studies show what the tissue *acts* like. Tracer-uptake imaging studies image the breast using special IV-injectable tracers; the rate and amount of tracer uptake inside the tissue are measured by a special camera outside the body. Since cancer cells take up much more tracer than normal cells, these tests can help distinguish cancer cells from normal cells.

Tracer-uptake tests are not very good at finding small tumors (under 1 cm), and they provide little information about the cancer's size, shape, or consistency. Getting one of these tests is like using a drug-sniffing dog, because while the test can help sniff out and lead you to the problem, it doesn't offer any details beyond that. Tracer-uptake tests have a number of different names, including molecular breast imaging (MBI), breast PET, BSIG, sestamibi, and others and are only used for:

- Evaluating a palpable mass or a mammographic or ultrasound abnormality that is of unclear significance
- Detecting tumors in women at high risk for breast cancer, particularly in those with dense breast tissue that makes normal testing difficult
- Evaluating the extent of tumor involvement in the breast as well as in the axillary (armpit) or internal mammary (under the chest wall) lymph nodes in women with a large breast cancer
- Assessing response to treatment after radiation or chemotherapy treatment, without having to do extensive surgical dissection

Tracer-uptake studies are not recommended for women at regular risk for cancer and are no substitute for mammograms for several reasons:

- They have no proven value as a screening test in any population.
- They are unable to detect calcifications, one of the earliest signs of curable breast cancer.
- These studies have trouble detecting very small cancers.
- Tracer-uptake studies use significantly more radiation to collect the images than a mammogram.
- They take a relatively long time to complete.
- They lead to more false positive results, associated with a higher biopsy rate, than mammography.

With more research and clinical use, these limitations should diminish and the technique's reliability should improve.

Positron Emission Tomography (PET) Scans

A PET scan involves the injection of a tracer, as described in the section on tracer-uptake studies. It can be used to evaluate increased cell activity anywhere in the body, including the breast, as just described, but most of the time PET scans are used for whole-body staging—to detect the presence and extent of metatastic disease. They can also be used to evaluate response to treatment. PET performs best like the detective dog described above, good at sniffing out trouble, but not so good at seeing any details about the cancer. That's why PET is often paired with CAT scans, allowing the strengths of both tests to synergize (working together enhances their total effect) and the weaknesses of each to largely cancel each other out. It's like hiring that detective dog in partnership with its master, the human detective.

The availability of PET scans is limited to medium to large hospitals. They are expensive, but if used in the appropriate clinical situations and preapproved, they are usually covered by most standard health insurance policies.

Digital Tomosynthesis

The goal of digital tomosynthesis is to provide clear images throughout the breast, one "slice" at a time. Imagine trying to read a twelve-line poem in which all lines are piled on top of each other (that's like a mammogram, in which all breast tissue is squashed into a pancake). Instead, digital tomosynthesis separates the lines of the poem so you can read them one at a time without missing a word.

Digital tomosynthesis creates a three-dimensional picture of the breast using X-rays. It is different from a standard mammogram in the same way a CT scan of the chest is different from a standard chest X-ray.

HOW DIGITAL TOMOSYNTHESIS IS DONE. The breast is positioned the same way it is in a conventional mammogram for digital tomosynthesis, but only a little pressure is necessary—just enough to keep the breast in a stable position during the procedure. The X-ray tube moves in an arc around the breast while about a dozen images are taken during a seven-second examination. Then the information is sent to a computer, where it is assembled to produce clear, highly focused three-dimensional images throughout the breast.

Early results with digital tomosynthesis are promising. Researchers believe that this new breast imaging technique will make breast cancers easier to see in dense breast tissue and will make breast screening more comfortable. Currently, however, digital tomosynthesis is available only for research purposes.

Chest X-rays

Chest X-rays are most commonly ordered for medical reasons not directly related to breast cancer, such as pneumonia, asthma, heart disease, diabetes, lung cancer, or asbestos exposure. A simple X-ray (two views: front to back and side to side) produces a picture of the entire chest. Its specific role for women with breast cancer is to

- Evaluate the small possibility that breast cancer may have spread to the lungs
- Assess the heart and lungs prior to general anesthesia or chemotherapy
- Evaluate upper respiratory tract symptoms (cough, fever chills, night sweats, chest pain) during treatment to rule out pneumonia (infection of the lung)
- Look for evidence of heart overload during or after taking medicines that can affect fluid balance and heart strength
- Check for a rib fracture or possible cancer involvement of a rib if pain occurs in a particular area of the rib cage

If your doctor needs any sort of detail regarding what is happening inside the chest, a CAT scan of the chest is in order.

Computerized Axial Tomography (CAT) Scan

A CAT scan is X-ray imaging of a series of cross sections of the body, which allows detailed study of a specific area. To get a CAT scan, you lie face-up on a moving table, passing through a doughnut-shaped machine that creates a composite, synthesized image of the part of the body being studied. The study is done with and without a contrast agent delivered through an IV to better visualize your tissues and organs.

CAT scans are not used routinely to evaluate breast conditions. They are more likely to be used to evaluate the rest of your body: chest, abdomen, pelvic area. They can provide important information in a number of different circumstances:

- Performing initial staging or periodic restaging, to check out the rest of your body for signs of cancer if you are at significant

risk of the cancer's having spread beyond the breast and adjacent lymph node areas (this is not routinely performed on people with as early-stage disease)
- Evaluating a particular sign or symptom—say, a CAT scan of the abdomen to investigate elevated liver enzymes detected by a blood test, or a CAT scan of the brain to find a reason for new, persistent, progressive headaches or double vision
- Assessing the extent of metastatic disease prior to treatment, and periodically during treatment to evaluate how the disease is responding

If your access to MRI is limited because of where you live or medical insurance restrictions, CAT scans may be used instead of MRI scans in a number of different situations in which MRI would typically be used first, if available, including evaluation of the brain, spine, and breast.

Bone Scans

Bone scans are obtained by injecting radioactive material into the blood system, where it is taken up by bone-making cells. Areas of intense bone activity (common in both cancer and arthritis) appear as dark patches on radiation-sensitive monitors. The greater the bone cell activity, the darker the image. Any activity in or next to the bone can produce dark spots on a bone scan, which are often referred to as "hot spots." Many different causes can account for hot spots on a bone scan, including recent or healing bone fracture, arthritis, and cancer. Distinguishing cancer from arthritis can be a challenge, but basically, cancer-related hot spots can occur anywhere within the bone, whereas arthritis activity shows up on the surfaces of bone joints.

Bone scans are very helpful in the care of people diagnosed with breast cancer. A baseline bone scan study may be done at initial diagnosis and staging for someone with invasive breast cancer who has:

- New or persistent worrisome back pain, or any other site of bone-related pain
- A significant risk for cancer spread (for example, if there is a large cancer in the breast with extensive lymph node involvement)

A negative bone scan (showing no signs of cancer) is very reassuring. An abnormal bone scan usually requires additional tests to further define the cause of the hot spots (for example, with plain X-rays of the bone or an MRI of the back). These extra tests are important to see if cancer is present, and if it is, to see if there is any abnormality that might cause a significant problem (such as involvement of the backbone, close to the spinal cord, or cancer in a weight-bearing bone, where there is a risk of fracture). For anyone who does have a positive bone scan showing the presence of cancer, a repeat bone scan can track response to treatment.

Bone scans are not recommended for women with early-stage or favorable types of breast cancer in the absence of symptoms because the risk of cancer spread to the bone is very low. There is also no need for repeat yearly bone scans in people with a negative baseline and in the absence of symptoms. The exam is expensive and time consuming, and it doesn't improve the quality of life or length of survival. (If bone metastases occur, finding them a little earlier by bone scan rather than waiting for active symptoms does not improve outcome.) Bone scans are unnecessary for women with noninvasive breast cancer.

DEXA Scan

A DEXA scan is used to measure the density of your bones, to determine your bone health and strength. As with growing older, various treatments for breast cancer can decrease your bone density (e.g., Arimidex, Femara, Aromasin) and increase your risk for osteoporosis and bone fractures.

Dual-energy X-ray absorptiometry, commonly known as a DEXA scan, uses low levels of X-rays and is quick and painless. A scanner passes over your whole body while you're lying on a cushioned table.

Using a DEXA scan to measure bone mineral density at the hip and spine is considered the most reliable way to diagnose osteoporosis and predict the risk of breaking a bone.

Your DEXA scan results come in two scores: a T-score, which is the difference between your bone density and the average bone density of a young, healthy woman, and a Z-score, the amount of bone you have compared to other women of your age and race. (If this score is very high or very low, you may need further tests.) Your doctor will help you interpret the results and understand what it means for your specific situation.

In general, doctors recommend that women sixty-five and older get a DEXA scan or other osteoporosis screening. But women may need to start screening earlier if they

- Are underweight
- Smoke
- Have lost height or developed stooped or hunched posture
- Have sudden back pain with no apparent cause
- Are older than forty-five and have broken a bone from minimal to no trauma
- Have a chronic illness

No matter your age, if you've been diagnosed with breast cancer and are postmenopausal, likely to enter menopause naturally or because of planned treatment (such as chemotherapy in a woman over forty years old), or likely to receive an aromatase inhibitor hormonal medication, your doctor will probably then recommend a baseline DEXA scan before you start treatment, and regular DEXA scans after completion of treatment (at about one-year intervals) until your bone health has stabilized as close to normal as possible. This will allow you to make sure your bones are staying strong and to take protective measures if you do start to lose bone strength.

Thermography

Thermography creates a heat map of the breast using a special camera on the skin surface. Cancer cells tend to produce more heat than normal tissue because they grow faster, have a higher metabolism, and require more blood flow. The procedure is noninvasive and involves no radiation.

Thermal scanning is not a screening tool for the early detection of breast cancer. It may be used to supplement information from a mammogram and help identify cancers that are close to the skin. But it has trouble finding small cancers and ones that are deep in the breast. Researchers are working on developing and testing new versions of thermography that someday may improve the test's accuracy and usefulness.

Blood Tests

Blood tests can assess the health of different organs and systems in your body. Blood tests include blood cell counts, blood chemistries, and cancer markers.

BLOOD CELL COUNTS. Immune cells can be significantly reduced by chemotherapy and, to a lesser extent, by localized radiation therapy. These immune cells are therefore measured before each chemotherapy cycle to make sure your body is able to tolerate the next dose of treatment. The cells might also be checked during a course of radiation, depending on how large an area is treated and whether chemotherapy is given at the same time. If your immune cells are significantly reduced, growth factors can be given to boost levels. (Neulasta is an example.)

Other blood cells that can be measured are your red blood cells—the cells that carry oxygen from the lungs to your body's tissues. Measurements of hemoglobin and hematocrit are a way of quantifying your blood's oxygen-carrying capacity. These measurements reflect the amount and concentration of the complex protein molecules in the red blood cells that carry oxygen from your lungs to your tissues. The number of platelets in your blood can also be counted. (Platelets are involved in the formation of clots to prevent bleeding.) All these cells can be reduced by cancer therapy, blood loss, and chronic illness. All blood cell counts are therefore closely monitored during chemotherapy. You may need transfusions or growth factors such as Procrit or Neumega to increase your red blood cell or platelet counts, respectively.

BLOOD CHEMISTRIES. Blood chemistries are used to evaluate the overall function of your organs by measuring the following:

- Levels of liver enzymes, special proteins that help conduct vital chemical reactions
- Bilirubin, a substance made by your liver that helps break down fat in your intestines
- Chemicals such as potassium, chloride, and urea nitrogen, which reflect the health of both the liver and the kidneys
- Calcium levels, which reflect your bone and kidney health

• Blood sugar, for people with diabetes and people who are taking steroids

CANCER MARKERS. If cancer is present and it is a type that produces a specific substance (usually a protein) that can be measured in the blood, that substance can become a "marker" for cancer. CEA, CA 15.3, CA 27.29, CA 125, and HER2 are examples of such measurable cancer marker proteins.

Some doctors consistently rely on markers as an early indicator of disease progression or recurrence, in order to find a local, curable tumor, or to assess response to chemotherapy. The clinical usefulness of these cancer markers, however, has some limitations. A marker test that registers normal does not prove that you are cancer-free, nor does an elevated test mean that you positively have progression or recurrence of cancer. Using markers to find metastatic cancer earlier has not yet translated into a survival benefit.

Biopsy

Biopsies are done for palpable lesions or for any lesion that looks suspicious on a radiographic study, palpable or not. Only about 20 percent of biopsies reveal a malignancy, which might suggest that many of the biopsies we do are unnecessary. In the United States, patients and physicians are generally unwilling to ignore a questionable image, because missing a breast cancer or delaying the diagnosis of a breast cancer is unacceptable, and a biopsy can be a relatively simple procedure. (It can, however, cost you considerable anxiety, apart from the economic cost.) In Sweden, where medical cost accounting is much stricter, 80 percent of biopsies turn out to be malignant because only the most suspicious lesions are biopsied.

Various biopsy techniques are available for diagnosing abnormal breast tissue:

NEEDLE BIOPSY. For palpable lesions, needle biopsy is the very least invasive and can be done in the doctor's office. Using a hollow needle, the surgeon obtains material from the area in question for microscopic analysis. Results are generally available within twenty-four hours.

STEREOTACTIC NEEDLE BIOPSY. This involves multiple core biopsies of a nonpalpable lesion using a hollow needle, with or without vacuum extraction. Placement into the area of concern is guided by an imaging technique (such as ultrasound, mammography, or MRI). After the tissue has been obtained, a small metal clip can be placed to mark the site in case the biopsy shows precancerous or cancerous cells and additional surgery is required.

INCISIONAL BIOPSY. In this type of biopsy, a small piece of tissue is taken from a lump to establish a diagnosis. This procedure is done if the needle biopsy is inconclusive and if the lump, mammographic change, or suspicious rash is too extensive or too big to be removed, or to be removed easily.

EXCISIONAL BIOPSY. This is an attempt to remove the entire lump of tissue. It is the surest way to establish the diagnosis without risk of missing the cancer (called a sampling error). If the lump is completely removed, the biopsy also has therapeutic value and can give you peace of mind. (The disadvantage of both needle biopsy and incisional biopsy is a possible inconclusive result because of sampling error; the advantage is a fast result.) Both incisional and excisional biopsies can be done in an outpatient surgery center.

If a surgeon is performing a biopsy on any area that can't be felt, it has to be localized using an imaging study. Once the area is found on an imaging test, such as mammography, ultrasound, or MRI, a special long, thin needle is placed in the lesion. When the needle reaches the lump, a collapsible hook at the end of the needle keeps the needle in place until the surgery is accomplished. (Local anesthesia can be used to reduce the discomfort.) X-rays are done of the removed tissue to verify that the abnormal area seen on the original X-rays is within the removed tissue specimen.

Tissue removed by the various types of biopsy is then examined with a microscope for cancer cells. Tissue is also processed for special tests to measure hormone receptors and the HER2 protein and gene.

Biopsies are not medical emergencies and can be scheduled at your earliest convenience. But for peace of mind, most people want their biopsies done as quickly as possible. Before proceeding with a biopsy, ask your doctor to show you the area of interest, discuss how and why the biopsy is to be performed, answer any of your questions, and arrange for you to sign any consent forms required.

Getting Your Test Results

Everyone wants to get test results immediately, and you should make it clear to your doctor that you want to hear any and all results. We discussed getting mammography results now or later on page 90. But don't assume that the results of other, more complex tests will be given to you as soon as they're ready. When your doctor orders a test, the doctor's staff or the test department's staff does the scheduling. Your doctor isn't likely to know exactly when the test actually gets done and when the results are available until the report comes into the office three to seven days later (depending on the facility and the kind of test ordered). Your doctor will share your results with you as soon as he or she has them.

Not every result, however, can be interpreted immediately. Often the information gained can't be understood until the results are combined with your medical history and the physical examination findings. That can mean that your doctors have to connect to discuss results and bring together whatever information is necessary to make an accurate interpretation. That equals more delay. Agony or not, sometimes you can't be spared that wait. At best, the likelihood is that it won't take a whole week.

Some doctors have a standing policy requiring all patients to come in to the office for all results, good or bad, so don't automatically assume the worst if you're asked to come in. But if you want results as soon as possible and your doctor's schedule is too busy to allow you to come in on the spot, you may opt for the results-by-phone system, whether the news is good or bad.

Getting Results by Phone

Whether it's a blood draw, CAT scan, pap smear, or biopsy, you leave your doctor's office or lab or hospital without knowing the significance of the specimen you are leaving behind. You go home to wait for a call that will tell you what your doctors have learned about you. How long should you wait before calling to get this information? What's the proper approach?

If you can stand it, give your doctor a week to get back to you. Sometimes, however, reports get sidetracked or sent to the wrong office. There are any number of reasons for delay. But if you're on the edge of your seat waiting to hear, and you don't—go ahead and call.

Scary-Sounding Test Results

You might receive a report that suggests a potential problem: "Your mammogram revealed findings that require evaluation. It is important that you follow up on this recommendation with your physician." In fact, the findings may be quite benign, related to past surgery and treatment, but until you make contact with your physician, you could be

---

CALLING FOR TEST RESULTS

To get your test results faster, call the doctor who ordered your tests. It always pays to be polite and patient and understanding. (You get more flies with honey than with vinegar.) "Is it possible that my results have come in and you haven't been able to reach me?"

When you call your doctor for those results, be prepared to let the receptionist know:

- What test you're calling about
- Where it was done
- The phone number of the facility
- When it was done
- Where you can be reached, including all your phone numbers and when and till how late at night to call
- Whether the doctor may leave a message on your voice mail or answering machine
- Whether the doctor may leave a message with someone else in your household if you're not available

To save yourself stress and phone-tag hassle waiting to hear back from your doctor, make an appointment for your doctor's call. To be realistic, allow a time frame between, say, one and three o'clock, arranging in advance that if you don't hear from your doctor by three o'clock, *you will call him or her back*. This way, you won't be stranded waiting, and you can plan to have someone around when you get the call—just in case.

going crazy with anxiety, particularly if the report arrives at a time when you can't reach your doctor.

Or you may receive a mammogram report that's more confusing than helpful—for instance, "Your mammogram showed no evidence of cancer," followed one sentence later by "Remember that a mammogram does not entirely exclude all cancer. Although mammography is the most sensitive tool available for the detection of breast cancer, it is not perfect and may fail to detect cancer in 10 to 15 percent of cases. If you have a persistent lump or other problem in one of your breasts, you should consult your physician for further evaluation." This language is designed to cover all possibilities, including protecting the reporting institution from being sued, but the report often leaves you worried and upset, and still dependent on your doctor's explanation.

Language for other kinds of reports can be equally scary or confusing. I had a patient with significant hip pain who received a note from her doctor that said: "Your CAT scan showed no evidence of cancer, just aseptic necrosis." Although the doctor thought he was being reassuring, my patient was terrified by the diagnosis of "aseptic necrosis," not knowing what it meant (deterioration of the bone due to causes other than infection and cancer). In any of these instances, try not to panic until you've had a chance to speak with your doctor.

Access to Medical Records

You have a legal right to all of your medical records, including your test reports and the tests themselves. Only you can authorize the release of records between hospitals or from a hospital to an individual. A personal letter, note, or signed form is required.

Make sure that the results of every test (positive or negative) have been secured and passed on to the physician who will act on those results. Once in a great while, test results get lost and no one is aware of the loss. So it's a good idea for you to keep track of all your records yourself.

Continuity of care is crucial. All new studies should be compared with prior ones, which are generally stored at the site where they were taken. Both old and new studies should be stored at one center. For example, if you change centers, arrange to have your mammography file moved with you.

If you are seeking a second opinion on your care, you will want the consulting physician to be able to go over your history, reports, tests, and records. You may want to carry your records with you if you want to be sure the consultant gets to see your whole file and chart. Most doctors want to see the actual X-ray films or studies on a compact disc, so get both the image and the report, or authorize the transfer of both via a trackable mailing service such as FedEx. For many other types of X-ray images, copied films are fine, but when it comes to a mammogram, the originals are the best way to evaluate subtle changes in the breast. Getting your hands on those originals may involve a test of your patience and persistence. Remember, they are films of *you* and you have paid for them. You have every right to them.

You are probably the best agent to cut through red tape and delay, and to collect all essential information. Clarify how, when, and where to get the material you want, and be sure you get the *complete* file. Make an appointment to pick up your records: "Thank you for getting them together for me. I will be there at two o'clock, promptly." You may need to assert yourself and be unnaturally persistent, yet still courteous and polite, says Claire Fagin, dean emerita of the University of Pennsylvania School of Nursing, a great patient advocate. "Nudge, nudge, nudge. Don't sit back and accept anything that fails to satisfy you. Speak up, protect your interests," she advises. No one else is as concerned as you are about your well-being. Keep informed about new tests and studies, and how they may relate to you and your ongoing care. Be your own strong advocate.

✣ Moving Forward

All along the way, from first diagnosis through the routine of your follow-up care, tests will give you the opportunity for early detection, a better understanding of new symptoms, and a way to measure response to treatment. Test results can sometimes create confusion— but often they can provide clarity and reassurance. And as medical advances march forward, tests of all kinds are likely to greatly improve.

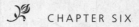

CHAPTER SIX

After Mastectomy: Re-creating a Breast— With or Without Surgery

I went through life looking terrible in clothes and feeling horribly self-conscious about my huge breasts. So when I had to have a mastectomy, I agreed only on condition that I could have reconstruction on the mastectomy side and reduction of the other breast at the same time. I had the belly flap, and between that tummy tuck and waking up with reasonably sized breasts, I made the best of a bad deal.

My new shape looks very nice in clothes, so no one can tell that my breasts have been removed. But I miss my nipples—they were a big part of my sex life and made my breasts look like breasts. In the next six months, my plastic surgeon is going to make me some new ones so they look sexy even if they don't feel sexy.

I've adjusted to being boobless, and can now enjoy a profound sense of freedom. No more tight bras, no more sagging; yes to running around without flopping and discomfort.

I was pretty flat-chested, but I'll tell you, it's amazing how the smallest breast turns into a mountain when there's nothing there next to it. I had to put something in my bra right away so I could feel normal again: a use at last for those stupid shoulder pads I always take

*out of my clothes. Slip 'em in, slip 'em out—just like my contacts.
I went back to work, and no one could tell a thing. That was very
important for me.*

✻ First Things First

You may have had or are about to have a mastectomy—by choice or for medical necessity. Whatever your age, marital status, sexual activity, or orientation, whether you work outside or inside the home, it's hard to know how you will react to the loss of your breast(s) and how important it will be for you to re-create a new breast(s). Even if you are clear and accepting that mastectomy will get you to a healthier and safer place, losing a breast is a big change and can be very upsetting.

It's very normal to feel anxious, uncertain, sad, and mournful about giving up a part of your body that was one of the hallmarks of becoming a woman: a significant part of your lovemaking, what made you look good in clothes, how you fed your babies. No one can ever take those memories and that legacy away from you. Moving forward, you now have the opportunity to shape and determine what you want to have happen next. But first you must do some careful thinking and delving into your feelings in order to figure out what is best for you. It's important for you and your breast cancer surgeon and plastic surgeon to discuss your options for breast reconstruction as well as alternatives, including prostheses or no reconstruction.

✻ Challenges

Consider Your Goals

This is a good time to stop and reflect: Are you open to not having reconstruction? How important is it to you to re-create your breast? As you review your options, here are some concerns and questions you might consider.

Medical priorities

- Are there medical considerations and priorities in your particular situation?
- Have your doctors offered you immediate or delayed reconstruction, both, or neither?

Self-image

- How much do you feel you need reconstruction to seem whole again?
- Have you thought about how you will appear in clothes, undergarments, and bathing suits?
- How much does it matter to you how others see you?

Function and comfort

- Is preserving your physical function and comfort your first priority?
- Will reconstruction help your intimate life?
- Will reconstruction interfere with your athletic activities and everyday life?

Practical considerations

- What are your personal priorities?
- Must reconstruction be now?
- How long can it wait?
- Can you live with "off-and-on" alternatives and be willing to pack your "stuff" when you travel?
- Do you want the option with the shortest surgery time and the shortest recovery?
- Do you want to get it over and done with now, no matter how long it takes—even if it requires extra time and effort up front?
- Are you undecided but want a short-term solution that won't limit future options?

Reconstruction: Goals and Expectations

Aligning your personal goals and medical considerations about reconstruction is key. There's the medical perspective: "The goal of reconstruction is to restore a breast mound and to maintain the quality of life without affecting the prognosis or detection of recurrent cancer," says

Dr. Peter G. Cordiero, a breast reconstruction specialist. But as you consider reconstruction, what matters most are *your* goals and expectations. What do you want and hope for?

Your reasons for reconstruction may not suit everyone. June's support group jumped on her when she suggested she was considering reconstruction to please a man. "No way! Guys come and go. Do it for yourself or don't do it!" For some women, though, doing it for a lover may be reason enough.

You don't have to be defensive or be judged about your decision. There's only one you, and you're totally entitled to your own set of reasons. Not every woman is convinced two breasts are necessary to feel complete. For some, less is more, less is acceptable, or less is less but still better than any substitute. Not having reconstruction may be your most flexible option: you can go breast-free, use a pop-in breast form, or change your mind and get surgical reconstruction in the future.

Betty, who had double mastectomies and no reconstruction, had no plans to shop for a prosthesis—or reconstruction. "This is the way I looked the first fourteen years of my life. I can handle it. But if I change my mind, or decide to wear a sexy dress from my former life, I can stick something into a bra or buy falsies."

If you choose not to replace or rebuild your breast(s), and if your choice is acceptable to you, that's great. But if you're seeking a breast substitute or reconstruction solution, the rest of this chapter will show you ways to satisfy your goals and expectations.

WHY SOME WOMEN CHOOSE RECONSTRUCTION

"I want to be able to wear my favorite clothes, have them hang right. Mostly I don't want an empty side reminding me of my cancer history every time I get dressed."

"I'm dating and I don't want the world to know I've had breast cancer; I want to look sexy, maybe show a little cleavage."

"I was fed up with searching about every morning for pieces of my body, to stuff into a brassiere that I never had to bother with before the mastectomy. I wanted to make my body as normal as possible and that's why I decided on reconstruction. My husband tried to talk me out of it: 'It doesn't matter to me,' he said. 'But it matters to me!' I told him. 'I'm doing it for me.' And I did, and I love it."

"As an opera singer, I sometimes wear seductive costumes. While I might be able to get away with a prosthesis, I don't want to worry about reaching for high C in an embrace with the tenor and have the damn thing pop out. It happened to another soprano I know. I don't want anyone knowing my secrets."

"I was set against two separate surgeries: mastectomy and then a reconstruction operation. 'A prosthesis will do me fine,' I said. But my husband said, 'I know you too well. You're not going to be happy walking around with a double D breast on one side and nothing on the other. Face the tough issues now and figure you'll have a longer time enjoying the new you.' I went for the dual surgeries and never looked back."

✄ Solutions

If you decide on some type of reconstruction, your ability to find the best solutions and make the best decisions for your specific situation will depend on how well each of the following options fits your lifestyle and needs.

- *Prosthesis.* An external breast form that's usually designed to fit inside a bra. Most popular is a plastic- or silicone-walled breast form filled with a silicone gel with the feel and weight of a natural breast. A customized prosthesis can also be made to stick to the skin with a special adhesive or magnet.
- *Implant reconstruction.* An implant consists of a silicone bag filled with fluid or gel (salt water, oil, or silicone), which is placed under the skin and muscle in the breast area to create a breast mound. An expander is usually put in place first to stretch out the skin and muscle envelope enough to accommodate the implant.
- *Tissue reconstruction.* A surgical procedure that uses your own tissue from one part of your body to rebuild your breast(s). If only a small amount of extra tissue is available for reconstruction, an implant might also be part of the process.

Prostheses: Breast Forms

An external ready-made breast form (prosthesis) is the fastest way to fill in the void where your breast(s) had been. The ability to slip into underwear and appear as you did before can be a big relief, particularly after suffering the loss of a breast and wrestling with so many big decisions. "I wanted to be with my friends and co-workers and not think they were eyeing my chest, wondering what had happened to me when I was out for cancer treatment."

When Ruth Handler, inventor of the Barbie doll, was looking for a prosthesis in the 1970s, her doctor told her to stuff some stockings into her bra. That wasn't good enough for Handler, who ended up inventing the first lifelike, natural-feeling artificial breast, called Nearly Me.

A trained volunteer from Reach to Recovery, a program of the American Cancer Society, can meet you in the hospital or at your home, bringing you all kinds of information along with a temporary breast replacement. (A list of local shops and services featuring specialty bras and prostheses is provided for your convenience.) In fact, many professional prostheses and bra fitters in specialty stores are breast cancer survivors themselves.

You can choose among surgical supply stores, pharmacies, custom lingerie or clothing shops (with the assistance of a trained fitter), or a private in-home service (usually at no extra cost). At a time when you're entitled to extra comfort and convenience, the opportunity to have personal service in the privacy of your own home is a marvelous treat. You can try out various samples under an assortment of your own clothes, from lingerie to sweaters to low-cut evening gowns.

When my mother was scheduled for a mastectomy, she arranged an appointment to check out breast forms prior to the operation, and had a suitable substitute on hand as soon as healing allowed for its use.

Types of Breast Forms

Prostheses come in many shapes, sizes, and materials: silicone gel, foam, or fiberfill interior; weighted or not. The ideal product has the shape, weight, balance, motion, and simulated nipple of the natural breast on the other side. Here are some of your options:

STICK-ONS. Ready-made products are matched to your natural size (one company, Amoena, offers eighty-six sizes). One product comes with stick-on adhesive patches that attach to the upper edge of your breast area, allowing you to go braless if you so desire. The adhesive patches last about one week before you have to replace them. But be cautious when applying adhesive to what may be particularly sensitive postsurgery skin, although most women have no problem. There is also a magnetic system consisting of a magnet that adheres to the skin with an adhesive patch and a magnet that is built into the back of the prosthesis. The breast form snaps onto the chest-based magnet to hold its position.

SLIP-INS. You'll probably want to buy two styles of prostheses.

- A lightweight model (polyfill or foam) is recommended for the initial postsurgery recovery period and is useful for informal leisure activities, especially during warm weather, and for swimming. (The product is machine washable.)
- A lifelike heavier silicone product (hand washable) is more aesthetically pleasing, and most women prefer it for day-to-day regular use as well as special occasions and intimate encounters.

Two shapes are offered: asymmetrical (one for the left side, one for the right) and symmetrical or pear-shaped (worn sideways to fill out the side, or straight up for center fullness and cleavage).

CUSTOM BREAST FORMS. If you're really prepared to splurge (and you may have to in order to pay for this style, which few insurers cover), you can buy a custom-made breast prosthesis, individually constructed to match the natural contours of your body and your other breast.

You may find the weight of the lifelike prosthesis—which is designed to replicate actual breast weight—intrusive and fatiguing, but the balanced weight it provides does help keep your shoulders even, your bra in position, and your posture straight.

Prosthetics of whatever type don't always come with instructions, however. "You have it in backward!" Lynn was told, months after she had begun using hers. Be sure to get full instruction about how best to

SPECIALIZED BATHING SUITS AND BRAS

Special bathing suits and bras designed for women who've had breast cancer are available from Lands' End, Sears, Nordstrom, or JCPenney catalogs, as well as small shops and department stores. Bobbie couldn't get over how well such a bra worked for her: "I can try on clothes in Loehmann's big open dressing room and nobody knows it's not me in that bra."

Most specialty bras and bathing suits come with a pocket to hold the prosthesis, or you can have pockets sewn into the ones you already own. "The pockets are great! I don't worry anymore about diving in and coming up to watch my breast filler floating off among the waves."

You don't have to be a skilled seamstress to manage the disguise yourself. I have a friend who is barely handy with a needle: she cuts up old shoulder pads and sews them into her bathing suits so that she never has to think about what's in place. (She finds the pads in inexpensive outdated thrift shop jackets.) You might also trim these shoulder pads for use in the pockets of your specialty bathing suits—or sew your own pockets from skin-colored T-shirt fabric into your ordinary bras and bathing suits.

use these options based on your specific situation, relative to your body type, the kind of clothing you like to wear, and the things you like to do.

Cost of Breast Forms

Prices of prostheses range from choices under $100 to high-quality products between $200 and $500 (size is usually not a factor). The custom-made model is considerably more expensive.

Breast forms generally last from two to five years. Salt water, chlorinated pool water, and hot tubs can damage the outer shell of the prosthesis, making it sticky (and more likely to collect dirt) and thinner (increasing the risk of rupture and leakage). You'd be wise to avoid using your more expensive form in any kind of water, if possible.

If you're applying for health insurance money to pay for a prosthesis, you may jeopardize the possibility of payment for surgical reconstruction at a future date. Some insurance plans won't pay for both. Be sure to check with your insurance company to find out exactly what it will cover for your recovery and rehabilitation. Most coverage allows for the cost of two special bras (with prostheses pockets) a year and a new prosthesis every two years.

It's important to obtain a doctor's prescription for your prosthesis in order to be reimbursed by your health insurer. Be prepared to defend your request. After all, the cost should be covered, since the loss of a breast is a side effect of breast cancer treatment (just like the cost of antinausea medicine is covered for nausea due to chemo). You can usually get this cost partially or completely covered if you are persistent.

Reconstruction with Surgery

Most women who are informed of the options by their doctors choose surgical breast reconstruction after mastectomy. (Surveys have shown that some doctors neglect to bring up reconstruction with their patients, and those patients are less likely to take advantage of reconstruction.) Breast reconstruction generally involves two phases: rebuilding the mound and re-creating a nipple/areola complex. Many women are satisfied with just the breast mound and forgo recreation of their nipples.

About two-thirds of women undergoing reconstructive surgery choose an expander/implant approach. Of the women who choose tissue reconstruction, most have the procedure done with belly tissue. If offered the choice, almost all women prefer immediate reconstruction during the same surgery as mastectomy.

Women who delay reconstruction typically do so for medical reasons (for example, if they have an aggressive cancer that requires an aggressive treatment plan) or for personal reasons (some women prefer to put off anything that's not completely necessary until their cancer therapy is done).

If you become dissatisfied with your choice of no reconstruction at the time of initial surgery, you can always change your mind later on. In fact, it's never too late to get reconstruction. Your health insurance policy, however, may have a time limitation, so be sure to check that out.

If you find you're unhappy with your reconstruction results, you can always choose to have the reconstruction revised—or it can be removed and you can go breastless, with or without a prosthesis.

Breast Mound Reconstruction with Implants/Expanders

Implants involve the least amount of surgery; slim, small-breasted women tend to do best with implants. In fact, many very thin women have no extra tissue anywhere on their body that could be used to make a new breast. An implant becomes their only reconstruction option.

Even if your breast cancer surgeon does a skin-sparing mastectomy, almost all women still require some expansion of the skin that remains after mastectomy, in order to prepare the pouch to later accommodate the implant and give the reconstructed breast a natural shape and position. (Think of how pregnancy slowly stretches the belly.)

The process of expansion takes about six months. A balloon-type device, called a tissue expander, is inserted under the chest muscle and skin, resting against the chest wall. Fluid is injected at regular intervals into a little button in the wall of the expander, called a port, which fills up the expander. This process (called hyperinflation) is continued until the expander stretches your tissues out beyond the size of implant in order to achieve a natural droop once the expander is removed and the implant is put in its place. Hyperinflation can cause significant discomfort by putting pressure on nerves and the rib cage.

All implants are made with a silicone bag, but they differ by the type of filling:

- Saline (salt water) filling
- Silicone gel filling
- Combination filling: silicone gel or vegetable oil in the outside chamber of the implant, saline on the inside

Silicone-filled implants were returned to routine use after several large studies showed no specific safety problem or health threat from the silicone gel. But the issues haven't disappeared entirely; some women may experience side effects from the silicone gel if it leaks out of its shell. If you remain concerned about the safety of silicone in your particular situation, saline-filled implants can be a reassuring alternative.

Implants also come in different shapes (teardrop or round), depending on the contour of your breast area. The surface of the implant may be smooth or rough—nothing you'd feel on the outside—but your plastic surgeon may have a preference for technical reasons. An implant normally lasts from ten to fifteen years, after which it can be replaced.

Breast Mound Reconstruction from Your Own Tissue

You may choose to have your breast re-created using your own tissue, transferred from another part of your body. This is described as autologous tissue reconstruction.

Tissue can be taken from several areas:

- Belly area
- The sides of the back (where some of us get "back fat" popping over our bra band)
- Buttocks and love handles
- Thighs

The borrowed tissue is moved into position either still connected to its blood supply or as a completely detached piece of tissue called a free flap. The tissue is then sewn into place where the breast had been. This can be done immediately after mastectomy or at a later time. The blood vessels of the free flap must be connected to a blood supply in the chest area using a special microscope.

BELLY TISSUE RECONSTRUCTION. There are three types of tissue reconstruction that use belly tissue to rebuild the breast. You have to have enough belly fat to be a candidate for a belly tissue reconstruction procedure.

Many women are pleased with their belly tissue procedure:

- It gives you a new breast mound that usually lasts forever (doesn't leak or need to be changed ten to fifteen years later).
- A belly tissue procedure provides a natural-feeling new "breast."
- It involves a fringe-benefit tummy tuck, removing excess belly fat or stretched-out postpregnancy belly tissues.

One woman I took care of waited a long time before she found her solution: "I was reborn. Ten years after a lumpectomy I had to have a mastectomy, and so I decided on the TRAM reconstruction [discussed below] and the doctor suggested I have reduction of the other side. Well, for years I'd thought about breast reduction—from a size double D—but I never could get up the courage for this elective surgery. You could call this a bonus: I lost my potbelly and I got two young breasts. I can wear any bathing suit I like, and I look great!"

But the abdominal tissue procedures are usually not feasible for everyone. Women who are unlikely to be candidates for this source of tissue reconstruction include:

• Thin women without enough extra belly tissue
• Smokers with compromised blood vessels
• People who have had multiple belly surgeries (Cesarean-section scars are usually not a problem)
• Women who plan on getting pregnant (the stretching of the belly during pregnancy may produce too much strain on the belly wall and the belly incision done for tissue transfer)

The *TRAM flap procedure* (named for the transverse rectus abdominus muscle) takes an ellipse of skin, fat, and muscle from the lower half of the belly and slides it up to the breast area through a tunnel under the skin. Even after the tissue is transferred, its blood vessels remain attached to their belly blood supply. The organs inside your abdomen are undisturbed. The transferred tissue is shaped into a breast form and sewn into place. If blood vessels have been cut, they are reattached by microscopic surgery to blood vessels in the chest area. The procedure takes about three hours per breast; if microsurgery is required, it can take hours longer.

PACKAGE DEAL: TUMMY TUCK

Most of the women I've taken care of are pleased to have a flat belly from the tummy tuck that happens after the extra belly tissue has been removed for breast reconstruction. Your tummy tuck scar and your refashioned belly button may take some getting used to, however. The long, horizontal tummy tuck incision extends from hipbone to hipbone, midway between your pubic bone and your navel. Your surgeon may need to create a new navel because after the abdominal area is reshaped, your natural navel may be stretched, distorted, or in the wrong place.

A second option is the *DIEP flap procedure.* DIEP stands for deep inferior epigastric perforator; this is the name of the main blood vessel that runs through the tissue that will be used to reconstruct the breast. Only skin, fat, and blood vessels are removed from the lower belly. In contrast to the TRAM flap, the DIEP does not usually involve any removal and transfer of muscle tissue. The DIEP flap comes with its own blood vessel, but it's detached from its original blood supply. Before the flap is sewn into place, its blood vessel must be connected to a blood supply in the chest area.

When it's available and offered by plastic surgeons experienced with this technique, the DIEP flap reconstruction is often preferred over the TRAM procedure, even though the surgery is more complex and takes more time. That's because no abdominal muscle is removed with the DIEP, resulting in faster recovery and greater abdominal wall muscle strength and function. Plus it tends to cause less persistent abdominal wall discomfort since fat tissue has practically no sensation (there are many more nerves in muscle tissue, which can feel pain if they are tampered with).

Another type of free flap belly tissue reconstruction procedure is the *SIEA flap*, which is named after the superficial inferior epigastric artery that feeds the flap. This is a flap that utilizes skin and fat from the abdominal area. The difference between the SIEA flap and the DIEP flap is that the DIEP flap requires a small incision to be made in the supportive layer of the abdomen as well as the rectus abdominis muscle (the long rectangular muscle that allows you to perform sit-ups). It runs from the rib cage down toward the pelvic bone. The SIEA flap does not

BELLY TISSUE RECONSTRUCTION: ONE-TIME OPPORTUNITY

The belly tissue can only be used once. In a situation where only one breast is reconstructed, both sides of the lower abdominal tissue are harvested and then used to match the opposite breast. When both breasts are reconstructed, the lower abdominal tissue is divided in half to reconstruct both sides. If your belly was already used for reconstruction of one breast, then you'd have to use another source for and method of reconstruction in the future if you were to have a mastectomy on the other side at some time later on. You could still consider reconstruction, using an alternative source of tissue, an expander/implant procedure, or a combination of both.

require these additional incisions be made. Both flaps have the advantage that no muscle is removed.

BUTTOCK TISSUE. Buttock tissue from the "love handles" on the sides of the hips or near the buttock crease can be used for breast reconstruction. The GAP procedure uses buttock skin and fat (no muscle) along with its gluteal anterior perforator blood vessel (thus its name, GAP), which has to be reattached to a vessel in the chest area with microscopic surgery. The rear-end scar (left by removal of the tissue) is concealed by clothing or inside the buttock crease. (Giving up some of your buttock tissue for reconstruction of your breast makes your butt smaller—for some a good thing, for others a disappointment.)

The amount of available buttock tissue may be relatively small—just enough to reconstruct a small breast. But if only a *very* small amount of tissue is available and you want something bigger, then an implant may also be employed.

This type of reconstruction is usually offered to women who do not have enough extra tissue from other sources (belly, back, thigh) or who are unable to use alternative sources of tissue for whatever reason (e.g., multiple abdominal surgeries may prohibit the use of a belly flap).

Buttock transfer surgery is technically difficult for a few reasons:

- It's a free flap: its blood vessel must be reconnected to a new blood supply, requiring the use of a surgical microscope.
- It requires significant changes of position during surgery: you're face-up for the breast surgery, facedown to harvest the buttock tissue, then face-up again to reconstruct the breast.
- It can take up to twelve hours in the operating room.

With more complexity, more can go wrong. Very experienced surgeons, however, generally have a low complication rate.

THIGH TISSUE. Plastic surgeons who specialize in the free flap technique may offer you another source of tissue for breast reconstruction: the gracilis muscle, from your inner thigh. This thin muscle starts at your pubic bone and ends along the inside of your upper leg. Its job is to help you bring your leg toward your body.

In contrast to free flaps from the belly and buttock that use only fat and skin, the gracilis flap is mainly a muscle—sometimes a little bit of skin is included. When it's moved up to the chest area to reconstruct the breast, its blood vessel has to be connected to a blood supply up in the chest area using a microscope (just like the other free flap procedures). After the flap is removed from the pelvic area, the incision is tucked into the groin crease, at the top of the thigh, where it's easily hidden.

This flap can make a small to medium-sized breast, but it may need to be combined with an implant to create a full medium size.

COMBINATION OF TISSUE AND IMPLANT RECONSTRUCTION: LATISSIMUS DORSI FLAP. The latissimus dorsi flap reconstructs the breast using the diagonal muscle (and surrounding fat) that's located

HARD TO GET: FREE FLAP TISSUE RECONSTRUCTION

The free flap reconstructions (DIEP, SIEA, buttock, thigh) are relatively complicated procedures, requiring extra training and taking much more operating room time than any other form of reconstruction—and often without significant additional payment to the surgeon. As a result, relatively few surgeons perform this procedure, so you may need to travel a distance to get it done and obtain health insurance coverage outside your local network.

If you want immediate free flap reconstruction after mastectomy, you'll need two surgeons who have privileges in the same hospital and who know how to work together: a breast cancer surgeon to do the mastectomy along with the breast plastic surgeon who is experienced with the free flap procedures. This can be a tough decision if you have to switch away from your current breast cancer surgeon in order to get the combined team.

Another option: you can stay with your current breast cancer surgeon and have delayed reconstruction with a free flap reconstruction surgeon at a later time. Or you can have the mastectomy with your breast cancer surgeon and have a local plastic surgeon give you a temporary immediate reconstruction using a tissue expander. This keeps all your options open. At a later time, the expander can be removed, and you can proceed with the expert breast plastic surgeon to get the tissue reconstruction of your choice, scheduled at your convenience. (But check with your health care provider in advance to be sure the second plastic surgical procedure will be covered/paid for.)

on the side of your back, behind the armpit. It's the muscle that helps you perform twisting movements, like swinging a golf club or turning a baby over on a changing table. The flap is slipped from the back to the front through a short tunnel under the skin. But because this muscle is relatively small and there is little body fat in that part of the back, an implant is almost always required in addition to the back tissue, depending on the desired size of the reconstructed breast. (The tissues can usually accommodate the implant without going through the expansion process.)

The latissimus flap can produce relatively good results and few complications, and many plastic surgeons favor this approach. But I'm not a real fan of this procedure:

- It may result in partial loss of strength or function of your back, making it challenging to lift and twist: certain swimming, tennis and golf strokes; picking up, turning, and manipulating heavy objects.
- It can cause visible soft tissue asymmetry of the back and a scar that might be hard to conceal in a bathing suit.
- It may produce an artificial-feeling breast: while the front tissue is soft and breastlike, the implant behind this tissue can feel firm and artificial.

In addition, the latissimus flap/implant combo is not a permanent option; you still have to have an artificial object in you, the implant, that only lasts ten to fifteen years (or less if it leaks or ruptures). (Other tissue reconstruction options rarely require an implant.)

Reconstruction Options after Partial Mastectomy or Lumpectomy

You may be seeking information about partial breast reconstruction if you are dissatisfied with the way your breast looks after having partial mastectomy (or lumpectomy, with or without radiation) for early-stage breast cancer. There may be a dent, distortion, or bulge near the area where breast tissue has been removed; the size or position of your treated breast may now be very different from the other side; you may have had severe healing problems after surgery, radiation, or infection, making you unhappy with the end result; connective tissue disease, like lupus or scleroderma, which interferes with healing after radiation, may not have been diagnosed until after radiation was given.

In spite of all these variables, you do have breast reconstruction options, but there is no general or standard approach. The best solution for you will have to be customized depending on the extent and nature of your prior treatments and your goals and cosmetic concerns. For example, a small dent in an otherwise nice-looking breast could be filled in with fat tissue obtained by liposuction of another area of your body that has extra fat. A significant dent or deformity might be filled in with tissue transplanted from your belly or side. A previously treated breast that's much smaller than the other side could be enlarged with an implant, or the larger side could be reduced and lifted to match. It's best to go to a plastic surgeon who specializes in breast reconstruction in order to get the benefit of his/her experience and judgment.

Most plastic surgeons will recommend that you wait at least six to twelve months after completion of your breast treatment before doing any plastic surgery revision. This allows your tissues to heal as completely as possible, so any distortion or asymmetry has stabilized.

Costs of Reconstruction

Reconstruction with an expander/implant costs the least; buttock free flap tissue reconstruction of both breasts is the most expensive. As I mentioned before, find out the costs and what your medical insurance company will pay for before you proceed. Some companies will pay for the entire procedure, even if it's years after the mastectomy. Other companies will pay only for reconstructing the removed breast, not additional "nonessential" procedures such as reducing the other breast to achieve symmetry.

If you meet resistance from your insurance carrier, be prepared to mount a strong case in advance of your surgery, with your doctor's support (a letter from your doctor is essential). Persistence should pay off, with additional pressure, if necessary, coming from your state or federal elected representative.

Side Effects of Breast Reconstruction

All surgery involves risk. Breast reconstruction involves slightly more than a 5 percent risk of one or a combination of the following:

- Infection
- Bleeding
- Chronic pain
- Disappointing cosmetic result
- Implant discomfort, rupture, capsule formation, shift out of position (for implant/expanders)
- Tissue breakdown, fat necrosis, healing problems, shrinkage (for tissue reconstruction procedures)
- Hernia at the tissue donation site (for tissue reconstruction procedures)

In general, the risks of plastic surgery reconstruction are higher if you already have medical problems and need to undergo more complex surgical procedures. We'll address general risks first, followed by risks specific for implant and tissue reconstruction.

Risks of Any Reconstruction

PAIN, INFECTION, AND BLEEDING. These may occur with any surgical procedure, particularly within the first month of surgery. These complications are usually self-limited and treatable or manageable.

- Bleeding usually stops on its own, but if it doesn't, your surgeon may need to stop the bleeding. Blood that collects under the skin (hematoma) is absorbed by the body over time—the larger the amount, the longer it takes. But a very large hematoma may need to be removed surgically.
- Infection usually responds to antibiotics; sometimes drainage of infected fluid is required.
- Postoperative pain is usually relieved by anti-inflammatory agents and careful use of pain medications. Persistent pain can be tricky to manage and is further addressed in Chapter 9.

Complications of plastic surgery are also increased by a long history of smoking, current smoking, diabetes, or obesity. Both nicotine and the effects of diabetes narrow the small blood vessels that heal and nourish the reconstructed tissue and protect it from infection. Many plastic surgeons will require the postponement of reconstruction until smoking and the need for nicotine patches have ceased and/or until blood sugars are under regular control.

Being significantly overweight can interfere with your ability to heal, increasing the risk of infection and tissue breakdown. It also increases anesthesia risks and heart problems. Some plastic surgeons will recommend delaying breast reconstruction until you get into a safer weight category.

RISKS OF ANESTHESIA. Prolonged anesthesia can affect short-term memory, the precision of your thinking and speech, and your ability to multitask. This side effect may be worse if you have other medical issues, if you stopped postmenopausal hormone replacement upon your diagnosis, and if you are older.

APPEARANCE. Even with the best plastic surgeon, there is no guarantee that you will be completely satisfied with the results of your reconstruction. Your rebuilt breasts may not live up to your expectations of size, position, angle, and balance. They may not be as soft or natural feeling as you had hoped. And the color and texture of transferred tissue and skin from the back, belly, and thigh are different from those of the natural breast.

Natural breast asymmetry is common. And breast reconstruction usually involves some asymmetry as well. Various factors affect symmetry:

• Results of your surgery (e.g., the amount of skin safely spared during mastectomy prior to reconstruction; the amount of tissue available to rebuild the breast; the length and location of scars)
• Illnesses or conditions that affect your ability to heal and recover (such as radiation, infection, scar tissue and capsule formation, smoking, obesity, diabetes)
• Change of weight after reconstruction

The tissue reconstruction site can gain weight along with the rest of the body—but it tends to gain less than your natural breast. There may also be some strain or discomfort in the reconstructed tissues because the weight gained fills in and around the area and can cause pressure and stiffness (like an overstuffed pillow). The skin envelope around an implant reconstruction doesn't gain weight, but there can be weight gain near the implant. Or if there's a natural breast on the other side, *it* might gain weight and look lopsided.

Whatever surgical procedure you settle on, there will be scars in the breast area and in the tissue donation site. For example, after belly tissue removal for breast reconstruction you'll have a scar from hip to hip and a newly altered navel position and appearance, as well as scars in the breast area. Scars do fade and recede over time in most women, but they don't go away. Some women have keloid formation (causing bumpy, raised, pink scar tissue along the incision line). Most scars, however, are generally located out of sight, even in a bathing suit or low-cut gown.

ALTERED BREAST SENSATION. The consistency or touch of a tissue reconstruction most resembles a natural breast, but while this newly transferred tissue may feel most natural to the toucher, you probably won't get much sensation from being touched.

Prior to mastectomy your breast area may have been an important erogenous zone for you. Most of the nerve endings responsible for the touch response of your breast were concentrated in the nipple area; the rest of the nerves were distributed evenly throughout the breast skin. But after the nerves are cut with mastectomy, the area usually becomes numb. The sensory nerves to the breast area have the potential to regrow, but the rate of nerve growth is extremely slow. Great patience is required.

Some sensation to the reconstructed breast area does occur, maybe for as many as half the women who undergo surgery. The sensation may feel good, strange, or unpleasant; fleeting, on and off, or continuous. Some women experience "phantom" sensations—as if the breast were still there.

If sensation is going to come back, some glimmer of feeling is most likely to emerge within the first year after surgery. (Chemotherapy can slow the timing.) If no sensation has returned by two years, it is very unlikely that any sensation will be restored. Instead, you may get sensation back *next to* the breast area. I had a patient who developed an erogenous zone in her armpit, which then took center stage in her foreplay.

Specific Risks with Implants

CAPSULE FORMATION ABOUND IMPLANT. Once an implant is in place, your tissues heal around the implant with a scar tissue capsule. Most capsules are soft to firm, but some women develop hard capsules that can distort, stiffen, and shrink the reconstructed breast and cause pain.

Radiation to the breast implant area increases the risk of scar capsule formation. Massage and exercises that move the implant up, down, and side to side may help reduce the risk of hard-capsule formation or soften a firm capsule that's already formed. But if you have a hard capsule that's not responding to these measures, surgical correction may be necessary. The implant and hard scar tissue are removed, then the pouch of skin that holds the replacement implant may need to be rebuilt with a combination of your tissues and a surgical tissue product, such as AlloDerm (made of a cell-free collagen framework from donated skin).

TISSUE BREAKDOWN. Sometimes the breast-area tissues have trouble healing from the pressure of the underlying implant or expander. The blood supply of the skin that remains after mastectomy could have been compromised by prior therapies such as surgery and radiation; preexisting conditions such as diabetes and/or years of smoking also can damage the small blood vessels that nourish the tissues and promote healing.

If tissue breakdown occurs, the dead tissue needs to be removed and the open area needs to be closed, either by natural regrowth of your own tissue or with surgical repair using special material such as Allo-Derm. Sometimes new skin (a skin graft) or new tissue (a tissue flap) needs to be brought in to cover or fill in the affected area.

PAIN AROUND IMPLANT. Some women experience pain and discomfort from the tissue expander, the implant, and/or scar tissue putting pressure on a nerve or other sensitive structure. A prescribed program of exercise, stretching, and massage—with or without anti-inflammatory medications—may relieve mild pain. Acupuncture, breathing exercises, yoga, and meditation can also be helpful. Significant pain may require additional measures, including physical therapy, evaluation by a pain specialist, more potent medications, and even surgery (see Chapter 9).

SHIFTING IMPLANT POSITION. Implants can shift position, riding up or down or to the side of the chest as the chest tissues that cover the implant nudge or squeeze it out of place. The direction of the shift depends on the mechanics and dynamics of how the tissues that surround the implant move around. If there's only a minor shift of position, and if the capsule surrounding the implant is soft to firm, then you may be able to massage the implant back into position. But if your implant migrates far and won't budge back into position, you may need a surgical solution to rebuild a reinforced pocket for the implant using your own tissue—and extra material as needed (such as AlloDerm)—to secure the implant back into its proper position.

LEAKAGE OF IMPLANT. The risk of an implant leak increases over time; most implants have some leakage after being in place for ten to fifteen years, although it's usually minimal. Significant leakage of an implant is detectable by loss of volume. A saltwater leak from a saline-filled implant is undetectable unless the implant collapses or loses volume. Underinflated implants can feel and appear wrinkled beneath the skin. When a silicone-filled implant leaks, the silicone collects next to the implant and shows up on special tests such as an MRI scan. A leaking implant should be removed—and replaced if you still want a breast form.

Fifteen years after getting implants, Elizabeth found that hers were leaking, although her breasts hadn't lost their shape. Their replacement was another trying experience, involving another recovery period, but six weeks later Elizabeth was back to her exhausting normal routine. "I'm as good as new. I'll be satisfied with another fifteen years." After thirty years Gena was ready to replace the original wrinkled implant she'd tolerated for some while; she was delighted with her fresh new breast, regretting she hadn't replaced it a few years earlier.

Specific Risks with Tissue Reconstruction

TISSUE BREAKDOWN. If the blood supply nourishing the reconstructed breast tissue is compromised in any way, part or all of the transferred tissue may not survive. The risk is higher with a free flap procedure because sewing tiny blood vessels together is tricky and takes a long time to perform. The seam between the vessels may narrow or leak. Breakdown of the flap—called "flap failure"—happens in about 5 percent of breast reconstruction cases; a plastic surgeon who is very experienced with free flap surgery will have the lowest risk of a serious complication.

LUMPS IN RECONSTRUCTED BREAST. Transplanted fatty tissue can form lumps (fat necrosis) that may or may not go away. They most commonly occur under the incision or the scar and usually don't affect the outside appearance of the reconstructed breast. You can feel them, and they may show up on a mammogram as lumps or a group of small calcifications (see Chapter 5 on tests). Over time, areas of fat necrosis may shrink or stay the same size; they don't usually get any bigger. That's in contrast to lumps due to cancer recurrence, which tend to get bigger over time. If you feel a worrisome lump, your surgeon may need to biopsy or remove it to establish that it's not cancerous.

MUSCLE WEAKNESS AT THE DONOR SITE. If a muscle is moved from its original location for breast reconstruction, it stops working as a muscle. It has a new job site and description: to fill in the new breast mound. As a consequence, the place where the muscle came from—like the back or the belly—may become weaker. For example, after the belly muscle is moved with a TRAM procedure, it will be much harder for you to do sit-ups. Another example: a pediatrician I know has trouble turning big babies over on the examination table after having a latissimus flap procedure on both sides.

HERNIA AND DISCOMFORT. Occasionally, there may be other problems: hernia (when a small portion of the intestine bulges out through a weakened area of the abdominal wall) or persistent pain or discomfort where the muscle was removed along the incision. Surgical revision of the hernia may be necessary; persistent pain needs to be evaluated and managed.

STIFFNESS AND LIMITED RANGE OF MOTION. Many women find it difficult to lift their arms for some time after breast, lymph node, and reconstruction surgery—making it hard to put on tops, brush hair, or use a hair dryer. "I could only wear shirts that buttoned into place. I also found a surgical camisole that was much more comfortable than a bra: no straps, no hooks. I could step into it, easy." Good practical advice (which is not always so easy to come by).

TABLE 6.1 Reconstruction Options

Implant alone

Timing: Immediate (only for small implant)
Length of surgery: 1 hour
Eligibility: Only for an occasional patient who has a lot of excess skin left over after skin-sparing mastectomy
Pros:
- Simple
- No extra scars
- Fast placement
- Immediate final results
- Unlikely to delay radiation and chemotherapy

Cons:
- Doesn't have natural breast consistency
- May have high position without natural droop
- Hard to customize size without initial use of expander
- Can dislodge, wrinkle, leak, encapsulate, cause pain
- Implant is not a permanent solution—it usually lasts 10–15 years
- Cosmetic outcome is often compromised by radiation

Tissue expander, then implant

Timing: Immediate or delayed
Length of surgery: 1–2 hours
Eligibility: Only for small or medium breasts
Pros:
- Simple
- No extra scars
- Fast placement

- Doesn't delay radiation and chemotherapy
- An option for smokers

Cons:

- Delayed final results
- Implant requires multiple port injections
- Second surgery required if expander is replaced by permanent implant
- Doesn't have natural breast consistency
- Can dislodge, wrinkle, leak, encapsulate, cause pain
- Implant is not a permanent solution—it usually lasts 10–15 years
- Mound tends to be round with little to no natural droop
- Cosmetic outcome is often compromised by radiation

TRAM flap

Timing: Immediate or delayed

Length of surgery: 3–8 hours, depending on the surgeon's skills and on whether the blood supply remains intact or needs to be reattached with microsurgery

Eligibility: Depends on belly size; not for smokers or anyone with a history of diabetes, vascular disease, or previous abdominal surgeries

Pros:

- Feels most like a natural breast
- Nothing artificial
- Tummy tuck can be used to create most breast sizes

Cons:

- Extra scars
- Longer surgery and anesthesia
- Longer recovery postpones radiation and chemotherapy
- Can cause fat necrosis, hernia, persistent breast and belly pain, abdominal weakness
- Can be done only once

DIEP flap

Timing: Immediate or delayed

Length of surgery: 5–8 hours

Eligibility: Depends on belly size; not for smokers or anyone with a history of diabetes, vascular disease, or previous abdominal surgeries

Pros:

- Feels the most like a natural breast
- Nothing artificial
- Tummy tuck can be used to create most breast sizes

Cons:

- Extra scars
- Longer surgery and anesthesia
- Longer recovery postpones radiation and chemotherapy
- Can cause fat necrosis, hernia, persistent breast and belly pain, abdominal weakness
- Can be done only once

SIEA flap

Timing: Immediate or delayed

Length of surgery: 5–8 hours

Eligibility: Depends on belly size; not for smokers or anyone with a history of diabetes, vascular disease, or previous abdominal surgeries

Pros:

- Feels the most like a natural breast
- Nothing artificial
- Tummy tuck can be used to create most breast sizes

Cons:

- Extra scars
- Longer surgery and anesthesia
- Longer recovery postpones radiation and chemotherapy
- Can cause fat necrosis, hernia, persistent breast and belly pain, abdominal weakness
- Can be done only once

Buttock area

Timing: Immediate or may be delayed

Length of surgery: 9–12 hours

Eligibility: Depends on size of buttock or hip; not for smokers or diabetics

Pros:

- Feels like natural breast
- Nothing artificial
- Bigger breast sizes possible
- Can be done more than once
- Alternative for women with multiple abdominal surgeries
- Minimal effect on function

Cons

- Long operation with more complications
- Higher risk of tissue breakdown
- Can be done only by plastic surgeon skilled in microvascular techniques

- Can cause fat necrosis
- Could delay radiation and chemo
- Pain and discomfort while sitting

Thigh (with or without an implant, depending on size desired)

Timing: Immediate or delayed

Length of surgery: 5–8 hours

Eligibility: Small to medium breast size, depending on the amount of extra fat in the inner thigh area

Pros:

- Provides a natural-feeling breast mound
- Incisions are easily concealed
- Alternative for women with multiple abdominal surgeries

Cons:

- Skin texture may be different from chest area skin
- Long operation with more complications
- Higher risk of tissue breakdown
- Done only by plastic surgeons skilled in microvascular techniques and this type of procedure (probably least common source of tissue utilized)
- Could delay radiation and chemo
- Pain and discomfort in the pelvic area

Latissimus dorsi with an implant

Timing: Immediate or delayed

Length of surgery: 3–6 hours

Eligibility: Small to medium breast size

Pros:

- Simpler operation than TRAM
- Excellent tissue viability
- Feels like natural breast tissue
- Alternative for women with multiple abdominal surgeries

Cons:

- Convalescence longer than implant but shorter than TRAM
- Can cause fat necrosis
- May cause discomfort, limit vigorous back and shoulder activity
- Can be done only once
- Healing may delay radiation and chemotherapy

Creating Symmetry with Your Other Breast

Your surgeon may recommend making your unaffected breast smaller and lifting it to help it resemble the perky new reconstructed breast. The nipple and areola position are moved up as well in this case. Over time, however, the natural breast may sag a bit, while the reconstructed breast tends to hold its upward tilt (a bummer in the buff, but unnoticeable in a bra).

Adjustment of your other breast may be done at the same time as your breast reconstruction. But most of the time, the final modifications are likely to come sometime after, when the reconstructed breast has healed and assumed a stable size and position.

This may be your opportunity for cosmetic surgery. If ever in your precancer life you considered breast reduction or enlargement, this is the moment to try to get what you want (as long as it's medically advisable). But before you go ahead with this additional surgery, be sure to find out who will pay for it: your medical insurance company or you.

Nipple Replacement or Reconstruction

You may choose to put a stop to the whole reconstruction project after your breast mound has been reconstructed—with or without a lift to the other breast. But many women take additional steps to replace or rebuild their nipples and areolas. Here are your choices:

- Apply removable thin rubber (polyurethane) semierect nipples to the surface (these are surprisingly lifelike in texture and color)
- Tattoo a look-alike
- Go for nipple reconstruction from transplanted tissue—fake or real, flat or "stick-out"

Nipple and areola reconstruction may use tissue from a number of sources:

- Local chest wall skin flaps
- Inside the upper thigh (the skin gets darker as you move from the knee toward the labia)
- The labia (the skin-fold lips of vulva, at the entrance to the vagina)

Removal of skin from the inner thigh or vulvar area, followed by nipple reconstruction, can be done as an outpatient procedure in less than two hours, under local anesthesia. All hair follicles should be surgically removed before the skin is formed into a nipple (if there is a lot of hair, this might be challenging for the surgeon). Inner thigh or vulvar discomfort usually resolves within a few weeks. "I thought about tissue transfer for areola and nipple. It was going to come from the inside of my thigh—but I have hairy thighs and I didn't want hairy nipples! Tattooing worked fine for me, especially when they made me a real stick-out nipple from nearby breast skin." Tattooing can provide custom color to match your other nipple in a twenty-minute office visit. (The color may need to be altered at a later visit.)

As in most tissue transfers, the reconstructed nipple has very little sensation. (Sensation in the vulva area is usually unaffected once the area has healed.) Avoid using part of your existing natural nipple/areola skin to re-create a new nipple/areola on the other side, because then both nipples will be numb. One of my patients was very upset to lose sensation in her nipples this way—they had been so much a part of her sexual pleasure.

Nipple replacement is done no sooner than a few months after reconstruction of the breast mound. You need at least this much time for the swelling to recede, any lumpiness to dissipate, and the rebuilt breast mound to settle into its "natural" sag so the nipple can be properly sited.

From Geralyn Lucas' book *Why I Wore Lipstick*:

> I miss my symmetry and I miss bikini tops and tank tops and I especially missed my nipple when my husband took me to St. Lucia to celebrate my last reconstruction surgery and we ended up on a topless beach. All of the European tourists were sunbathing topless but I didn't have the courage to take off my bathing suit top. It would have involved too much explaining and I was tired.

When Geralyn tells her mother about her reluctance to go for any more reconstruction (for her nipple), her mother goes ballistic

> and calls constantly to nipple-nag. She even left me a desperate cell phone message saying she was sitting next to a woman on

the Metroliner, they got to talking and the woman told her she just finished her breast cancer treatments and had just gotten her nipple done. My mom is telling me it looks fabulous, and the woman is screaming into the phone that she loves her nipple—no one can tell which one is real.

MEDICAL PRIORITIES AND TIMING CONSIDERATIONS

Every woman is unique, and medical advice varies greatly depending on medical and timing considerations. There are also logistical issues when coordinating your two surgical teams—a breast cancer surgeon to perform removal of the breast(s) and a breast plastic surgeon to reconstruct the breast(s).

Early-Stage Breast Cancer

If you are diagnosed with early-stage breast cancer and choose or need a mastectomy, immediate reconstruction is the most common choice. "I want to go into that operating room asleep, have the doctors do what they must, wake up, and have it all over, with *something* sitting on my chest. If I can't have tissue reconstruction, I want that expander in place and on its way, because it'll be six months before I'm where I hope to be."

Such a combined procedure requires complex coordination of both breast cancer surgery and plastic surgery teams (on the same day, at the same time and hospital—where they all must have the credentials and privileges in order to practice) and may result in scheduling delays. Surgeons' offices are used to jumping through hoops to get this done, but they do need time and flexibility to make it happen.

Intermediate-Stage Breast Cancer

If your diagnosis is intermediate-stage cancer, you may require prompt chemotherapy or radiation, or both, after mastectomy (unless treatment was completed before surgery). These medical priorities may have an impact on the timing and type of reconstruction.

Locally Advanced or Inflammatory Breast Cancer

If you were diagnosed with locally advanced cancer or inflammatory breast cancer (a large cancer in the breast with skin breakthrough or involvement or extensive lymph node involvement), most doctors would recommend that you delay any complex breast reconstruction for a few reasons:

- **Delay of anticancer treatment.** The extra plastic surgery may require extra healing time that could delay necessary chemotherapy and radiation.
- **Radiation side effects might increase.** A breast implant can distort the relationship between the tissues of the chest wall region that need radiation and the tissues underneath that should be protected. For example, if the fully filled expander or implant pushes the chest wall down closer to the heart, it may be more difficult to protect the heart from potential side effects of radiation therapy. A partially filled tissue expander (containing about 150 cc), however, is usually enough to maintain the skin envelope and serve as a space holder without delaying treatment or increasing radiation complications.
- **Monitoring high-risk areas.** The breast-area tissues—particularly the leftover pouch of skin that had surrounded the breast—are at high risk of recurrence and must be monitored carefully because of the advanced stage of local disease. Reconstruction can make it harder to detect and manage recurrences.

Whatever your situation, work with your team of doctors to design a customized plan, including the sequence of treatments and restorative procedures. For example, a possible sequence is: (1) chemotherapy, (2) mastectomy and breast reconstruction with a DIEP flap and a breast reduction on the other side to achieve symmetry, (3) nipple/areola reconstruction, and (4) tattooing of the right rebuilt nipple to match the color of the left side.

❧ Moving Forward

You will want to get opinions from each of your cancer doctors and your plastic surgeon to help you select the best options for your specific situation. But an objective and comprehensive review of all your reconstruction options is best obtained from a plastic surgeon who has experience performing all the options under consideration (for example, a plastic surgeon who does only expander/implants or latissimus dorsi flaps with an implant is unlikely to give you the best advice regarding a DIEP-type reconstruction).

Learning from other women who have had breast reconstruction is enormously helpful. A great place to go is Breastcancer.org's discussion boards on reconstruction, where women from around the world are ready to listen to your concerns, share their experiences, offer their personal wisdom to help you find your best solutions, and provide support while you're going through the process.

In counseling my patients, here are the priorities we usually set up together:

1. Effective anticancer therapy has right of way over all other factors.
2/3. Your ability to fully function with comfort after recovering from the procedure (to swim, play golf, do yoga—whatever you like).
3. Aesthetics: the way the reconstruction feels (in terms of consistency, since the reconstructed breast rarely has sensation) and looks (size, shape, and symmetry).
4. All the practical considerations: duration of reconstruction, cost, and availability of the procedures. Are you committed to a permanent solution (like a tissue reconstruction) without any foreign object in you (like an implant), or are you set on the simplest procedure (like an expander/implant) with an extended benefit (ten to fifteen years, but not permanent)? Do you have access to the specialized breast plastic surgeons who know how to do the flaps? Can you cover the costs of the procedures? Can you get enough time off from work to have the surgery and recover from it?

There are no guarantees that you're going to get just what you want. All you can do is make the best decisions you can at each step along the way, with the best information available to you, so you can get on with your life.

CHAPTER SEVEN

Ongoing Therapy: Hormonal, Herceptin, and Other Treatments

I thought chemotherapy was the last step. Now you tell me about tamoxifen, which goes on for years. What about its side effects? Is it worth it? Do I really, honestly, need it? Will my treatment ever end?

As I near the end of my five years of hormonal therapy, I'm afraid to give it up. It's my security blanket. I'm going to ask my doctor to keep me on it.

The first half of Herceptin therapy went much better than I expected. Will the rest be just as easy?

I'm not a medicine-person. I much prefer nontraditional therapies to stay healthy.

❧ First Things First

The goal of ongoing therapies is to get rid of cancer cells anywhere in the body that might be left behind after your main treatment with surgery, chemotherapy, or radiation is over. Ongoing treatment may be given on a daily basis (hormonal therapy), once every three weeks (Herceptin), or taken over a week every few weeks (oral chemotherapy). It aims to change the environment inside your body, making it hostile to

cancer cell growth and friendly to your normal tissues. That's how benefits are maximized and side effects are avoided or minimized.

Your customized plan of ongoing medical treatments—prescribed
by your doctors, with your participation—will depend on:

- The stage and nature of your situation with breast cancer
- Past treatments and how you responded to them
- Other medical conditions
- Personal considerations and circumstances

For women with early-stage disease, most of these ongoing treatment
decisions will be made up front, when the rest of your treatment strategy
and plans are worked out. For women living with breast cancer, changes
in treatments may be required due to progression of disease on a prior
treatment program. A change of therapy may also be necessary because
of unacceptable side effects for women with any stage of disease.

Ongoing complementary therapy may also be part of your recovery
and wellness plan.

✤ Challenges

Understanding and accepting the reason for ongoing medical therapy is one of your biggest challenges: your remaining risk of developing a new, recurrent, or progressive breast cancer after completing
your initial treatments. The next big challenge is deciding whether
more treatment is both necessary and reasonable. Talk to your doctor
about these important issues. It's important to prepare for this critical
discussion, so write down your questions (put the most important ones
at the top), make sure to have a long enough appointment time (one
hour is best; a half hour is the minimum), and bring someone with you
as a second set of ears and to take notes (see page 48 in Chapter 3).

More Is Not Necessarily Better

Subjecting yourself to potential new side effects on top of lingering side
effects from treatment you've just completed is probably one of the *last*

things you really want to do. Watch out for three myths that can have a profound effect on how you view the prospect of ongoing treatments:

- Myth one: More treatment is automatically better.
- Myth two: The more side effects, the more effective the treatment must be (and the flip side: the better you feel, the less effective the treatment).
- Myth three: A pill form of medication taken at home is automatically less effective than one delivered intravenously in the doctor's office.

These myths can misguide your thinking. Here are the facts:

- Fact one: Less treatment may give you greater overall benefit and fewer side effects. For example, combining Arimidex with tamoxifen was less effective and produced more side effects than Arimidex alone, according to a major study by the National Surgical Adjuvant Breast and Bowel Project.
- Fact two: Some of your most effective therapies may have the fewest side effects. The more a treatment targets just the cancer and spares normal tissue, the greater its benefits and the fewer its side effects. For example, hormonal therapy targets hormone receptors in hormone receptor–positive breast cancer. The targeted therapy Herceptin works against the HER2 receptors in HER2-positive breast cancer.
- Fact three: Some medicines given by pill can be just as effective—if not more so—

A LIMIT ON SYMPATHY

One of the challenges of ongoing therapy is wearing out the goodwill from family members, friends, and co-workers. Extra help, accommodations, flexibility, and support at home and at work may be harder to come by as time passes. Resentment may lurk. You may even be expected to "pay back" past favors or time off. Most women feel discouraged, frustrated, angry, and maybe depressed by these expectations. This book will provide you with a range of solutions to help handle the emotional and physical package deal that can go along with ongoing treatment. (See more about support in Chapter 2.)

than some medicines given by IV. For example, hormonal therapy is usually equally if not more effective against hormone receptor–positive breast cancer than chemotherapy. (Both may be recommended in some situations.)

As you think through your ongoing treatment options and decisions, it's important to base your decisions on facts, not myths. This will lead to better decisions, less fear, greater quality of life, and maybe even longer survival.

Putting Ongoing Treatments in Perspective

It can be a struggle to make a whole other set of treatment decisions after you've been worn out by the initial treatment. Many women I take care of find it helpful and comforting to think of ongoing treatment in one of these ways:

- *An occupation.* Initial treatment with surgery, radiation, and chemotherapy can feel like an ambush when your body is swarmed from all sides and you're caught in the middle. Ongoing therapy is like the occupation after the initial takeover, the quieter therapies to establish calm after the storm. Your quality of life will depend on what the occupiers are like (gentle, strict, or militant) and how you get along with them.
- *Heavy-duty housekeeping.* Keeping your home clean and comfortable requires daily maintenance, discipline, and the occasional ambitious project. You would prefer a clean, organized, uncluttered body, too, but living with vigorous regular housekeeping in the form of ongoing treatment can be annoying. For women living with disease, new treatments for areas of spread are analogous to dealing with big projects around the house: attacking the attic, garage, or basement. The extra work can wear you out and land you on your back for a stretch, but if the new treatment works against the big things, you'll be very satisfied with the results.
- *An insurance policy.* You "buy" into an ongoing therapy "insurance policy" in case any cancer cells were left behind after initial treatment. You hope you don't need the insurance, but it's good to

have in order to lower the risk of recurrence and increase your peace of mind.

No matter how you view ongoing therapies, you need to think of them as powerful solutions to fend off breast cancer recurrence. The focus of this book is on your recovery after initial treatment is over and on your quality of life during ongoing therapy. So we're going to skim over most treatment decisions and focus mainly on how you manage the challenges and enjoy day-to-day life during ongoing therapy.

Solutions

One or more ongoing medical therapies may be recommended after your initial treatment is over, such as hormonal therapy, targeted treatments (such as Herceptin), or chemotherapy (for example, Xeloda). In this chapter, we will focus primarily on hormonal therapy, since this starts up only after your initial treatment is over and because you take it for an extended period of time (five years or longer).

For information to help you deal with your initial treatments, or to get updates on new hormonal treatments that emerge after this book is in print, turn to Breastcancer.org. There you can find 24/7 research news and the most up-to-date medical information.

Hormonal Therapy: Overview

Hormonal therapy is an important option for anyone with hormone receptor–positive breast cancer (cells that have either estrogen receptors or progesterone receptors present, or both), including women of all ages, with any stage of disease.

- ***Early-stage invasive disease.*** Hormonal therapy can reduce the risk of recurrence of the original hormone receptor–positive breast cancer. It can also reduce the risk of a new, unrelated breast cancer in either breast.
- ***Recurrence of a prior cancer.*** If the cancer comes back and is

hormone receptor–positive, hormonal therapy may still play an important role.

- *Advanced (metastatic) disease.* Hormonal therapy can shrink and further limit the spread of metastatic hormone receptor–positive breast cancer

Hormonal therapy can also reduce the risk of ever getting breast cancer in women who've never had breast cancer but who are at increased risk for developing the disease. These women may be at high risk because of a strong family history of breast cancer, a known breast cancer gene abnormality, or a prior breast biopsy showing an overgrowth of irregular cells (atypical ductal hyperplasia).

How Hormonal Therapy Works

About 60 percent of breast cancers have receptors for the hormones estrogen, progesterone, or both. The growth of these hormone receptor–positive breast cancers depends on the presence of estrogen. Hormonal therapies work to reduce the effect of estrogen on the body so that it can no longer promote the growth of hormone receptor–positive breast cancer cells. Without estrogen, the cancer cells are unlikely to grow.

The different hormonal treatments block hormone receptors, eliminate hormone receptors, or lower estrogen levels in the body. Each one has slightly different benefits and side effects.

HORMONAL THERAPY IS NOT HRT

Hormonal therapy against breast cancer is the opposite of hormone replacement therapy (HRT), used to reduce menopausal symptoms.

Hormonal therapy reduces the presence or effect of estrogen.	HRT adds estrogen to the system, to make up for the lowered estrogen production that accompanies menopause.
Hormonal therapy reduces the risk of hormone receptor–positive breast cancer diagnosis and recurrence.	HRT increases the risk of breast cancer.

Types of Hormonal Therapy

All four major kinds of hormonal therapy have a shared goal: to get rid of or inhibit the growth of hormone receptor–positive breast cancer by reducing the amount of estrogen in your body or by blocking the effects of estrogen on breast cells. Here is how each class of treatment works.

Aromatase Inhibitors

This powerful hormonal therapy works by reducing the amount of estrogen produced by fat and muscles in postmenopausal women. The three main aromatase inhibitors are Arimidex (anastrozole), Aromasin (exemestane), and Femara (letrozole).

Selective Estrogen Receptor Modulators (SERMs)

These medicines work by blocking estrogen receptors. Tamoxifen is the most common example. It has both estrogenic and antiestrogenic effects. It blocks estrogen receptor activity in the breast—like musical chairs, it sits in the place that estrogen would have taken in the estrogen receptor. In addition, it can have a very weak estrogenic effect in other organs such as the endometrium (where it thickens the uterine lining), liver (lowering blood levels of cholesterol), and bone (helping to increase density and strength).

Another SERM, Evista (raloxifene), used for treatment of bone loss

---

KNOW YOUR HORMONE RECEPTOR RESULTS

- **Positive.** Receptors for estrogen and/or progesterone are detected in a significant number of the cancer cells in the breast cancer tissue.
- **Negative.** Receptors for estrogen and/or progesterone are *not* detected in a significant number of the cancer cells in the breast cancer tissue.
- **Borderline positive.** A low number of receptors for estrogen and/or progesterone are present, falling barely within the positive level. There may still be a role for hormonal therapy.
- **Quantity not sufficient (QNS).** The tumor is too small to permit adequate testing for hormone receptors. (These small tumors, however, commonly behave as though they were estrogen receptor–positive.)
- **Unknown.** Hormone receptor test results have not yet been sent or the test has not yet been completed. Make sure your doctor arranges to get this test done.

in postmenopausal women, was found to reduce the risk of breast cancer in women without a history of breast cancer. It has no proven role as a breast cancer treatment, however.

Estrogen Receptor Downregulators (ERDs)

An ERD works by destroying estrogen receptors. With no receptors available, estrogen is unable to turn on cancer cell growth. Faslodex (fulvestrant) is the only ERD so far.

Ovarian Shutdown or Removal

This hormonal therapy approach eliminates the major source of estrogen in women before menopause: the ovaries. There are three ways to stop the ovaries' production of estrogen:

- *Medicines.* Zoladex (goserelin) and Lupron (leuprolide) are medicines that tell the brain's hormone control center to stop the ovaries from producing estrogen. They are given by injection once a month or every few months.
- *Surgery.* Oophorectomy removes the ovaries, which dramatically lowers the amount of estrogen in the body.
- *Radiation.* Low-dose radiation to the ovaries, sometimes called ovarian ablation, can also stop estrogen production. This method of shutting down ovarian function is rarely used in the United States.

You and your doctor will choose the treatment that is right for you by balancing the benefits and side effects of each hormonal therapy, then comparing one treatment approach against the others (e.g., SERM versus aromatase inhibitors, or Zoladex versus removal of the ovaries).

Side Effects

Side effects differ among the categories of hormonal therapy, although all of the hormonal medicines have some side effects in common. Some are brief, mild, and manageable (although annoying). Serious side effects rarely occur.

Predicting and identifying the cause of side effects can be confusing. Lingering side effects from chemotherapy are often experienced during hormonal therapy. And any individual can have her own unique reaction to any particular treatment. Benefits, risks, and personal comfort all have to be factored into the treatment choice that you and your doctor make. The list of shared side effects and the comparison table of side effects below give you an overview of what you might expect.

Side Effects Common to All Hormonal Treatments

Each of the hormonal therapies can produce the following shared side effects:

- Hot flashes
- Mood swings
- Vaginal dryness
- Other menopausal symptoms, including fertility problems
- Weight gain
- Reduced energy
- Depression, anxiety, panic attacks
- Nausea and bloating
- "Flare reaction" or burning pain in bones (metastatic cancer only)

But not all women experience all or even any of them.

There are also possible side effects that are specific to the different types of hormonal therapy, described in Table 7.1.

Talk to your doctor about balancing these various side effects against the benefits you hope to achieve with hormonal therapy. Other sections of this book will address both the challenges and solutions of many of these side effects; for example, there are chapters on fatigue, menopausal symptoms, and fertility.

Before you can make any final decisions on the benefits and side effects discussed so far, you also have to weigh in other medical considerations.

TABLE 7.1 Treatment-Specific Side Effects

Type of Treatment	Side Effects
SERM (tamoxifen, Evista)	• Increases risk of uterine cancer (< 1 percent of women) • Increases risk of blood clots and stroke • Causes irregular menstrual periods • Slightly increases risk of cataracts
Aromatase inhibitor (Arimidex, Femara, Aromasin)	• Weakens bones, increases risk of fracture • May cause muscle and joint pain and stiffness • Increases cholesterol levels • Increases risk of blood clots and stroke (but less risk than SERMs)
ERD (Faslodex)	• Weakens bones, increases risk of fracture • May cause swelling at injection site • May produce stomach symptoms, headache, back pain
Ovarian shutdown/removal (Zoladex, radiation, surgery)	• Brings on early menopause • Weakens bones, increased risk of fracture • May increase cholesterol levels • Causes permanent infertility if ovaries are removed

Other Health Considerations

You may have other health concerns, unrelated to breast cancer, that might influence your choice of hormonal therapy as well as your health care during hormonal therapy. These health concerns include:

• *A personal history of blood clots.* If you have had blood clots, your doctor will probably want you to avoid tamoxifen. But if you are premenopausal, your history of blood clots was not serious, and tamoxifen is an important part of your care, your doctor may recommend taking a blood thinner (such as baby aspirin) along with tamoxifen. Shutdown or removal of the ovaries is another approach.

- *Serious osteoporosis.* If you are postmenopausal, you should check your bone density with a DEXA scan (bone density test) prior to choosing hormonal therapy. This is because some hormonal treatments can weaken bone strength. Some women may find out from their first DEXA scan that they already have osteoporosis. If this happens to you, your doctor may steer you right away to tamoxifen—rather than an aromatase inhibitor—and also put you on a bone strengthening program. But if being on an aromatase inhibitor is a high priority, then an aggressive bone-strengthening program is needed. If you don't respond to the bone strengthener or you've had broken bones already, your doctor will likely recommend tamoxifen over an aromatase inhibitor.

- *Arthritis.* A common condition in women with or without a diagnosis of breast cancer, arthritis involves inflammation inside the joint space between two bones. Aromatase inhibitors can cause new joint and muscle pain and stiffness mostly around the joints. If you already have significant arthritis or significant joint and muscle discomfort (for example, fibromyalgia), hormonal therapy and in particular the aromatase inhibitors may make your existing aches and pains worse. Your doctor may modify hormonal treatment recommendations accordingly.

- *Uterine concerns.* Tamoxifen is associated with an increased—but still very low—risk of uterine cancer in postmenopausal women who have not had a hysterectomy. (If you have had your uterus removed, this uncommon but serious side effect is a nonissue.) So if you take tamoxifen, it's extra important to follow up regularly with your gynecologist. New vaginal bleeding after menopause—with or without tamoxifen—requires immediate medical attention. If you have a history of uterine cancer, however, tamoxifen is usually avoided even though you no longer have a uterus.

Making a Decision: Factors to Consider in Choosing a Hormone Therapy

Hormonal therapy can produce remarkable benefits with relatively few side effects in many women. Still, there are factors you must sort out and pros and cons you must weigh before you decide on hormonal therapy.

You and your doctor will carefully evaluate your particular situation, including:

- Factors about the cancer that can influence the benefit from hormonal therapy relative to other forms of treatment, such as tumor grade (grade I means slow growth, grade II means moderate growth, and grade III means fast growth). For example, you may derive your greatest benefit from:
  ~Chemotherapy (if hormone receptor–negative, high-grade)
  ~ Hormonal therapy (if hormone receptor–positive, low-grade)
  ~ Both chemo and hormonal therapy (if hormone receptor–positive, high-grade)
- Your medical history, including other significant health concerns and conditions
- Your menopausal status and personal preferences
- The balance of potential benefits and side effects of the hormonal treatment choices under consideration
- The impact of your other health concerns on these benefits and side effects

HOW MUCH BENEFIT?

In general, hormonal therapy reduces the risk of recurrence by about 50 percent in women with hormone receptor–positive breast cancer.

Here's what that number might mean for you. If your risk of recurrence is 40 percent and hormonal therapy can reduce it to 20 percent (a 50 percent drop), that's a very significant benefit. If your risk is 15 percent and hormonal therapy can reduce it to 7.5 percent, does that improvement make it worth taking hormonal therapy? How about a 4 percent risk decreased by half to 2 percent? Is that worth it to you? Were there no side effects to consider, the answer would be easy, but you have to balance the magnitude of the benefit against the risk of uncommon serious side effects such as endometrial cancer and pulmonary embolism as well as relatively common side effects such as hot flashes or muscle and joint stiffness and discomfort. There is also the cost of the medicine.

This discussion takes time, care, attention, and a great deal of thought. Start with the doctor who knows you best, but make your final decision only after consultation with a medical oncologist (the doctor with the most expertise in prescribing cancer-fighting medications).

You need to speak up and voice your concerns and preferences. Your doctor's recommendation will be based on your input, clinical guidelines, experience, and judgment. Over time, review and reaffirm or modify your decision with your doctor, depending on how things are going.

Sequence and Combinations of Therapies

Hormonal therapy may start before or after other treatments. Usually it comes last, after surgery, chemotherapy, and radiation. Hormonal therapy might come before other treatments to shrink a large cancer in the breast or lymph nodes. In women with metastatic disease, it might be the only form of ongoing therapy. Hormonal therapy is not given at the same time as chemotherapy because it can make chemo less effective, but it can be given together with Herceptin (trastuzumab) after chemotherapy is completed.

Interference with your body's ability to convert tamoxifen into its most active form, endoxifen, might keep you from getting the essential benefits of the medication and potentially lead to a higher recurrence rate. The main enzyme (a special protein that converts one chemical into another) that activates tamoxifen is called CYP2D6. There are two ways to limit CYP2D6's ability to work:

- *Having an abnormal CYP2D6 gene.* About 10 percent of people have a faulty CYP2D6 gene. As a result, their CYP2D6 enzyme's ability to activate tamoxifen is limited. These individuals are likely to attain greater benefit from another form of hormonal therapy. You can ask your medical oncologist doctor to check your CYP2D6 gene using a blood test or a swab of cheek cells from inside the mouth.
- *Taking medications that block CYP2D6 function.* There is a whole list of medications that can inhibit CYP2D6 activity, dropping the amount of available activated tamoxifen (endoxifen) by about half, thereby limiting the effectiveness of tamoxifen. Thus you should avoid taking strong and moderate inhibitors of CYP2D6 while you're on tamoxifen (see Table 7.2). Of note: the CYP2D6 enzyme is not needed to activate Evista (raloxifene), a sister medicine to tamoxifen that is used to reduce the risk of developing hormone receptor–positive breast cancer in postmenopausal women.

Even with a faulty gene and taking medicines that might block CYP2D6—tamoxifen usually provides some benefit. But if you've finished or are still taking tamoxifen and you're concerned about whether you've gotten or are getting its full benefits based on this information

---

TABLE 7.2 Medicines to Avoid While Taking Tamoxifen

The following medications can block the effectiveness of tamoxifen by inhibiting the CYP2D6 enzyme.

Strong Inhibitors

Generic Names	Brand Names
Bupropion	Wellbutrin
Fluoxetine	Prozac
Paroxetine	Paxil
Quinidine	Cardioquin

Moderate Inhibitors

Generic Names	Brand Names
Duloxetine	Cymbalta
Sertraline	Zoloft
Diphenhydramine	Benadryl
Thioridazine	Mellaril
Amiodarone	Cordarone
Trazodone	Desyrel
Cimetidine	Tagamet
Terbinafine	Lamisil

Not Inhibitors

Generic Names	Brand Names
Venlafaxine	Effexor
Citalopram	Celexa
Escitalopram	Lexapro
Fluvoxamine	Luvox

Source: Indiana University, http://medicine.iupui.edu/clinpharm/COBRA/ TamoxifenGuide.pdf

Note: This table is not a complete list and it is subject to change as medicine advances.

---

about CYP2D6, talk to your doctor about your specific situation. As medicine marches forward, new knowledge emerges. You can't change past treatment decisions, but you can make more informed decisions about current and future treatments that can benefit you.

It appears to be acceptable to give hormonal therapy together with radiation. Some doctors remain concerned that it might make the radiation less effective—as is true of hormonal therapy given with chemotherapy. Here is the basis of their concern: Cancer cells are most vulnerable to chemotherapy and radiation when they are actively growing. But if hormonal therapy makes the cancer cells inactive, then taking it at the same time as chemotherapy or radiation might make the cancer cells harder to eliminate.

So far, retrospective studies (looking back on treatments that have already been given) don't appear to show any loss of benefit when radiation is given together with hormonal therapy. However, there has not yet been a well-planned clinical trial to properly answer this question. Until this concern is resolved, I prefer to postpone hormonal therapy until radiation is over. This short delay—at most two months—doesn't seem to cut into hormonal therapy's effectiveness for a treatment that's usually given for five or more years.

Separating the treatments also makes tolerating the radiation a bit easier and helps distinguish possible side effects (not an option when two new treatments are started at the same time). If you've just finished chemotherapy, a short delay before starting the next medicine regimen can make recovery easier. But all this said, if your doctor thinks it's critical for you to start hormonal therapy ASAP, proceed accordingly.

Starting Hormonal Therapy

There's generally no rush to start hormonal therapy. Since you will be taking this therapy for five years and sometimes longer, delaying its start by several weeks is usually not a big deal. (If you have aggressive disease, however, your doctor may want you to start your hormonal therapy right after chemotherapy, and continue it during radiation.)

Perhaps you've planned a vacation to celebrate the completion of your main treatment. If your disease is not aggressive and your doctor concurs, then go and have fun; start your hormonal therapy upon your return. It's never a good idea to begin a new medicine when you're traveling away from home. Or maybe you need extra time before you feel ready to take hormonal therapy. That's okay, too. But don't put off hormonal therapy for more than a few months; it's important to move ahead with your decision so you don't lose the benefits of the treatment.

How Long Do You Take Hormonal Therapy?

The preferred length of time for adjuvant hormonal therapy ranges from five to ten years. If you are starting hormonal therapy for early-stage disease, your doctor will usually prescribe tamoxifen or an aromatase inhibitor (or one and then the other) for the first five years. If you have completed five years of hormonal therapy, your doctor might recommend that you extend your treatment with one form of hormonal medicine or another.

For women with metastatic hormone receptor–positive disease, hormonal therapy continues as long as it is working for you. If it's keeping the cancer under control with acceptable side effects, there is no time limit.

The length of hormonal therapy may be shortened if you have difficult-to-manage side effects with a major negative impact on your quality of life. Your doctor may suggest that you switch to another hormonal therapy, to see if it's easier for you to tolerate. But if you experience a serious side effect, such as a blood clot to the lung, your antiestrogen medicine will be stopped immediately. (If it's critical for you to stay on hormonal therapy, however, your doctor may restart hormonal therapy together with a blood thinner.)

Switching Hormonal Therapy

A significant number of women end up switching from one type of hormonal therapy to another, because another hormonal medicine may appear to be more effective or have fewer side effects (or both). Here are some examples of situations that might lead you to switch:

Greater Potential Benefit

If medical breakthroughs show that another drug is more effective for your particular type of breast cancer than the drug you are currently taking, you may change from your current therapy to the one that may have superior benefits. For example, after two to three years of tamoxifen, postmenopausal women may switch to an aromatase inhibitor for the rest of their five-year course of hormonal therapy (rather than staying on tamoxifen for the full five years). For premenopausal women with aggressive breast cancer who continue to menstruate on tamoxifen, your doctor may recommend switching over to a combination of ovarian shutdown or removal together with an aromatase inhibitor. More is not always better, however. For postmenopausal women, there is no advantage to doubling up treatment with tamoxifen and an aromatase inhibitor.

Medication Failure

Cancer cells may have figured out how to grow despite the medication. They may have even learned to thrive on it. If your cancer comes back, enlarges, or spreads while you are taking one form of hormonal therapy, that particular medicine should be stopped. Stopping the medicine alone, however, is only a partial therapeutic step. Another form of hormonal treatment is usually required—and possibly other treatments as well.

For women with metastatic hormone receptor–positive disease, switching to another form of hormonal therapy is necessary if the one you're on stops working. Different hormonal therapies are often given over time (for example, first tamoxifen, then an aromatase inhibitor, next Faslodex). Your doctor's treatment recommendation will depend on your response.

Changing Circumstances, Changing Treatments

You may be diagnosed with breast cancer when you're premenopausal, but over the course of your treatment you may become postmenopausal. Now you're eligible for an aromatase inhibitor. Or you may have had a hormone receptor–negative breast cancer upon initial diagnosis, but then you developed a new, different breast cancer that is hormone receptor–positive. So a medication that may not have been right for you at one time may become appropriate for you as your medical situation changes.

Fewer Side Effects

You're experiencing unpleasant or unacceptable side effects on one hormonal medicine, so you're seeking another medication that's safer and easier to tolerate. For example, fewer hot flashes but more muscle and joint discomfort tend to occur on aromatase inhibitors relative to tamoxifen. Choice of treatment partly depends on whether you experience these side effects and how much they affect your quality of life.

You may also experience serious unacceptable side effects on one medication, forcing you to switch to another. Safety is a major concern in any of your health decisions. Examples of this include a diagnosis of endometrial cancer or a blood clot while on tamoxifen, or bone fractures due to osteoporosis unresponsive to bone builders while on an aromatase inhibitor.

Extended Treatment

You may have finished a full course of one hormonal therapy and you want to extend your treatment by switching to another type. For example, after five years of tamoxifen, postmenopausal women may be able to get additional benefit from switching to an aromatase inhibitor for five more years. But for women with early-stage disease who have finished five years of an aromatase inhibitor, it's unclear whether more hormonal therapy would be beneficial (ongoing studies are evaluating this important question).

More Affordable

The high cost of one hormonal therapy may cause you to switch to a more affordable option. A medication that is still under patent, such as some of the aromatase inhibitors, will be more expensive than another type of hormonal therapy for which the patent has expired, such as tamoxifen. Also, brand-name medications cost more than their generic versions; for example, Nolvadex (brand name for tamoxifen) is more expensive than the generic tamoxifen citrate.

If it's important for you to stay on an expensive hormonal medicine and its cost is a serious issue for you, apply to the pharmaceutical company that produces the medication for a discounted price. (For example, Astra-Zeneca makes Arimidex and Zoladex, Novartis makes Femara, and Pfizer makes Aromasin.)

Lower-cost sources of high-priced medicines are becoming increasingly available, too. Check Internet, buying clubs (Costco, BJ's, Sam's Club), and advocacy membership groups such as AARP. And be careful to avoid websites that sell counterfeit drugs.

Medicine Works Only When You Take It

You get the best results with hormonal therapy when you take the medications as prescribed, year after year. That means sticking to both the prescribed daily dose and the recommended length of treatment. The reality, however, is that many women have trouble continuing hormonal therapy for the full five years of treatment. One study, co-authored by Dr. Ann H. Partridge at the Dana-Farber Cancer Institute in Boston, showed that 23 percent of patients missed taking tamoxifen more than 20 percent of the time. The study also found that adherence rates declined with years of treatment, from 87 percent in the first year to only 50 percent by the fourth year.

Missing a dose of hormonal medication every now and then probably doesn't make a big difference. But if you regularly miss doses of hormonal therapy, you're unlikely to get the benefit you need. Plus, it's harder for your doctor to judge how the medicine is really working for you. If you remain disease-free, great! But if the cancer returned, it would be unclear if it is due to a medication failure or a failure to take the medicine properly.

If side effects of hormonal treatments are bothering you, talk with your doctor or nurse right away. Don't suffer in silence—this will just make you less likely to stick to the treatment in the long run. And never stop taking your medicine without telling your doctor—you'll lose the protection it provides and create a disconnect with your doctor.

❧ Moving Forward

The bottom line: Ongoing therapies could prove to be your biggest investment in your future. But they only work if you take them. Making a treatment decision is relatively easy (although it can feel huge at the time); the hardest work is implementing your decision. It takes a lot of courage, determination, resources, resolve, and dedication to swallow that pill each and every day, and to keep going back to your doctor's office as needed.

Understanding the necessity of ongoing treatment is the only way to get the drive and determination to stick with the plan. But as you move forward, make sure to give yourself credit, incentives, and rewards for working so hard to be healthy.

PART THREE

Coping with Side Effects of Treatment

CHAPTER EIGHT

Fatigue and Loss of Energy

Exhaustion hits hardest after chemotherapy—not during. No one told me what to expect. I was totally unprepared.

My fatigue was indescribable—and that's a big part of the problem: you can't point to a place and say, "See, here it is." I lay in bed much of the day, out of sorts and unable to concentrate on anything for more than a few minutes at a time. Nothing shows, and some of the people around you begin to think it's all in your head. Even you may begin to think so. But fatigue is all too real! S-l-o-w-l-y things got better, but it was a year before I felt like myself again.

First Things First

Fatigue is the most common, nagging, and debilitating side effect of the breast cancer experience. Fatigue is very different from the way you get tired from performing your job, running errands all day, or overseeing your home and your kids' lives. When you're tired, it's usually after a day's activity; you get some sleep, and the next day you feel better. Fatigue is not so cause-and-effect: it's due to a whole bunch of things over time, and it doesn't go away with just rest and sleep.

Fatigue feels like a total lack of energy, a weakness in your whole body, and sometimes a loss of interest in people and things you normally like to do. You don't feel normal; you don't feel good. "I wanted to keep going—but I couldn't do anything." "My mind keeps making appointments my body can't keep."

During treatment, your body is working overtime to defeat the cancer, handle the effects of treatment, and run basic body functions, such as walking, eating, and going to the bathroom. Your body needs to conserve its precious energy for this work and shut down other activities that aren't absolutely necessary. The result is fatigue, making it hard to attend to ordinary obligations at home, at work, or in your community. Everyone's path is different: for some fatigue is worse during treatment, while for others it's worse after, when accumulated effects take their toll.

After treatment is completed, fatigue can still hang on—with the added burden that you have to struggle to catch up with everything you had to put on the back burner.

℘ Challenges

Emotional and Psychological Causes of Fatigue

Uncertainty

Dealing with the uncertainty that accompanies breast cancer diagnosis and treatment can drain all energy from even the toughest person. Always the questions: Will this work? What if it doesn't? What next? Each test begets another question, followed by an answer that raises another question. The fear and anxiety of recurrence refuse to leave. "It's like hanging your life up on the line and watching it dry out." Exhausting!

Depression

Fatigue can make you feel depressed even if you're truly not. Not knowing why you feel washed out week after week can bring anyone down. On the other hand, depression can be a cause of fatigue. The breast cancer experience—including the side effects of breast cancer medications—can deepen feelings of depression.

Stress

When you're enveloped by fatigue, many ordinary stresses seem— or are—worse now: your job, your marriage, your children, and your financial situation. Any one of these problems can wear you down. As hard as it may have been to deal with these issues before diagnosis, it's harder to manage them now when you're worn down by fatigue.

Physical Causes of Fatigue

Surgery and Anesthesia

Fatigue from surgery depends on the type of surgery and length of anesthesia required. If you had lumpectomy alone with local anesthesia, then fatigue is probably minimal. Longer and more complex surgeries—such as mastectomy, lymph node dissection, and tissue flap reconstruction—require longer anesthesia. In general: the longer the anesthesia (and the older and heavier you are), the greater the fatigue that follows. If, for instance, you had a ten-hour surgery involving mastectomy and free flap reconstruction, you may feel zonked for a few weeks—even a few months—afterward.

Further compounding fatigue from surgery, a stay in the hospital means that doctors, nurses, and other staff will be in and out of your room all day and night, making it hard for you to get solid rest. Add the disruption of your body's normal rhythms, nausea, pain medication, constipation, and bloating, and fatigue can hit hard.

Chemotherapy

During a course of chemotherapy, fatigue may come on full force when your immune system is at its lowest. This often leads to anemia—a low count of red blood cells or a low level of hemoglobin (the special molecule inside the red blood cells that picks up oxygen in your lungs and delivers it to the cells and tissues of your body). Because oxygen gives your body energy, being anemic means the amount of oxygen that reaches the cells of your body is reduced, so you feel much less energetic.

When your immune cell counts are low, the risk of fever and infection goes up, and fatigue tags along for the ride. The longer the infection and the higher the fever, the more exhausted you're bound to be.

With each successive cycle of chemotherapy, you feel increasingly knocked down. Maybe after the first cycle you bounced back, but by the time you get to your last cycle, you won't bounce back as far or as quickly. Your body may not feel the full effect till the middle or end of chemotherapy—at which point you're thrust into early menopause, and the chemo effects plus the changes that accompany menopause fully hit home. This is one reason fatigue can actually worsen after treatment. In addition, much of the supportive care that is given during treatment—steroids, blood count growth factors, IV fluids, and lots of medical attention, as well as family support and compassion— disappears as soon as treatment is completed, further increasing your fatigue.

Radiation

If your treatment up to this point has been confined to surgery, you may feel like you're on your way to recovery—until you move into the next phase, radiation. If you've just completed chemotherapy, you'll probably already be experiencing fatigue. This is the point when many of my patients tell me they feel like a one-hundred-year-old woman crawling out of bed in the morning.

Radiation to just the breast area usually involves minimal fatigue. But if the nearby lymph nodes are also being treated or if radiation is given to other parts of the body where there is spread, your fatigue will probably be worse. This fatigue can slowly build up over the course of radiation and linger for a month or longer after treatment is completed. The physical demands of daily treatment will only increase your fatigue; the inconvenience of going back and forth to receive treatment five days a week, for weeks in a row, is a major commitment and can disrupt your life.

Hot Flashes

When hot flashes blast on and off throughout the day and then wake you up at night, they drain your energy and rob you of a good night's rest. If this continues day after day, night after night, fatigue quickly sets in. (See Chapter 14 for more on hot flashes.)

Steroids

Steroids may be given along with chemotherapy to avoid an allergic reaction and to ease other side effects. While you may feel very energetic on steroids, when you taper off the steroids your energy is likely to fizzle. Weathering these highs and lows can wear you thin.

In addition, moderate to high doses of steroids can interfere with sleep. Steroids given over an extended period of time can also weaken muscles, particularly in the hip and shoulder areas, which adds to your overall fatigue.

The good news is that only a short course of steroids is typically used during breast cancer therapy. After steroids have been stopped, fatigue will usually go away as your body readjusts to its normal state.

Weight Gain

You may find yourself eating more to ease nausea, or putting on weight as a side effect of treatment. Suddenly you're twenty pounds overweight and your self-image sinks through the floor. Not surprisingly, you then tend to be less active, and you may give up all efforts at exercise. The less you move, the less you feel like moving, and the easier it is for the pounds to build up and slow you down further.

Other Medical Conditions: Hypothyroidism, Sleep Problems

A number of different medical conditions contribute to fatigue. An underactive thyroid gland (hypothyroidism) makes your metabolism run slow. Thus your body doesn't burn food fast enough to give you the energy you need. Hypothyroidism is a fairly common preexisting condition, but occasionally it can be a side effect of treatment. Other preexisting medical conditions can make you fatigue-prone, including Lyme disease, fibromyalgia, and chronic fatigue syndrome. And some women have seasonal affective disorder, causing extremely low energy levels during the darkness and cold of winter.

Sleep problems that block your ability to get a good night's sleep can also cause significant ongoing fatigue (see Chapter 15).

It's also important to remember that fatigue can be dangerous. When you're feeling less than 100 percent, you're more likely to fall or have an accident. You and others can be hurt. Have you ever fallen asleep at the wheel or backed up the car without seeing someone right behind you? Have you ever been tired and tripped on something you didn't see going down the stairs? For your safety— and many other reasons—it's important to work on ways to manage fatigue.

✿ Solutions

There's no magic pill that will cure fatigue. It requires more than one solution because it usually involves more than one cause. Below are suggestions and guidelines that have helped my patients.

Listen to Your Body, Check Your Energy Gauge

Are your expectations for yourself set too high? Are you too used to being a dynamo? Do you think you have to be Superwoman, pushing your career, covering the home front, and signing up for community events as well? It's time to reset your priorities. Maybe your body is telling you, *Stop!* Listen to your body. Give yourself a break. "My job right now is to finish my chemo and let go of the other things that deplete my energy."

First and foremost is a Zen-like suggestion. Fatigue *is*, so accept it, don't fight it. Fatigue is a signal to you that your body needs to recover. Try not to do more than you need to. Meditate. Try yoga; gentle postures may get your body loosened up. Try massage to ease muscle tension. Rest and recover on your way to managing fatigue.

Address Contributing Medical Conditions

You should get your body checked out for any medical condition that may be contributing to your fatigue, as many are not obvious or visible—and most are treatable. Let your doctor know that you've reached your limit and need help. If your doctor doesn't respond well to your concern about these problems, find a doctor who will.

Fatigue due to low immune cell counts will improve with time after treatment, good nutrition, and growth factors such as Neupogen or Neulasta. Most infections are effectively treated with the appropriate antibiotics. Anemia from iron deficiency can be treated with iron; anemia caused by slow red blood cell production might improve with Procrit. Anemia from bleeding involves identifying the source of the bleeding (for example, stopping a medicine that may be causing bleeding). Blood transfusions can increase your blood counts immediately. Low platelet counts, which can contribute to bleeding, can be improved with the use of a growth factor called Neumega—and if necessary, platelet transfusion.

Hypothyroidism is easy to diagnose and remedy: a blood test, results within a week, and one pill a day. If depression is an issue, treatment by individual therapy and/or medication is essential. Lyme disease, fibromyalgia, and chronic fatigue syndrome require medical evaluation and management.

Consider Medication

If your energy is nonexistent and you can barely manage your daily tasks, your doctor might consider the use of a prescription stimulant medication, such as Ritalin, Dexedrine, Provigil, or sometimes simply caffeine. You will need to seek out a doctor who is familiar with the use of these medicines for fatigue (your primary care doctor or a neurologist). You must also consider possible side effects of these medications, such as irritability, nervousness, mood swings, and insomnia.

Conserve and Allocate Your Energy

Think of your energy level as a precious bank account that must be kept balanced. Whenever you exert yourself and take energy out of your energy bank, you have to balance it with rest and relaxation. Every "yes" to a new task or responsibility has to be balanced by a "no, thank you" to another demand. Saying no may be a new tactic—one you can and must learn.

Keep your priorities in check and schedule those must-do activities during the times of the day when you have the most energy. Plan rest and recovery for when your energy is lowest. And protect your good spirits: do what you enjoy. One expert suggests you focus on something good. "I made a list of things that make me feel good, and when I'm feeling bad, I pick something from the list." Do what *you* want to do, not what others think you should. That includes saving your energy for the people you care about most.

Manage Your Stress

Get a handle on what is stressing you most—job, family, money—and try to figure out how to make things better. If you haven't yet learned that it's okay to ask for help, now is the time to explore that option. (See Chapters 2, 4, and 19.)

E-HELP

Make it easy on yourself: use Breast-
cancer.org's organizer in the online
community or Lotsahelpinghands.com.
Put someone in charge of organizing
these jobs who is able to email re-
quests, errands, and schedules. Then
you can stay out of the loop until you
recover some of your old zip.

Even with help from devoted
friends and family, you may find
you have to hire some help to do
what you feel must be done. Most
important, do what you can and let
the rest go. (I regularly hand out
prescriptions that say "Give up the
housework.")

For some people, scheduling a
dedicated time to seek solutions
to the issues that are causing you
stress can be helpful. If worries about your illness, treatment, or
recovery persist, make an appointment with your doctor to discuss them
and come up with a plan to manage them further.

Rest

Regular rest is absolutely critical to your health. Protecting and cherish-
ing your sleep will require discipline on your part and cooperation from
the people (and pets) with whom you live. Your best rest happens at
night; little pick-me-ups in the form of naps may be essential for some
people at some times, but they don't solve the real problem of restorative
sleep. In fact, too long a nap during the day can spoil your sleep that
night.

Falling asleep may be a challenge. Chapter 15 will provide a range
of suggestions and solutions for a sound night's sleep.

Exercise

Rest needs to be balanced with activity. Every practitioner who treats
fatigue prescribes some form of exercise; start with a little bit at first so
you don't wear yourself out. Walking is the easiest choice for most people. Amble along your favorite street; walk to the house of a nearby
friend, or bring a backpack and go to the local grocery store for fresh
fruit and something for dinner. Work up to a pattern you can live with:
ten minutes three times a week, then half an hour, then possibly a full
hour per session. Try to build up to some activity every day. How about

a gym? You might love strolling on a high-tech treadmill. Or swimming. Or an elliptical trainer or NordicTrack: "I got on that NordicTrack, first to music, then to silence—and I got to feeling great."

Rather than sit and talk on the phone, walk and talk with your family and friends so you keep on the move. A few friends and I meet up regularly at the local school's track and walk and talk for about an hour (the time flies by). Or I walk while I talk to my sister in another city by cell phone. And once a week, I walk to the store for milk and a few groceries.

It may be worth it to you to engage a personal trainer for enough sessions to get you going and to stick with a plan. If that's too much of an expense, try to find a good friend who will commit to an exercise program with you.

You'll find you sleep much better on the days you exercise. Exercise also reduces hot flashes and anxiety, making it less likely that they will wake you up at night.

Eat and Drink Well

Proper nutrition can help keep your energy level steady—without highs that jazz you up or lows that bring you down. And eating and drinking well, along with physical activity, will help keep your bowels moving; sparing you undue stress and keeping you comfortable.

To figure out your best sources of "fuel," it can be very helpful to meet with a nutritionist or dietitian. (This kind of consultation might even be covered by your health plan.) For more on eating a healthy diet, see Chapter 17.

Balancing Light and Darkness

If your energy is low during darkness or the short days of winter, you can take steps to enhance lighting during the day and extend this brightness into the evening. Open your curtains and drapes to let in as much outside light as possible during the day. Leave a few key lights on throughout the day, so when it's gloomy outside you're greeted by a warm, welcoming light as you move around the most commonly used rooms of your home. (Motion-activated fixtures and low-energy bulbs such as

LEDs and compact fluorescents conserve energy as well as electricity costs.) When it's time to rest or sleep at night, start the ritual of turning off all lights and closing all curtains in and near your bedroom.

✄ Moving Forward

Although there is no time limit to how long fatigue may last, my rule of thumb is that after you finish treatment, fatigue tends to hang on at least as long as the time from diagnosis through the end of treatment. So if diagnosis and surgery took two months, followed by six months of chemo, it will likely take at least another eight months after you finish chemo for the fatigue to go away. Complete recovery from major surgery alone often takes six months. But fatigue related to breast cancer treatment has been known to go on for years. If you've done all you can and you are still fatigued, get professional help. Meanwhile, watch your energy bank account and keep up your anti-fatigue program. You may need to accept your reduced energy level as one aspect of the breast cancer experience. Things can get better, especially if you're prepared to turn to a resource person who can step in and help where and when you most need help. "Even a pile of unpaid medical bills can be managed," says Irene Card of Medical Insurance Claims. Capitalize on what energy you do have at the moment, and look forward to improvement in the future.

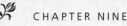

CHAPTER NINE

Understanding and Controlling Pain

Usually I'm good at handling pain, but I was in such pain that I really needed the morphine. The nurse came in to say, "We don't have the kind of morphine you need. You'll have to wait till morning. There's nothing more I can do," and she left. But I couldn't stand it, and I started to cry. Another nurse heard me, and went and found something that helped. That experience was the worst. Later on, I found out that someone always has a key to the pharmacy, but I was in no condition to demand anything. I was just lucky the second nurse heard me and understood how much pain I was in.

The swelling and pain in my hands and feet after the chemo I had is so bad! A so-called side effect. I'm walking on my heels and I have Band-Aids all over the cracks on my fingers.

Anytime something hurts, I think the cancer has come back.

I don't know if I should take pain medicine around the clock or wait till the pain comes back so I know I really need it.

❧ First Things First

If you have had breast cancer, you divide all kinds of pain into cancer-related pain and non-cancer-related pain—and knowing that most pain has nothing to do with cancer may not reassure you. The physical and psychological overtones of pain can be overwhelming. I'm always getting calls from patients worried about a new pain and what it means. I can understand their fear; past experience has taught them how vulnerable they are. The best way for me to be the most helpful is to make an immediate distinction between non-cancer-related and cancer-related pain.

Non-cancer-related pain results from repetitive overuse, strenuous new activity, injury, aging, other medical conditions, and side effects from treatment. Treatment-related pain may come from surgery, radiation, or chemotherapy. You may feel pain and soreness in the breast area after breast surgery and radiation, or mouth sores after chemo. Treatment-related pain usually doesn't stir up fear of recurrence as other pain does—probably because you know to expect it—but it still carries its own psychological weight: it's a persistent reminder of the breast cancer treatment you've been trying to put behind you. And it is *pain*, whatever the cause.

Pain you can't attribute to anything, pain that *might* be caused by cancer, is the pain that really worries you. The fear of cancer recurrence or progression grows—and you think about dying. And one of the greatest fears of dying is being in pain, so there you are in a vicious circle. Reassurance can't come soon enough; a visit to your doctor may be necessary to break the cycle of anxiety. In most cases your fear will be unfounded.

Both cancer pain and non-cancer-related pain can be acute or chronic. Acute pain is intense and distressing, and lasts a few days to a couple of weeks; chronic pain is persistent, is less dramatic, and varies in degree. Acute pain scares you, you deal with it, and it's over. Chronic pain, on the other hand, can limit what you do with ease from day to day; it may leave you weak, helpless, dependent on others for the simplest things, uninterested in much of anything, and feeling isolated from friends, from places you love, and from the precious rough-and-tumble of your normal life.

You may have only one kind of pain, or it may be a bunch of different kinds of pains—with or without a preexisting tendency or condition (like arthritis or fibromyalgia). However simple or complex the pain, the only way to rise to the challenge is to understand its causes so you can work with your doctor to find the most effective solutions.

You don't have to suffer forever. Pain can be treated and alleviated. Pain medications and treatments have become increasingly sophisticated and effective, with better delivery systems, new products, and information, and awareness of how to use pain relief with fewer side effects. With customized treatment and improved communication, most people can be relieved of most, if not all, pain.

৶ Challenges

All pain, regardless of its source, is felt by your sensory nerves, which then transmit the pain messages to your brain. All through your body things happen that could be experienced as pain—but only if there is a nerve there to detect the painful episode and report it to your brain.

If you've had a mastectomy, the nerves in the area may no longer be working, and numbness results. You could have a muscle spasm or a rash in that area and not feel anything. On the other hand, if you have a hypersensitive nerve in the area and someone barely bumps you, it could feel like a football tackle. So the best way to understand the various causes of pain is to start by looking at the role of the nerves in each situation.

Nerve Pain

Nerves are sensitive structures that almost always make you feel pain or discomfort when they've been disturbed. Some women develop a hypersensitivity to touch within the area of surgery, because of damage to the fine nerves of the skin (which lie just beneath the surface). This effect usually improves slowly over time, as the nerves grow back. But some extra sensitivity can flicker on and off or persist with lessened intensity. (This condition can make it very uncomfortable to wear a prosthesis after a mastectomy.)

Pain can be caused by a non-cancer-related problem *near* a nerve, when:

- Tissue is removed, irritating nearby nerves
- Swelling builds up pressure in the area, from lymphedema, infection, surgery, or radiation

NEUROPATHY OF LOWER ARMS AND LEGS

Pain of the hands, forearms, feet, and lower legs, called neuropathy, is relatively common in people receiving taxane chemotherapy—Taxol (paclitaxel) and Taxotere (docetaxel). It is due to the effect of chemotherapy on the nerves that supply sensation to these areas—and it can be severe, interfering with your normal day-to-day functioning. "I had stabbing pains shooting up my legs, weakness in my knees, pins-and-needles sensations in my feet. Sometimes I woke up feeling like a bunch of bees were stinging me. I took pain medication here and there to deal with the tough days and nights, and I managed to work throughout my treatment."

Once the cancer medication has stopped, this nasty side effect can get worse for a few months (particularly once the steroids that go with chemotherapy have stopped). Then it slowly improves over a long period of time. It may ease up in a little over three months, get noticeably better by six months, and be much better by one year. Occasionally this pain remains significant for longer than a year.

Tenderness and a burning sensation in the hands and feet can be caused by the chemotherapy Xeloda. This nerve-related side effect goes away soon after the medication has stopped (for more information, see page 181).

You can also get pain from a non-cancer-related problem that *directly affects* the nerve:

- Surgery cuts, stretches, or bruises a nerve
- Radiation irritates or damages a nerve
- Scar tissue wraps around, squeezes, or pinches a nerve
- Chemotherapy affects nerve growth and repair

Cancer-related pains can also affect nerves. Breast cancer can cause nerve pain by growing around, along, and into nerves in areas within the body and spinal cord, or into the nerve tissue that makes up the brain.

Nerves that are upset or damaged can be hypersensitive and produce any of a whole range of symptoms: itching, burning, tickling feelings, stabbing or shooting sensations, pains, a sensation like bugs crawling across the skin. Nerves grow very slowly, so it will take a number of months, possibly six, before sensation starts to return to normal. Some types of chemotherapies, like Taxol and Taxotere, interfere with nerve maintenance, repair, and regrowth. So if you've had surgery followed by these chemotherapy agents, most of the nerve healing doesn't happen till the chemo is well over. But nerves are usually not fully forgiving—they often hold a grudge and will continue to cause occasional discomfort for years to come.

Shingles

Shingles is the reactivation of the herpes zoster virus (the same virus that causes chicken pox) in a particular nerve pathway, most commonly in the face and chest areas, with moderate to severe pain. This is non-cancer-related nerve pain, and it is not uncommon in women with breast cancer.

This viral infection usually shows up as a red rash with small blisters in a band over the skin, which often becomes extremely painful. The rash may be barely visible (or, on occasion, totally absent), but the pain hangs on. Shingles can go away within a few weeks of treatment or last for months—depending on the severity of your symptoms, other medical conditions you're dealing with, and the strength of your immune system.

Arm, Shoulder, Underarm, Breast Area, and Chest Wall Pain

Many women experience a strange mixture of numbness and pain in the skin, muscles, and supportive tissues of the arm, armpit, and breast area after surgery and/or radiation to these structures, as well as with chemotherapy delivered to the whole body.

Armpit Pain

Lymph node removal can cause numbness, soreness, and fullness in the armpit, and sometimes numb and tender feelings along the inside of the upper arm. Armpit discomfort often comes as a surprise to most people, and furthermore, it's usually worse than any breast area pain. That's largely because the armpit is a very busy area, with lots of nerve activity. Before surgery you probably never paid much attention to your armpit, so any discomfort there grabs your attention and becomes an insistent reminder of your condition. Over time, armpit area discomfort tends to ease up significantly and may even go away completely. (See Chapter 10 for ways to ease swelling and stiffness.)

Breast Area Pain

After a lumpectomy with or without radiation, the biopsy area may be tender and numb. Shooting discomfort is common, particularly in the nipple area—the most sensitive part of the breast. You may also get a heavy, achy, sore feeling in the breast, particularly if you are big-breasted and have had radiation. These symptoms resolve over a period of six months to a year but sometimes can persist longer.

Numbness and pain after mastectomy with or without reconstruction largely depend on the extent and types of these surgeries and if other treatments were also given (such as radiation and chemotherapy). For example, if you had a TRAM procedure for breast reconstruction, your belly and chest may hurt for some time. A tissue expander put in place after mastectomy can produce significant discomfort when the skin and muscle overlying the implant are stretched and the chest wall underneath is put under pressure. (See Chapter 6 for more information about reconstruction.) An extensive mastectomy with or without reconstruction can cause a burning sensation in the breast area and armpit. The underlying chest wall and muscles can feel stiff and sore with extra activity such as lifting, heavy vacuuming, and twisting.

Muscle, Joint, and Bone Pain

Common non-cancer-related causes of soreness, aches, and stiffness of the arm, shoulder region, breast area, and rib cage (including the little joints on each side of the breastbone) include:

- Surgery to breast area and underarm lymph nodes with or without reconstruction
- Radiation to breast area and underarm lymph node region
- Lymphedema (swelling) of the arm (see Chapter 10)
- Chemotherapy
- Hormonal therapy

Ongoing pain can lead to reduced range of motion and weakness that can last for weeks or months.

Muscle and Joint Discomfort

The main non-cancer-related cause of persistent overall muscle and joint stiffness throughout the body is from shifts of your body's internal hormonal environment due to:

- Stopping postmenopausal hormone replacement therapy upon being diagnosed with breast cancer
- Stopping steroids after chemotherapy is done
- Early onset of menopause after chemotherapy
- Ongoing hormonal therapies (especially with an aromatase inhibitor such as Femara, Arimidex, or Aromasin)

JOINT AND MUSCLE DISCOMFORT FROM AROMATASE INHIBITORS

About one-third to one-half of women will experience joint pain or stiffness while on an aromatase inhibitor, most likely due to low estrogen levels as a result of the treatment. This may be either a new symptom or a worsening of prior symptoms.

Most symptoms occur in the arms and legs—especially involving hands (finger joints), wrists, shoulders, knees, feet, and ankles. Some women will experience pain and stiffness of multiple joints, others of just one joint. These symptoms can start after a few days to a few months on the medication (1.5 months on average). The symptoms are usually mild to moderate. The discomfort may improve or stabilize—but it can also last the whole five years that you're on the medication. Less often, this side effect may be seen in women on tamoxifen.

Of the people suffering joint pain who sought evaluation by a rheumatologist (a doctor who specializes in muscle and joint problems), most were diagnosed with:

- Tendinitis: inflammation of the tendons that connect muscle to the bone
- Tenosynovitis: irritation of the sheath that surrounds the tendon
- Osteoarthritis: inflammation and breakdown of the cartilage cushion between the bones of a joint
- Bursitis: inflammation of the small fluid-filled sacs that lubricate and cushion pressure points between your bones, tendons, and muscles

> • Carpal tunnel syndrome: narrowing of the small opening in the wrist
> structure through which important nerves pass through to the hand
>
> You may experience one or more of these conditions for the first time or
> you may experience worsening of one of them from a preexisting condition.
>
> A number of factors are associated with an increased risk of developing
> joint pain and stiffness while on an aromatase inhibitor:
>
> • Prior chemotherapy (especially with a taxane, such as Taxol or
> Taxotere)
> • Prior hormone replacement therapy
> • Being either very thin or significantly overweight
> • High levels of hormone receptors on tumor specimens

In addition to aches and pains from hormonal changes, you can also get sore muscles and stiffness from these non-cancer and cancer-related sources:

• Holding your body rigid and straight to avoid pain from movement or at an awkward angle to guard a painful area from getting bumped
• Overworking your arms and shoulders by using a walker to get around
• Overstraining out-of-shape muscles when you resume regular and/or newer activities after your main pain is successfully treated

Bone Pain

Bone pain is a common side effect of medicines taken during or after chemotherapy that increase the bone marrow's production of immune cells (for example, Neumega or Neulasta).

Bone pain can also result from breast cancer spread. The framework of the bone is destroyed around the area of cancer spread, weakening the bone, irritating nerve endings, and causing pain. In addition, nearby muscles may be overworked and strained as they compensate for the pain. For example, swiveling one hip each time you walk to take pressure off the other, painful hip can lead to added discomfort.

Pain in Hands and Feet

Pain of the hands and feet, called hand-foot syndrome (the fancy medical term is erythrodysesthesia), can be a disabling side effect of various chemotherapies, including Xeloda (capecitabine), 5-FU (fluorouracil), and Doxil (doxorubicin). This syndrome starts out with redness and swelling of the palms, fingers, soles, and toes. But then the normal friction of using your compromised hands and feet can make the soreness and tingling worse, and can also lead to cracking and peeling of the skin.

Any or all of these symptoms can make it difficult if not impossible for you to perform normal daily activities, including brushing your hair, wearing your usual shoes, and touching anything that's warm or hot. Symptoms develop over time while on the medication and they generally resolve within a few weeks after the medication is stopped. Some residual sensitivity may persist, however. (See pages 197–199 for ways to minimize and deal with this challenging problem.)

Abdominal Pain

There are many kinds of abdominal pain. The most common non-cancer-related types are due to lingering treatment side effects:

- Constipation, gas, or diarrhea from pain or medications
- Abdominal wall discomfort after extra belly tissue is taken for breast reconstruction (see Chapter 6)
- Belly pain radiating from the back, due to shingles
- Blockage of the bowel caused by severe constipation or because of scar tissue around the bowel, signaled by crampy belly pain and bloating followed by nausea and vomiting (this condition requires immediate evaluation and emergency management)

Cancer-related types of abdominal pain in women with advanced breast cancer include:

- Enlarged lymph nodes in the center of the abdomen invading or pushing on nearby organs and nerves

- Liver pain (in the upper right and side of the abdomen and sometimes the right shoulder) when the liver is distended with cancer, stretching the capsule covering that surrounds it
- Belly pain that radiates from the back due to cancer involvement in the bones of the back
- Pain from blockage of the bowel caused by cancer

Mouth, Throat, and "Down There" Pain

Treatment-induced mucositis is characterized by swelling and shallow ulcers of the cells that line the mouth, throat, rectum, and vagina. A lump in the throat, sores in the mouth, and painful swallowing are common symptoms. Vaginal mucositis causes pain, discharge, and sometimes itching, plus it can burn when you pee. (If you have this, forget about sex until it clears up.) Rectal mucositis can really hurt when moving your bowels—particularly if you are constipated.

Mucositis can be caused by:

- Chemotherapy (such as with Xeloda)
- Side effects on the esophagus from radiation treatment to neck or chest area
- Yeast infections (thrush) resulting from the suppression of the immune system or an imbalance of bacteria and yeast (for example, with the use of chemotherapy, steroids, or antibiotics). They can be recognized by a thick white coating of the mouth or throat or a cottage-cheese-like or pasty white discharge from the vagina.

As unpleasant as this side effect is, mucositis is temporary and very treatable (see the "Solutions" section of this chapter).

Other Pain Syndromes

The descriptions of the most common causes of pain listed above are by no means all-inclusive. If your pain doesn't fit any of these descriptions, it doesn't mean that your pain is bizarre and that there is no way to relieve it. Talk to your doctor and nurse about it, to obtain the necessary

PAIN IS NOT PUNISHMENT

If you are deeply religious, pain may shake your faith in God: "Why are You making me suffer this way? What have I done to deserve this? How can this be part of Your plan?" Follow this up with guilt for doubting God plus all the "woulda, coulda, shouldas" about things you maybe could've done differently, and you probably end up feeling depressed on top of everything else. Even if you're not at all religious, you may ask yourself very similar questions, wondering why you have been "chosen" to suffer.

There is an important take-home message here: *don't let pain punish you any more than it already has*. There is no personal reason or message from God to explain why you are experiencing pain. No one elected you to suffer; you weren't singled out for this "honor." It happened; that's it. Now is the time to take action and pursue effective ways to reduce your pain and maybe even become pain-free. You have the same right as every other human being to live free of pain. And we doctors are here to see that it happens.

evaluation in order to figure out what is causing the pain. You'll then be able to work out a treatment plan together that you'll reassess with your doctor at regular intervals.

Major Obstacles to Pain Relief

Fear of Pain

Pain sets off the cancer alarm in your head. Your worst fears are triggered. Ask you doctor and nurse if you are dealing with a non-cancer-related or cancer-related pain so you can know sooner rather than later what you're up against and start finding the best solution.

Isolation

Severe pain can be so disabling and so powerful that it can imprison you in your bed, hopeless and depressed. It can even keep you from getting to your doctor and nurse for a proper evaluation and treatment.

Myths About Pain and Treatment Effectiveness

You may have heard the myth that pain medications interfere with effective cancer treatment. Don't believe it! You can get pain management at the same time you get effective anticancer therapy—they don't compete or interfere with each other's efficacy (except in very specific situations, such as medicines that block tamoxifen activation; see Chapter 7). Make *both* cancer treatment and pain relief your top priority. And fear not—pain medications are not likely to cover or conceal any important sign or symptom you need to report in order to get the best anticancer care.

Fear of Addiction

The "old days" of undertreating pain are history—or should be. Fear of addiction and dependency on painkillers, an "I can take it" stoicism, and contempt for pill-taking self-indulgence are outdated notions. There's nothing virtuous about suffering with pain, and addiction is not an issue for people taking pain medication for real physical pain. (Emotional pain also deserves and requires effective treatment—but with different tools and strategies.) Addiction is when your life is all about living for drugs. Medication—a medical approach—is when you use medicines to live your life. People often confuse the development of tolerance and the need to increase medication to maintain pain relief with addiction. There can be a normal and expected physical dependence on pain medication, after weeks or months of treatment, that can involve withdrawal symptoms if it is stopped. But these problems are nothing to be ashamed of and can be solved medically once the pain has been successfully managed.

Solutions

Communication Is Crucial

Your pain is invisible to other people, so if you don't tell your doctor that you're in pain, you can't assume your doctor will know about it or provide you with relief. Taking an active role in your care by reporting all symptoms, asking about new treatments, and making suggestions helps your doctor and nurse help you. If you feel your doctor is not taking your pain seriously enough, find a doctor or a pain management team who will. Many hospitals have special pain programs with doctors, nurses, and complementary care team members trained in the specialty.

ONE MAIN DOCTOR, ONE COMBINED PLAN

This chapter has a lot of information about pain relief from common pain problems—but it's not a how-to-do-it-all-yourself chapter. Use the information to better understand the source of your pain so you can work with your doctor and nurse to become pain-free. The more you know, the more effectively you'll be able to speak up for your best care. If there is a symptom in this chapter that seems to apply to you or there is a medication that you think may help you, ask your doctor or nurse about it.

Remember, have one physician in charge of your pain medications. More than one doctor prescribing pain medications can be confusing and even dangerous. If your care is transferred from one group to another or from one hospital to another, the new team must talk to the old team, and a new physician must be established as the primary caregiver when it comes to your pain medications.

Your doctor may recommend other practitioners to give you the benefit of various conventional treatments combined with complementary medical therapies, such as acupuncture, meditation, visualization, distraction, hypnosis, yoga, Reiki, shiatsu, and biofeedback for mild to significant chronic pain.

Communication also means your listening to what your body has to tell you. Don't let cancer fear warp your thinking, convinced that your pain comes from recurrent or progressive disease. Many types of pain have nothing to do with cancer. Pain is a by-product of life's wear and tear, and as we've explained above, it can be a side effect of cancer therapy.

Disclose Financial and Physical Limitations

Don't be embarrassed to tell your doctor or nurse if you're having trouble paying for your medications—you can usually get effective medications to fit your budget.

Along with being honest with your doctor about your finances, be just as straightforward about any physical limitations. Tell your doctor exactly what you are physically capable of doing—if, for instance, you prefer pain medication in a patch that gets changed once every three days over a pill if you cannot swallow without difficulty or are bedridden and have limited assistance. In that case, medication delivered automatically by a subcutaneous pump may be another option.

Describe Your Unique Situation

Before an effective treatment plan can be designed for you, you must be able to describe and characterize your pain for your doctor and nurse as accurately as you can. The best way to get started toward your pain solution is to figure out and provide partial or complete answers to the following questions:

- Where does it hurt? Does it start in one place and stay there, or does it move around to other spots?
- What does the pain feel like? Sharp, dull, hot, cold, aching, throbbing?
- Were there any precipitating events? A fall, discontinuation of long-term steroids, resumption of activity after prolonged bed rest, or strain from compensating for a problem elsewhere (such as sore shoulders from using a walker)?
- How bad is the pain, on a scale of 0 (no pain) to 10 (the worst pain you can imagine)?
- How long does the pain last? When does it start? Is it constant, intermittent, fleeting, the same throughout the day, or worse at a particular time?
- What makes it get worse? A certain position or movement, particular foods, lying on a hard surface, cold or rainy weather, feeling upset?
- What makes it get better? A particular position, time of day, medication?
- Do you have any other symptoms associated with the pain? Sweating, anxiety, palpitations, depression, insomnia?

Designing a Strategy to Relieve Pain

The next step is to work out the solution to your pain problem. There is a large and evolving assortment of pain therapies that can effectively relieve pain, alone or in combination. Specific sites of pain suggest specific localized treatments; diffuse pain requires general treatment.

The following pages offer several basic approaches to managing pain.

Utilizing Pain Medicines

Effective use of pain medications should operate on the following principles:

- Plan for continuous round-the-clock pain relief, rather than intermittent, as-needed pain relief.
- Only accept a medication that you are able to take; if you are unable to swallow or you have nausea, find a non-pill form of treatment.
- Start medications at the low end of their power to relieve pain; increase the dose based on how pain symptoms respond to the medication.
- Combine medications when appropriate to take advantage of the synergy between medications and to address the multifaceted nature of the pain.
- Change medication if it fails to relieve your pain after you have used it to its therapeutic potential. Try any new medication for at least a week before you give up on it and try another. If you are taking a combination of pain medications, try to change only one at a time.
- Address other medical and psychological conditions that can affect how you experience pain. Treat or prevent side effects. Manage anxiety that you might get from or in anticipation of pain.
- Keep the solution to your pain problem simple, within your budget, and compatible with your lifestyle. For example, avoid multiple medications that must be taken frequently but at different times of the day

In addition, make sure your doctor knows about any allergies you may have, so you can avoid any medication to which you are allergic. In fact, it's a good idea to mention your allergies anytime your doctor is about to prescribe medication for you. Allergies to codeine and morphine are not uncommon. Bear in mind, however, that there is a significant difference between an allergy and a difficulty in tolerating the side effects of a particular medication. For example, nausea is a side effect, not an allergic reaction.

Plan Based on Pain Intensity

Most pain medication regimens start with acetaminophen or non-steroidal anti-inflammatory medications (NSAIDs) and add an opioid (narcotic) medicine as needed.

Acetaminophen and NSAID dosages have an upper limit, because too much can cause kidney and liver damage, or worse. Narcotics on the other hand, can be given in increasing doses, side effects permitting, without a comparable upper limit. There are many choices of medications in each group (see the pain medications table below). Your doctor and nurse must monitor you closely to balance benefits and side effects.

Medicines to Manage Mild to Moderate Pain

NSAIDs include over-the-counter and prescription drugs that help reduce inflammation and pain (see sidebar). The non-NSAID acetaminophen helps reduce pain, fever, and hot sensations but doesn't reduce inflammation.

PAIN MEDICATIONS

Non-Narcotic Medications

Over-the-Counter

NSAIDs
Ibuprofen (Advil, Motrin)
Naproxen (Aleve)
Aspirin (Ecotrin)

Other
Acetaminophen (Tylenol)

Prescription

NSAIDs
Choline magnesium trisalicylate (Trilisate)
Ketorolac (Toradol)
Etodolac (Lodine)

COX-2 Inhibitors
Celebrex (use restricted by FDA)

Narcotics

Morphine, sustained or immediate release (MS Contin, Oramorph, Kadian, MSIR, Roxanol)

Hydromorphone (Dilaudid)

Oxycodone, sustained or immediate release (Roxicodone, OxyIR)

Fentanyl (Duragesic, Actiq)

Meperidine (Demerol)

Methadone (Dolophine)

Narcotic/Non-Narcotic Combinations

Acetaminophen and oxycodone (Percocet, Tylox, Roxicet)

Aspirin and oxycodone (Percodan)

Acetaminophen and propoxyphene (Darvocet)

Acetaminophen and hydrocodone (Vicodin, Lortab)

Among these medicines, I usually start with acetaminophen and never exceed the maximum dose recommended by the manufacturer. Mild but persistent discomfort, such as breast and underarm surgery pain, can usually be managed by acetaminophen or an NSAID alone.

If these medicines are unable to control all your pain, the next level of medications combine acetaminophen or an NSAID with a narcotic, offering more pain relief through synergy between the medicines, with fewer side effects than if you took a narcotic alone to control your pain. Combined medications within this group (see sidebar) are all fairly similar, and which one you start with depends on what your doctor and nurse recommend and what you tolerate best.

Of these various combinations, I usually start with Percocet because it works well and it has a long history of use. I usually avoid aspirin, because it prolongs bleeding. How you and your doctor choose one medication over another depends on various factors, discussed in the next few sections.

Adjust Dose or Drug Type Until Pain Is Gone

If the pain is not controlled with the initial dose. I usually increase the dose until the pain is controlled or until the maximum dosage of acetaminophen or NSAID is reached. The dosage of any pain medication containing acetaminophen or an NSAID is limited because excessive amounts can damage the kidneys, liver, or GI tract and can cause thinning of the blood, ringing in the ears, and other significant problems.

If the safe limit of a medication has been reached but pain persists or progresses, you can continue with the maximum dose of acetaminophen and either separately increase the dose of the narcotic you have been taking (such as oxycodone) or replace it with a stronger narcotic (such as morphine or Dilaudid).

Medicines to Manage Moderate to Severe Pain

There are many choices for relief of moderate pain. Acetaminophen and the usual NSAIDs remain useful; a stronger NSAID, such as ketorolac, can be used for treatment of acute moderate to severe pain (like after surgery), but only for a few days because it carries a higher risk of side effects than the other NSAIDs.

All of the narcotics (see list in sidebar) are powerful pain relievers, but they have significant side effects proportional to the amount of medication taken, including constipation, lethargy, nausea, and dry mouth. Still, these side effects are usually more tolerable than the pain, and most can be managed. They come in a wide variety of forms: pills, liquids, suppositories, intravenous preparations, patches, and even a lollipop. The essential difference in treatment of moderate and severe pain is the dose of narcotics required to relieve your pain.

Problems with Pain Management

Variable, Constant, and Progressive Pain

If the pattern of your pain is variable and no set dose works, your doctor may suggest a variable dose of one short-acting narcotic (like Dilaudid). Or she may recommend a longer-acting narcotic to cover the background mild to moderate pain and use a short-acting one for episodic, more intense breakthrough pain.

Persistent, steady, predictable pain is easier to control; the choice is usually one of the extended-release morphine preparations, a Duragesic patch, or methadone.

If your pain worsens and your condition declines, you will need an augmented but simplified regimen, such as the longest-acting oral morphines, the Duragesic patch, or continuous morphine by intravenous drip or subcutaneous pump.

Keep in mind that you may need to try several different pain medications before you find the one that gives you significant pain relief. Don't lose hope—just keep the dialogue going with your doctor and nurse so they can better understand your pain and tailor your treatment.

Managing Side Effects of Pain Medication

If you experience side effects from pain treatments, let your doctor know, and indicate which side effects you are willing to tolerate and which ones you find unacceptable. For instance, one patient may say, "I'll accept a little sleepiness if I can get complete pain relief." Someone else may insist on a clear mind above all, with pain relief secondary.

Here are some of the common and challenging side effects of narcotics:

- Lethargy and drowsiness
- Confusion (sometimes disorientation and delusion)
- Nausea and loss of appetite
- Dry mouth and dehydration
- Constipation
- Slowed breathing
- Urinary retention
- Slow response time (you should not drive while on narcotics)

The side effects you experience depend on your sensitivity to each medication and the way you take it. Smaller, more frequent doses of medication may produce fewer side effects than higher doses taken less often. Your doctor can change your medication or its dose with the hope of finding a more tolerable level or drug. Or you may decide to continue with the medication and dosage you're on because it controls your pain and you're prepared to cope with the side effects. (You may require additional medication to handle those side effects.)

Accident Prevention

Also, keep in mind: if you are not 100 percent yourself, be careful about your and others' safety. When you're in pain and/or taking pain medications, you're more likely to fall, injure yourself, or have a car accident. It's vital that you avoid multitasking and take accident precautions while on these medication. See Chapters 8 and 13, addressing fatigue and mind fog, for more on preventing accidents.

Many of the complementary therapies that focus on "mindfulness" train you to be present in the moment—mindful of how you're feeling and thinking and how your inner self is interacting with your outer world. These mindful skills are extremely useful in staying safe and avoiding accidents.

Complementary Therapies

Complementary therapies such as meditation, hypnosis, distraction, visualization, biofeedback, acupuncture, yoga, breathing techniques, and massage can do wonders to reduce your pain—mild or severe—with or without pain medications and conventional medical procedures. Here are just a few examples:

- Meditation and self-hypnosis are simple forms of focused concentration. To get started, you might:
  - ~Enter an imagined world—floating, perhaps, on a tropical ocean—for a self-altering experience.
  - ~Focus your attention on one or two thoughts, and put everything else in your mind outside your field of concentration. You can use a special word or phrase, like a mantra, to focus your thoughts.
  - ~Concentrate on the pain itself, either willing it outside the boundary of your concentration field or imagining the part of your body in pain as being warmer, cooler, or lighter.
- Music, in whatever style you prefer. "I felt best listening to Mozart—it was like healing sunshine." "Pavarotti's high C's sent chills up my back, taking me to another planet." "The Boss— that's who I need now!" Listen to any music that makes you feel good and takes your mind off the pain.

These techniques can help you "filter the hurt out of the pain," competing with the pain messages traveling along your nerve cells and bombarding your brain. You alter and reduce pain perception, and occasionally you may be able to eliminate the pain altogether. Relaxation is also part of the self-hypnosis process: as muscles relax and tension eases, pain lessens. All of these powerful techniques require practice and adjustments over time. Meditation for instance, is not as easy as it sounds—keeping your mind focused on one image takes effort and practice.

Management Based on Specific Pain Syndrome

The solutions offered in the first part of this section focus primarily on the intensity of your pain regardless of its cause. What follows will tell you how to tailor your pain management based on the underlying cause of your pain.

Nerve Pain

Depending on its cause, nerve pain may respond best to one or a combination of the following therapies and practical modifications:

- NSAIDs alone may control mild pain; a narcotic may be added for more significant pain.
- Steroids relieve swelling and pressure on the nerve tissue.
- Neurontin (gabapentin) is a medication that works directly on nerve function. It can help with nerve pain in the hands and feet after taxane chemotherapy. (This medication will not interfere with tamoxifen's effectiveness.)
- Radiation therapy can shrink or eliminate cancer that's pressing on nerves.
- A TENS (transcutaneous electrical nerve stimulation) unit is a small, portable device that emits low-voltage vibrations that interfere with the pain message your nerves are sending from somewhere in your body to your brain. It works best for a specific site of pain that is mild and persistent.
- A ReBuilder unit amplifies nerve signals to retrain and reset the nerves' and brain's responses to pain. For example, for the treatment of neuropathy from taxane chemotherapy, you may apply the device's electrodes to your lower legs 10 to 30 minutes

a day. The ReBuilder is prescribed by a physical therapist and is available at www.rebuildermedical.com or by calling 866-725-2202.

• A nerve block involves numbing just the painful nerve by injection of a medicine that surrounds the nerve. This is usually performed by an anesthesiologist.

• Surgery can release a nerve if it's trapped or pinched by tissue that can be safely lifted or removed. A surgeon may actually cut the nerve causing the pain, but only if the nerve can be safely sacrificed.

The art of nerve pain management requires an integration of these therapies and lifestyle considerations, with adjustments all along the way, to maximize your pain relief and your ability to function independently and well.

Shingles

Treatment for shingles—a viral infection that affects the nerves—requires prompt initiation of antiviral medications such as famciclovir (Famvir), valacyclovir (Valtrex), or acyclovir (Zovirax) along with pain medications such as steroids, NSAIDs, narcotics, or Neurontin (gabapentin).

Arm Pain, Stiffness, and Swelling

Special considerations in the management of a tender, swollen arm caused by lymphedema are described in Chapter 10.

Breast Area and Chest Wall Pain

Pain in these areas responds to pain medications, but any underlying cause of pain must be addressed as well. Here are just a few examples:

• Infection can cause pain and must be quickly treated with antibiotics.

• Recurrent cancer in the breast area can cause significant pain, which often responds to treatment of the cancer with radiation and medicine therapy (chemotherapy, hormonal therapy, and/or targeted treatments) combined with pain medication.

Numbness, tenderness, and nerve-related pains after cancer treatment tend to improve over time. But until they do, they should respond to acetaminophen or NSAIDs, and if necessary one of the medications for nerve-related pain. Occasionally a TENS unit or a ReBuilder can help.

Muscle and Joint Pain

Back muscle strain responds to a few days of complete bed rest, doctor-supervised use of NSAIDs and muscle relaxants (such as Valium), massage, heat or cold applied to the surface (depending on the type of problem and status of your circulation), and strengthening of the muscle groups with guided regular exercise followed by stretching.

Muscle and joint discomfort while on aromatase inhibitors is common and deserves effective pain management so you can lead a full and independent life and stay on this important anticancer therapy.

AROMATASE INHIBITOR–RELATED MUSCLE AND JOINT PAIN RELIEVERS

If you are experiencing significant muscle and joint stiffness and discomfort while on an aromatase inhibitor, talk to your medical oncologist to get help with your symptoms. There are a number of solutions that might help you reduce your symptoms, ranging from various activities to supplements to medications.

- Activities
  - ~ Regular exercise—water aerobics, swimming, or walking
  - ~ Stretching
  - ~ Yoga
  - ~ Rest
- Supplements
  - ~ Calcium and vitamin D
  - ~ Glucosamine and chondroitin
  - ~ Omega fish oil
- Complementary medicine
  - ~ Acupuncture
  - ~ Massage and Reiki

- Medicines
  - ~ NSAIDs, including COX-2 inhibitors
  - ~ Acetaminophen
  - ~ Narcotics
  - ~ Antidepressants, such as Cymbalta (duloxetine)
  - ~ Antiseizure medications, such as Lyrica (pregabalin)
  - ~ Bisphosphonates

Until you try a particular activity, remedy, or treatment, you won't know if it will work for you. Some of these treatments are proven and others are unproven—but all are presented in case you happen to respond to an unproven therapy or have no response to a proven type.

Coordinate these treatment options with your primary physician, one of your cancer doctors, or a pain specialist. For additional care to address significant joint and muscle problems, ask for a referral to a rheumatologist (a doctor who specializes in this area). If your symptoms mostly relate to preexisting severe arthritis in a particular joint, such as one or both knees, and your symptoms were worsened by taking an aromatase inhibitor, talk to an orthopedic surgeon who specializes in knees to see if the severity of your joint disease makes you a candidate for joint replacement.

If you get inadequate relief from these measures, talk to your medical oncologist about your hormonal therapy options. These may include:

- Sticking with the current hormonal therapy and increasing pain management measures.
- Taking a one- to two-month treatment break from your current hormonal therapy medication to figure out how much of your symptoms are due to the aromatase inhibitor and how much may be related to other potential causes (for example, long-standing arthritis).
- Restarting the same medication (you might experience fewer symptoms the second time around—possible but unlikely).
- Trying a different aromatase inhibitor. If the same symptoms occur, consider switching to tamoxifen.

Stopping the aromatase inhibitor on your own without working with your doctor is a bad option: you don't want to lose the important benefits of hormonal therapy. Persistence and patience are the keys to a positive solution to this challenging problem.

Bone Pain

Bone pain due to immune cell boosters (such as Neulasta) will resolve as soon as the treatment is finished, but while you are suffering from it, acetaminophen or an NSAID can help ease the discomfort. Immobilization or limited use of a painful area, such as wearing a sling until radiation to a painful shoulder metastasis has been completed, is sometimes helpful.

Pain from breast cancer that has spread to the bone can respond to a range of therapies. An anti-inflammatory agent with or without a narcotic can make a big difference until cancer therapy procedures succeed in controlling the basic cause of the problem. Radiation therapy is the most effective treatment of specific painful bone metastases, providing substantial or complete pain relief in over 85 percent of people for a significant period of time, without the sedation and constipation associated with narcotic pain medication. And a bisphosphonate medication (for example, Zometa) can help reduce bone pain, strengthen the bones, and reduce the risk of new spread to bone.

Hand-Foot Syndrome

There are many critical and practical steps you can take to reduce the severity of redness, soreness, swelling, tingling, or tenderness of your hands and feet beyond the pain medications that have so far been described. Here are some tips that are likely to make a big difference:

Avoid friction and heat
- Avoid exposure to hot water (in the sink, bath, shower, hot tub).
- Use the dishwasher; limit washing anything by hand. (Use thick rubber gloves for anything you hand-wash.)
- Stick to short warm showers or baths.
- Arrange for someone to wash your hair—or treat yourself to a salon.
- Avoid cooking with high heat.
- Use insulated cups with a cardboard cuff for hot take-out beverages.
- Avoid vigorous rubbing when using lotions or creams.
- If you are overheated, place your hands and feet on a thin towel

on top of a cold surface—like a cold pack or a bag of frozen
peas—for fifteen to twenty minutes at a time.

Avoid extra pressure on your hands and feet
- Limit the length of time standing on your feet.
- No running, jogging, aerobics, jumping, power walking, or
  long walks.
- No weight lifting.
- Avoid use of garden, household, or power tools that require a
  tight grip or strong pressure.
- No handstands, downward-facing dog, or plank positions
  during yoga.
- No moderate or heavy lifting.
- Wear soft, comfortable bedroom slippers.
- Wear open-toe shoes (for maximum air circulation) and shoes
  that don't rub; wear socks if it's cold.
- Wear mittens, not gloves, for less friction.

Moisturize your skin
- Gently apply a moisturizer. Try olive oil spray, Aveeno,
  Lubriderm, Moisturel, Eucerin, Aquaphor, Biafene, Udderly
  Smooth, or Bag Balm. (Don't apply these moisturizers to cracked
  areas, however, without your doctor's guidance.)
- Apply strips of Xeroform dressings (gauze laden with ointment)
  or apply Silvadene cream to cracked areas after consultation
  with your doctor.

Seek pain relief
- Over-the-counter medications such as acetaminophen can ease
  the discomfort related to hand-foot syndrome.
- A balanced diet and good rest will make a big difference.
- Some practitioners recommend taking vitamin B_6 (pyridoxine)—
  but talk to your doctor before taking any vitamins during
  chemotherapy because they might interfere with the effectiveness
  of your treatment.
- Your doctor may recommend taking a narcotic, such as Percocet,
  for a short period if you experience severe symptoms.

If the hand-foot syndrome continues and you still require ongoing treatment with Xeloda, your doctor may suggest a reduction in the daily dose of your cancer medication, or possibly a treatment break.

Diarrhea and Gas

Diarrhea and gas resulting from chemotherapy or abdominal-area radiation are managed with a change to a low-residue diet (no fresh fruits or vegetables, limited fiber) and the use of a medication such as Pepto-Bismol, Imodium AD, Lomotil, or Bentyl. Diarrhea following a long course of antibiotics needs to be evaluated first with a stool sample because it may be the result of a *Clostridium difficile* infection that is treated with still another kind of antibiotic (Flagyl).

Constipation Management

Constipation from pain and pain medications will respond to changes in diet, supplements, and medications. To avoid constipation when you're on pain medication:

- Drink lots of liquids.
- Follow a high-roughage diet that includes fresh fruits and vegetables and bran.
- Use daily stool softeners such as Senokot, Colace, or mineral oil.
- Use bulk-formers, such as Metamucil and Citrucel (You must be sure to take in plenty of fluids while using bulk-formers; otherwise, they can jam up and create an even worse problem.)

If despite all these steps, your bowels have slowed to a halt, you'll need to take additional steps to get things rolling again.

- Add one of the following medications to make your bowels move faster: Dulcolax tablets or drops, Milk of Magnesia, Haley's M-O, or your favorite over-the-counter brand. Or use mineral oil, which works as a stool lubricant.
- Then, if there is still no action after one to two more days, ask your doctor about the following bowel stimulants:

Dulcolax suppositories, magnesium citrate (looks like a small bottle of soda), senna extract (X Prep), MiraLAX, or lactulose. A Fleet enema will both stimulate bowel action and lubricate the stool.

• If there is still no action, you should have your caregiver perform a rectal exam to see if the cause of your constipation is impacted stool (hard stool plugging up your rectum). This requires urgent medical attention to loosen and remove the blockage, get your bowels moving again, and help you feel better.

Painful Abdominal Lymph Nodes or Liver Involvement

Abdominal pain due to cancer in enlarged lymph nodes or the liver is typically addressed with anticancer medications (chemotherapy and targeted therapies) along with pain medications.

If despite anticancer medicines abdominal lymph node or liver disease has not budged or has grown, and if the pain remains uncontrolled and progressive, radiation may offer relief. A painful growth in the liver may respond to an internal procedure performed by an interventional radiologist.

Painful Mouth and Swallowing

A combination of diet changes, medications, and common sense is required to treat pain due to mucositis, which is characterized by inflamed and ulcerated linings of the mouth, throat, rectum, and vagina.

Avoid irritating food and drinks (those that are very hot, spicy, acidic [tomato sauce, orange and grapefruit juices]), caffeinated, or very dry. Stick to soft, wet, slippery foods and drinks: cold yogurt with honey or applesauce (try Greek-style yogurt just before meals to coat the passageway and ease discomfort), baby foods, or pastina (tiny pasta balls) in a stew with chicken or vegetable broth.

Medications to ease mouth and throat discomfort include easy-to-swallow or easy-to-use preparations; try over-the-counter NSAIDs in liquid form. Prescription options include Carafate suspension, 2 percent viscous lidocaine mixed half and half with Maalox or Mylanta and swallowed slowly before meals or as needed to numb the mouth and throat, or liquid Tylenol with codeine. Your doctor may also have his or her own favorite throat-numbing "cocktail."

Speak Up, Get Help

It is likely that you will need to speak up and ask for (or even demand) what you need to control your pain. When Richard was visiting his wife in the hospital at night, she was in real pain. The nurse told them, "That's all the doctor has ordered for you." Richard said, "Well, then, find the doctor and have him order more. I'm not leaving my wife's side till she gets more medication. I'm not going to let her suffer all night, and I'll raise hell if necessary." His wife got the medication she needed.

In the Hospital

Reach out for help if you are in significant pain and:

- The nurse says she can't give you more medication (politely request that the nurse page the doctor on call).
- The doctor is tied up or doesn't answer within a half hour (ask to have the doctor paged again, or ask to speak to his/her nurse practitioner).
- You're getting no response from your immediate caregivers (demand to speak to the patient ombudsman or patient relations advocate).

You'll be letting your caregivers know how much you're hurting, and that you're not going to let them put you "on hold." Someone should be able to find a doctor to help you get better pain relief. Make it happen. I can't emphasize this enough: Speak up for yourself. Forget docile. No more "good girl." Don't lie there quietly in pain.

At Home

Reach out if you have new or uncontrolled pain.

- Call your doctor through his or her answering service or through the hospital, and ask to have a prescription called in to a pharmacy that delivers. (Narcotic prescriptions, however, can't be called in; someone has to hand over a written prescription and pick them up.)

- If you can't get anybody and you have new excruciating pain, go to the emergency room.
- If you're enrolled in hospice, call your hospice nurse.

Covering the Cost of Pain Treatment

Prescription Medicines

Cost is an important factor in choosing pain medications. A pill is generally the cheapest form of medication. Most of the medications available today cost approximately the same for equivalent pain relief over a defined period of time. For example, one Kadian tablet is approximately twice the cost of MS Contin, but it lasts twice as long. The cheapest narcotic is methadone, which is also very effective and long lasting, but it's hard to adjust the level up and down for acute or variable discomfort.

Whenever possible, I give my patients samples to try out any new prescription medication before they fill a big, expensive prescription that might not work for them. If samples are not available (narcotic samples are very hard, if not impossible, to get), I suggest they ask their pharmacist to fill only part of the prescription they are going to try—for example, asking for just ten pills of the sixty prescribed. If the pills work, they go back and get the balance.

Your choice of pharmacy can save you money. You can use a mail-order pharmacy, or shop through AARP (the American

FILLING YOUR PRESCRIPTIONS

Call your doctor during the workday, if possible, for pain relief prescriptions, suggestions, complaints, and renewals. Have your pharmacy name and phone number in hand. Note that federal law forbids filling most narcotic prescriptions without a form *in hand*. If you are in severe pain, your pharmacy can dispense a seventy-two-hour supply of narcotics based on a verbal order from your doctor, as long as your doctor gives the pharmacist a written prescription for that seventy-two-hour supply within forty-eight hours. There is more flexibility for people in hospice.

The law also stipulates no refills on narcotics. So every time you run out of medication, you need a new prescription form in hand. At the least, you can ask your doctor or nurse to call in the prescription so it's ready when you show up with the actual prescription slip, saving you some time and frustration.

Association of Retired Persons) if eligible. Buying in bulk can be cheaper, too, but remember, you save money with a bulk order only if you are sure you will use the medications. If you use a mail-order pharmacy or buy your medications through AARP, you may need two prescription forms from your doctor: one to take to your local pharmacist for a small supply to hold you over until the larger order arrives, the other to send away for the larger order. You may be able to expedite your mail order by asking your doctor to fax the prescription to your supplier.

Over-the-Counter Medicine

Ironically, over-the-counter medications (OTC) may end up costing you more money than prescription medicines because they are not usually covered by health insurance plans. To save at least some money, go for the generic or store brands, such as acetaminophen instead of name-brand Tylenol. If your employer offers a tax-advantaged medical flex spending account, using it for OTC drugs can help you cut costs.

Some American Cancer Society chapters will help pay for pain or antinausea medications. Some insurance companies will pay for OTC medications if they are ordered by a doctor's prescription.

Procedures

The cost of specific pain-relieving procedures and therapies—radiation, chemotherapy, anesthesia, and interventional procedures—is generally covered by most health care plans, but you may need to obtain precertification.

If you have already elected the hospice benefit under Medicare, you are usually eligible for palliative treatment *only if* adequate relief is not obtained from pain medication. (The decision to start the hospice benefit requires that you agree to give up definitive treatments; your health insurance resources are then applied to a full range of supportive care services.) Health maintenance and insurance organizations are likely to require a strong letter from your doctor to justify the reason for one of these expensive palliative treatments. Be advised: your hospice business advisers may try vigorously to discourage you from this therapy because the cost of the particular treatment may be subtracted from their fee.

✣ Moving Forward

Successful pain management requires careful attention to other aspects of your physical and emotional health that affect how you experience pain. Are you nauseated? Depressed? Exhausted? Paying attention to and managing these other symptoms can make treatment of your pain much more effective at lower doses, with fewer side effects.

Don't forget: pain medications work only if you take them, if you take the right ones, and if you take enough of them. Above all, you must have your doctor's prescription and individualized recommendations before you try any of the suggestions in this chapter. For more information about pain, you can contact the American Pain Society (847-375-4715 or www.ampainsoc.org/people). Breastcancer.org's online community is also a vital resource.

CHAPTER TEN

Swelling (Lymphedema), Stiffness, and Skin Changes: Prevention and Management

I just finished radiation treatment and my boob is pink, puffy, and painful. I won't let my husband near it! Why didn't anyone tell me this could happen?

I was taking the roast out of the oven and my hand bumped the side wall and gave me a nasty burn. Within hours my hand swelled up like a water balloon. After antibiotics and two tubes of Neosporin, most of it went away—now just the back of my hand is still puffy. I wear a special glove to control the swelling and people just assume I have carpal tunnel problems.

My skin is so dry and rough and itchy. Between the scratching and the flaking, I feel like a dog with fleas.

My armpit is numb and sore and swollen, and hangs over my bra. It's not pretty and I'm so uncomfortable!

I had no trouble with my arm on the side of my surgery, not for ten years. Then I went on a hike in the middle of a hot summer day and between poison ivy and sunburn my arm swelled to double its size. It took three months to go back down. Now I'm worried it will happen again.

✣ First Things First

As doctors, we do our best to inform you of any potential side effects of each treatment. At best that's a good guess or an interpretation of other people's experience relative to yours. Sometimes the person we'd expect to experience persistent side effects escapes them entirely, and the person we'd least expect to have a problem gets hit with the worst-case scenario. Most of the time, the things that spark and aggravate side effects can be identified and understood, improved, or managed.

Your risk of developing significant lingering swelling of the arm, armpit, and breast area sometime in the future ranges from 5 to 35 percent—depending on the status of your breast cancer; the type, amount, and extent of all treatments received (surgery, radiation therapy, chemotherapy); and other medical conditions that may affect your tissue's ability to heal and repair itself.

Other symptoms in the breast, arm, and underarm areas can also occur, including:

- Stiffness
- Discomfort
- Limited range of motion
- Weakness
- Skin changes

LYMPHEDEMA TRIGGERS

New and existing medical conditions, what you do, body positioning, and things you wear can trigger or aggravate swelling and stiffness. Triggers to watch out for are:

- Infection: through a cut in the skin or a torn cuticle, or following a dental procedure (bacteria circulate in the bloodstream and can cause infection in compromised tissue)
- Trauma: injury, burn, bug bite, poison ivy (or other such rash), cut, broken arm, excessive exercise

- Obstruction of free flow of lymph fluid:
  - ~ Wearing tight bras (with or without underwires) that exert extra pressure on your tissues and can trap fluid in the armpit and in the lower part of your breasts
  - ~ Carrying around a heavy handbag over your shoulder (can increase arm swelling)
  - ~ Sleeping on top of your affected arm or on your stomach (prevents drainage of fluid out of the affected areas)
- Running a marathon, walking an extended distance with your arm in the downward position and swinging like a pendulum (backed-up lymph fluid is forced down your arm)
- Too high a temperature in a hot tub or too long a time in a hot tub
- Long flights, with the changes in air pressure
- Being very overweight or gaining a lot of weight
- Blood circulation compromised by smoking, diabetes, heart failure
- New diagnosis of connective tissue disease involving difficulty with healing
- Extensive breast cancer in the lymph nodes, unrelated to treatment
- Blood clot in the axillary (underarm) vein

Having one or more risk factors doesn't mean that swelling and stiffness will inevitably happen. Conversely, some people develop lymphedema without even one risk factor.

Some of these risks can be almost eliminated, and others can be modified or improved. For example, you can avoid a hot tub, use an oven mitt, and make sure your diabetes is under control. In the "Solutions" section, I'll show you how many day-to-day adjustments can lower your risks.

The major focus of this chapter is the swelling and stiffness of the arm, armpit, and sometimes the breast area, called lymphedema (*edema* means "swelling"). Lymphedema results from backed-up lymph fluid caused by disruption and scarring of the fluid drainage pathways called lymphatics.

Extent and Duration of Lymphedema

Lymphedema can affect all or part of the arm and/or breast—such as the hand, the wrist, the area below the elbow, or the upper arm. The whole breast area may be involved, or just the area around the surgery or the very bottom of the breast. Occasionally the swelling is confined to the armpit.

Most cases of lymphedema are barely noticeable and are neither disabling nor unduly uncomfortable; however, others are much more severe. Although episodes of lymphedema may be transient, once an episode occurs, the condition tends to persist or recur, and to vary in degree. The episode may resolve spontaneously, or it may resolve only if treated quickly. Episodes may last for days or weeks. Some women experience symptoms for the first time years after treatment is over.

If you've ever had a bout of swelling, you're at higher risk of having another episode. If your edema lasts for months, it's likely to be permanent, but even the most severe cases can be substantially improved with ongoing treatment.

The longer you are free of lymphedema, the greater your chance of

SCAR TISSUE AND SIDE EFFECTS

Scar tissue is the way your body repairs itself—a stiff type of healing tissue like a combination of spackle, grout, and industrial glue. Normal scarring holds the tissues together without limiting function. A large amount of scar tissue—because a large area needed to be filled in or excess scar tissue resulted from a problem with the body's healing and repair mechanisms—can lead to stiffness, reduced range of motion, weakness, and discomfort. Scar tissue, in other words, is rarely a perfect replacement for what's been removed.

Only certain types of cells in the breast and lymph node regions have the capacity to regenerate. For example, your body can make brand-new blood cells and vessels to nourish your healing tissues, but it cannot make new lymph nodes, breast tissue, or muscle out of scar tissue. Some functions can never be completely recovered.

Even as your tissues are healing and regenerating (completely or partially), you must manage, adjust, and adapt to the new ways your body now works and feels. You have to develop patience, and deal with the frustration you experience when debilitating side effects keep you from living your life as you'd hoped and expected.

avoiding it altogether, because your body has probably learned how to reroute any excess buildup of lymphatic fluid. On the other hand, the more lymphedema you have and the longer you have it, the harder it is to reduce your arm back to its original size.

ꙮ Challenges

You might think of lymphedema of the arm and breast area as a plumbing problem. All fluids in your body must circulate: the fluid that comes into a part of your body eventually has to flow out of that body part; otherwise it would overfill with fluid and create serious problems.

Blood travels from your heart to your arm, armpit, and breast areas within arteries and capillaries (the small blood vessels that connect arteries to veins). As the blood percolates through the capillaries, oxygen, nutrients, and a clear, colorless fluid called lymphatic fluid (aka lymph) pass through the capillary walls into the tissues of your arm. Veins carry the used, nutrient-emptied blood back to the heart and lungs, and another type of vessel, thin-walled lymphatic channels, carries excess lymphatic fluid (rich with protein and waste products) from the tissues back into circulation. The protein in lymphatic fluid helps hold on to water. As long as the protein is moving inside the lymphatic channels, the fluid will stay in the channels and leave the area.

Lymphatic fluid is propelled up your arm and across your chest by contractions in your muscles and the walls of the lymphatic channels; valves within these lymph vessels keep fluid moving in a forward direction. The lymphatic channels pass through bean-shaped structures called *lymph nodes* (located in the arm, neck, groin, and other regions), which filter out bacteria, cellular debris, and toxic substances from the lymphatic fluid. The trapped debris is broken down and discarded.

Removal of lymph nodes and associated scar tissue formation can disrupt or block the flow of lymphatic fluid. The overflow of fluid then seeps into the tissue. If the protein stays in the tissues or in backed-up lymphatic channels, water builds up in the area. Lymphedema is the result.

SENTINEL NODE REMOVAL LESSENS LYMPHEDEMA RISK

Limited underarm lymph node removal, guided by the sentinel lymph node tracer technique, is associated with a lower risk of lymphedema than a full axillary lymph node removal procedure.

Sentinel node tracer detection technique identifies the main lymph node that can indicate whether cancer cells have spread from beyond the breast. To do this, dye is injected into the region of the tumor, and the first lymph node(s) it drains to—the "main" lymph node—is identified and removed. If the main lymph node (or nodes) is clear of cancer cells, removal of more lymph nodes is usually unnecessary. With most lymph nodes still in place, lymphedema is unlikely to occur. However, if cancer cells are detected in the main lymph node, the regular lymph node removal procedure usually follows.

The sentinel lymph node removal technique removes about one to three lymph nodes, in contrast to about fifteen nodes removed with regular lymph node removal procedures. The lymph nodes that are left behind take over the work of the removed nodes. The armpit has a variable number of lymph nodes: some women have only five; others have more than forty. This variation can also affect your risk for lymphedema.

Breast Cancer Can Cause Lymphedema, Stiffness, and Discomfort

Breast cancer itself is an uncommon cause of arm lymphedema. It can occur when the cancer affects many underarm lymph nodes. In such a case the cancer cells clog up the lymph node filters, and the lymph fluid gets backed up, causing uncomfortable swelling in the area.

Breast cancer cells can also clog up the lymphatic channels inside the breast, blocking free flow of lymph drainage out of the breast. The result: the breast enlarges and stiffens, and the skin turns red. This is called inflammatory breast cancer. Breast cancer cells can also form a rash or nodules under the skin, making part of the breast swollen and firm.

Breast Cancer Treatment Increases the Risk of Lymphedema

As long as the amount of fluid coming into the tissues is the same as the amount leaving the tissues, everything is fine—no edema. But when the flow of fluid in these channels gets disrupted with the removal of the lymph nodes, the fluid must be diverted to other channels.

The remaining lymphatic channels can generally handle this extra re-routed fluid in addition to their regular workload.

But without adequate drainage, the lymphatic fluid can back up and accumulate in the spaces between the cells of the soft tissues of your arm, armpit, and breast area—skin, fat, muscle, nerves, blood and lymphatic vessels, and connective tissue—resulting in lymphedema in the arm, armpit, or breast area. The lymphatic drainage system can also be significantly compromised when operating at its maximum capacity: it gets pushed past its limit when infection, sunburn, bug bite, poison ivy, or something else causes extra fluid to collect in the arm or breast area tissues.

Arm and Armpit Edema

Treatments for breast cancer that may increase the risk of lymphedema, stiffness, and discomfort of the arm and armpit include:

- Lymph node dissection (with mastectomy or lumpectomy)
- Radiation
- Chemotherapy

The risk of lymphedema depends on the number of fluid drainage channels working after all your treatment is over. The more lymph nodes are removed, the higher your risk (since lymph nodes serve as filters on the lymphatic channels, and each time a node is removed, fluid drainage can be disrupted). Radiation to

ARM LYMPHEDEMA: NOTICEABLE AND UNCOMFORTABLE

A swollen arm after breast cancer can affect how you feel and function. You may find it:

- Leaves your arm looking swollen and unattractive
- Alters your self-image
- Interferes with your routine activities and what clothes you can wear
- Serves as a troubling reminder of the disease you've tried to put behind you
- Makes your arm feel heavy, with less sensation, particularly in hot weather
- Can be very painful
- Can make you feel hot
- May require continuous medical care, expense, and inconveniences
- Can cause thickening of the skin, stiffness and hardness of the arm, and leakage of fluid from minor injuries

the lymph nodes can increase scar tissue that impedes fluid drainage of the arm, whereas radiation to the breast area doesn't significantly increase this risk. The breast area treatments, however (partial or full mastectomy with or without reconstruction and radiation), can increase the risk of swelling in the armpit and breast area. The more chemotherapy you have had, the harder it is for your body to completely heal itself. Some types and doses of chemo affect healing more than others.

Breast Area Swelling

You might develop swelling, fullness, and stiffness of the breast area after any type of breast treatment or procedure, with or without:

- Partial or complete mastectomy
- Lymph node removal
- Chemotherapy
- Radiation
- Reconstruction

The amount of swelling you get tends to increase with added amounts and types of treatments. Extra pressure on soft tissues can block free drainage of fluid, leading to a buildup. A breast expander and implant can put extra pressure on your chest wall; the scar tissue capsule around the implant can harden the tissues even more, restricting fluid drainage.

Severe Breast Lymphedema and Scarring

Rarely, a woman may experience a severe reaction to breast radiation or be left with extensive scar tissue after a large infection that leaves behind a hard, red, painful, shrunken breast that doesn't get better—and may get worse. Your doctor might describe this excessive scarring as "fibrosis." This problem is most likely to happen to someone who has a known or not-yet-diagnosed connective tissue disease (such as lupus) in which the immune system attacks the soft tissues of the body (skin, muscles, cartilage, sheaths, ligaments, etc.), and there's a limited ability to repair tissue damage (caused by the immune system, radiation, infection, or another kind of insult).

If you have had severe shrinkage and scarring of just the breast for a year or more as a complication of radiation or a past infection, and it's been unresponsive to conservative measures such as antibiotics, steroids, or hyperbaric (high-pressure oxygen) treatments, you may be a candidate for removal of the affected tissues by full mastectomy (no skin sparing is possible), followed by tissue reconstruction (to cover just the removed area or to rebuild a breast). See Chapter 6, "After Mastectomy." Only a highly skilled plastic surgeon who specializes in breast reconstruction should be considered to do this kind of surgery for you.

Other Breast Area Changes

Redness

Mild to moderate redness (brisk redness) is a common side effect of radiation to the breast. Brisk redness from radiation is most likely to result if your radiation was designed to give a full dose to the skin of the whole breast area (for example, after mastectomy) or if a small area of the skin gets a relatively high dose (for example, within a skin fold or from concentrated partial breast radiation).

These tissues often get bright red within the first few weeks after radiation is over, sometimes peeling (like after a sunburn) or forming a blister. If chemotherapy is given around the same time, the reaction may be more pronounced.

After brisk redness resolves over the next few weeks following treatment, the skin may go back to its normal color. Or there may be a mixture of pink and pale color changes, tanness, and occasionally telengiectasias (thin squiggly tiny red lines that look like spider legs). In addition, any freckles or moles that may have been in the radiation treatment area might turn darker by end of treatment and stay dark for a long time. Usually they eventually peel off or lighten up.

The most common reason for new or recurrent skin redness of the breast is infection, which requires your doctor's immediate evaluation and antibiotic treatment (such as Keflex or Cipro). Other causes include:

• Certain chemotherapies given following breast area radiation
  that can reactivate redness—called "radiation recall"

SKIN WHISKERS: SUTURE ENDS

A few weeks after any kind of surgery, you may notice little suture (i.e., thread) ends sticking out of your incision like a whisker. The suture may have been there since surgery—but hasn't fallen off yet. Or, the suture may have been on the inside and now your body is trying to eject it. It's safe for sutures to stay inside you, but when they're sticking out they can irritate the skin and increase the risk of infection. If there's no redness or pus around suture whiskers, you have nothing to worry about; the suture ends will usually work themselves out. But you should call your doctor if there is any sign of infection (pinkness, tenderness, swelling, warmth around the "whisker") or if it's uncomfortable or annoying.

- Psoriasis, activated by the irritation of radiation or other treatments, usually in a woman who already has a history of psoriasis
- Reactivation or new diagnosis of a connective tissue disease associated with healing problems
- Cancer recurrence

Dry Skin

Lingering skin dryness is common, particularly in the winter months when the air is dry. Dryness should respond nicely to moisturizers; try something natural and pure, without fragrance, such as cocoa butter or olive oil.

Remember that irradiated skin is more sensitive to sunburn, even if your treatment is years past. Protect your skin from the sun with a lotion of SPF 30 or higher, reapplied frequently, as well as full cover-up. (A T-shirt alone is inadequate protection, having an SPF of only 8.)

Breast and Skin Surprises: Stiffness and Thickening

Scar tissue stiffens healed areas. Swelling fills up your tissues, causing firmness, pressure, heaviness, and a pulling sensation. Your skin may also feel thick or leathery.

These breast texture changes may resolve relatively quickly or may take years—two to three years is not uncommon. As the breast area softens up, don't be surprised to feel a new area of firm tissue where the prior surgery was performed; it's been there the whole time, but it was "buried" within the general swelling and firmness that linger after surgery and/or radiation. This buried area may continue to soften and become less tender over time.

The muscles behind the breast can feel stiff, particularly when you work them repetitively and hard—such as after vacuuming a big room, scraping burned food off a pan, or playing tennis for the first time in a long time. I've had a number of patients page me, scared to death, about a breast lump they felt in the back of their breast after restarting rigorous upper-body exercise. Each of these lumps turned out to be a small bruise in the muscle from the strain of heavy exercise.

You may feel stiffness in your rib cage when taking deep breaths while exercising. You'll feel it more when you reach, stretch, or sleep on your chest (there is less give in the skin, and the breast may no longer be there to cushion your chest wall).

Altered Sensations

Nerves regrow very slowly; that's why it takes a number of months, possibly six, before sensation starts to return. As the nerves regrow, you may get all sorts of odd sensations in the area—shooting, sharp, dull, hot poker, aching, itchy, crawling—as well as heightened sensitivity to touch, heat, and pressure. Even after the nerves heal and settle down, they always hold a grudge. Thus, any of these funky feelings can come back and surprise you. They are nothing to worry about, but can be an unpleasant reminder of your breast cancer experience. (For more on pain and discomfort, see Chapter 9.)

❧ Solutions

Prevention is the best strategy against lymphedema, stiffness, and discomfort of the arm, armpit, and breast areas. If you already have or have had arm or significant breast edema, you are at higher risk for a return of this condition in the future, but you can substantially reduce this risk by being attentive and taking special care of yourself.

WINGED-OUT: SHOULDER BLADE

Occasionally during lymph node removal, a minor nerve that keeps your shoulder blade in position in your back is damaged. If this happens, you may notice that your shoulder blade sticks out slightly with certain movements of your arm. This nerve may not regenerate, but the altered shoulder blade position is unlikely to result in any disability of motion or function. It may look a little funny, but chances are you're the only one who notices.

It's important to avoid any strenuous activity that can strain or injure your muscles—like lifting heavy children and moving furniture or heavy boxes. Repetitive, resistance-oriented movement in the at-risk arm, like weight lifting, should only be done with expert guidance and with very gradual increase in weights and level of resistance. Wearing a custom-fitted elastic sleeve on the at-risk arm while weight lifting may be recommended for women without lymphedema, and it is critical to use for women with lymphedema.

Skin Care: First Line of Defense

The skin acts as a barrier to infection, so any break in this barrier can spell trouble. Burns, chafing, dryness, cuticle injury (such as hangnails), cracks, cuts, splinters, and insect bites are immediate risks for infection.

Here are two long lists of important dos and don'ts to incorporate into your lifestyle:

Your do list
- Do moisturize your skin frequently and regularly, with fragrance-free lotions such as Aveeno, Moisturel, Eucerin, Vaseline Intensive Care, cocoa butter, Aquaphor, or your own favorite brand, to make your skin supple and prevent cracking. (For green products, go to www.ewg.org and search under "Consumer Goods.")
- Do keep your hands and arms extra clean, but don't use harsh soaps such as Ivory (despite Ivory's advertised image as a gentle soap), Irish Spring, or Dial. Use Dove instead.
- Do use rubber gloves when you hand-wash dishes or clothes.
- Do wear protective gloves when you garden or do outside chores.
- Do wear oven mitts when handling hot foods.
- Do use an electric razor instead of a safety razor.
- Do use insect repellents that won't dry out the skin, such as Avon's Skin So Soft, which includes a moisturizer. Avoid brands that contain a significant amount of alcohol. (Any ingredient that ends in *-ol* is a type of alcohol.)
- Do apply antibiotic ointment to any insect bites or torn cuticles (as long as you are not allergic to its contents).

- Do protect your arm from sunburn with sunscreen, minimum SPF 15; SPF 30 is preferable.
- Do use a thimble when you sew.
- Do rest your arm on a soft surface in an elevated position whenever possible (get in the habit).
- Do control your blood sugars very carefully if you have diabetes, to minimize the danger of small blood vessel damage and infection.
- Do wear compression bandages on the affected arm when flying in airplanes if you've already had arm edema.

Your don't list
- Don't smoke; smoking constricts the small blood vessels, adversely affecting the flow of fluids in the arm.
- Don't take unusually hot baths or showers.
- Don't go from extreme hot to cold water temperatures when you bathe or wash dishes.
- Don't go into high-heat hot tubs, saunas, or steam baths.
- Don't carry heavy objects with your at-risk arm, especially with the arm hanging downward.
- Don't carry heavy shoulder bags on the affected side.
- Don't wear clothing that has tight sleeves or that restrains movement.
- Don't wear your watch or other jewelry on your affected hand or arm.
- Don't use a heavy breast prosthesis after mastectomy. (It may put excessive pressure on alternative routes of lymphatic drainage that are already doing double duty; find a lightweight model or make one yourself.)
- Don't consume large amounts of salt because it makes your body accumulate excess water.
- Don't drink much alcohol. Alcohol causes blood vessels to dilate and leak extra fluid into the tissues.
- Don't get manicures that cut or overstress the skin around the nails. A manicure that is done in a safe manner, protecting the skin's integrity, is okay.
- Don't permit blood pressure testing on your at-risk arm.

- Don't get tattoos on the at-risk arm or breast area.
- Don't permit any piercing of the skin for injections, blood draws, vaccinations, or acupuncture on the at-risk arm or breast area. (Don't trust anyone, not even your personal physician, to remember which is your at-risk arm.) If you have had breast cancer in both breasts, blood should be drawn from your nondominant arm. In an emergency (e.g., a car accident), if an IV needs to be started, let them do what they need to do to establish an intravenous line as soon as possible.

TAKE ACTION RIGHT AWAY

With or without existing swelling in your arm or breast area, it is urgent that you take care of any burns, cuts, rashes, or new signs of infection.

- **Infection management**
  - ~ Start antibiotics under the direction of your physician.
  - ~ Call your doctor's office during the day, or page your doctor at night or on the weekend through the office or hospital operator to get the evaluation and treatment you need.
  - ~ Have at hand the phone number of a pharmacy that is sure to be open when you ask your doctor to call in the prescription.
  - ~ Be sure to let your doctor know if you have any allergies to antibiotics. (Don't depend on your doctor's memory of your history.)

Immediate Treatment Required: New Swelling, Infection, Burns, Cuts, Rashes

It's important for you to be alert for any signs or symptoms of infection in your hand, arm, shoulder, and breast area, such as:

- Fever
- Redness
- Swelling
- Warmth
- Tenderness

Infection, redness, warmth, and tenderness in the area can escalate quickly, moving up or down the arm or beyond the breast area. Call your doctor as soon as you suspect any trouble. You should be seen in the office right away—a phone evaluation is not sufficient. Immediate use of antibiotics is usually required. If

you have arm edema and a significant infection, intravenous antibiotics and admission to the hospital
may be necessary.

Even in the absence of any
clear signs of infection, you may
still need to start antibiotics if you:

- Already have edema or
  diabetes (with or without
  edema present) and you've
  just experienced an injury to
  the swollen area
- Just developed new onset
  of edema

- **Burn**
  - ~ Cover burns with Silvadene
    cream and a clean nonadher-
    ent dressing.
  - ~ Periodically cleanse the area
    and reapply the cream and
    bandage.
- **Cuts**
  - ~ Keep any cuts or abrasions
    clean: wash the area two to
    three times a day with a solu-
    tion that's half peroxide and
    half water.
  - ~ Apply antibiotic ointment and
    bandage.

Under these circumstances, your doctor may start antibiotics right
away (such as penicillin, Keflex, or Cipro), because infection is one of
the only completely reversible causes of arm edema, and side effects of
a short-term course of oral antibiotics are usually minimal. Not every
insult requires oral antibiotics, however: for example, a tiny cut on your
finger with only a little swelling might be treatable just by soaking your
hand in warm (not hot) water several times a day, followed by the application of topical antibiotics.

Proper treatment also requires careful reevaluation to make sure
that the treatment is working and that the infection has gone away completely. Do not stop antibiotics early when you see the signs and symptoms go away. The full course of antibiotics, ten to fourteen days or
longer, is always required.

Without prompt and complete treatment, swelling can start or
progress and eventually become intermittent, persistent, or progressive.

Managing Ongoing Swelling, Stiffness, and Discomfort

All therapies for chronic edema require a commitment to a modified
lifestyle. Nonurgent care for edema takes many forms.

You can usually control lymphedema, stiffness, and discomfort and improve your strength and flexibility with expert care coordinated by your health care team. Basic management and prevention guidelines must be the bottom line of your lifestyle.

Seek Expert Care

The health care professionals who specialize in the management of arm edema problems are physical medicine doctors (physiatrists), physical therapists, occupational therapists, and exercise specialists. But don't assume that anyone in these specialties is automatically an expert in the management of breast and arm lymphedema, stiffness, and related issues. Ask about experience and references before you let *anyone* work on your edema problem.

Most metropolitan areas have physical and occupational therapists whose practice is dedicated to managing the physical side effects of breast cancer treatment. If you can't find a therapist with this expertise and experience, look for a general physical therapist or physical medicine doctor in a rehabilitation center or department who has experience taking care of women with breast cancer. The National Lymphedema Network (NLN) has lists of specialists all over the world on its website at www.lymphnet.org. The NLN can also be reached at 800-541-3259 or 510-208-3200.

Put Gravity to Work

If you are experiencing any degree of arm lymphedema, you'll want to take steps to ease the drainage of lymph fluid from the affected arm back into circulation.

TRACKING YOUR PROGRESS

Your physical therapist, physician, and nurse can follow your progress through various treatments by regularly documenting the swelling of your arm and comparing it with your unaffected arm. There are two main ways to measure arm lymphedema: circumference and volume.

- The circumference of both arms is usually measured at three points: at the wrist and 10 cm above and below the inside elbow crease.
- The volume of your arm is assessed by placing each arm into a water chamber. The amount of water your arm displaces equals the volume of your arm.

These readings are recorded in your chart and tracked over time.

- Keep your hand and elbow higher than your heart (and ideally higher than your shoulder), maybe with a decorated crutch as an armrest. (But don't bear weight on it.)
- Get into the habit of keeping your arm in an elevated position whenever possible. If you rest it on a hard piece of furniture, such as the back of a chair, keep a pad under your elbow, or whatever part of your arm that rests on the furniture.
- Don't put pressure or tension on the arm or armpit area.
- Don't hold your arm up without support for very long, since this will strain your arm muscles and can cause additional swelling.

Compression Sleeves and Wrapped Bandages

Compression sleeves—elasticized sleeves custom-fitted to your arm—are a long-standing therapy device. They can be used on their own or in conjunction with manual lymphatic drainage or mechanical drainage.

When using a compression sleeve, all stitching and seams should be parallel to the length of your arm; the pressure of the sleeve (or bandages) should be a little tighter at the bottom without digging into your wrist or hand, and then gradually a little less tight as it approaches the shoulder. This helps keep a degree of pressure in the upward direction, to help propel the fluid back into circulation. To prevent the sleeve from rolling down—which diminishes its effectiveness—apply a water-soluble adhesive lotion under the top of the sleeve. (Soap and water removes the adhesive when you want to take off the sleeve.)

Buy two sleeves and alternate their use, washing them in lukewarm water every two to three days (dry flat, don't wring); they'll last much longer if you have two and treat them with care. Since most sleeves stretch over time, you may need to replace them about every six months. (Get a prescription from your doctor to help cover the cost through your insurance plan, though you may have to battle for this payment.)

An appealing solution to the sleeve issue was devised by Rachel Troxell and Robin Miller, who formed a company called LympheDIVAs that sells attractive patterned sleeves, softer and moisture wicking, to make the best of this uncomfortable condition. Call 866-411-DIVA or visit www.lymphedivas.com. Prices run under $100.

A roll of specialized elastic material (*not* an Ace-type bandage), along with padding material, is an alternative to the sleeve and is relatively easily modified to your needs. It should be applied first by a trained therapist, who can then show you how to apply it yourself. Be careful to apply it with the right pressure gradient and without too many underlaps and overlaps, or you will get little puffy areas of extra fluid from insufficient pressure next to areas of indentation from excessive pressure.

Sleeves and bandages each have pros and cons. Both are hard to apply since you only have one hand and arm to work with. The sleeves tend to be a bit easier to apply with even pressure, and you can use them comfortably during your daily activities. But they cost more than bandages, and they generally provide only enough support to keep swelling from getting worse, not enough to reduce it. And if you have excessive swelling for whatever reason, the custom sleeve may be too small for you. Bandages are more adaptable, but they are bulkier and more cumbersome, and take longer to apply.

Light exercise combined with a custom-fit compression bandage (use an old one for swimming) is a very effective way to pump lymphatic fluid back into circulation. The force of the contracting muscles against the firm binding of the bandages helps drain the lymph. (For this approach to work best, the bandage needs to be applied correctly, as described later.)

Safe Exercise

Part of deciding what activities you can safely pursue depends on how much the sport means to you, along with how it affects your arm. I encourage my patients to be active, but also to be cautious. There is no one-size-fits-all recommendation for all women. Any advice should be customized to your needs. And check with your doctor before undertaking any exercise program.

It's very important to seek the expert care and guidance of a physical therapist working with your doctor who can chart your progress and get you safely moving and grooving with a program tailored to your needs and ability. Throughout your workout program, your team can monitor your arm lymphedema status. If your edema worsens, the use of weights should be immediately discontinued and your situation reevaluated. Be careful before blaming it on the weights. The increase in edema could also happen because you've stopped doing something that was helping to control it (like manual lymphatic drainage). Or maybe you did something to increase your edema, such as tanning.

SWIMMING. The safest and, in my opinion, best exercise for arm and breast area lymphedema is swimming: dog paddle, breast stroke, crawl, side stroke, back stroke, and water aerobics. Swimming, like walking, keeps the circulation of body fluids at maximum efficiency. Plus the deep lung action that goes along with vigorous exercise is believed to create a suction effect, encouraging the return of lymph fluid to the heart and promoting lymph flow. (But before getting wet, be sure to moisturize your skin to protect it from the drying effects of chlorine or salt water.)

WALKING. Walking with elbows bent, fingers pointed to the sky, and arms up in front of you (at the level of the shoulder and above), swinging with the rhythm of your walk, is the best positioning to facilitate drainage of lymph flow. You can get tired of this very quickly, however (that's when you really figure out how much your arms weigh and how weak and out of shape you might be—argh). Limit the time your arms are swinging down by your sides, as this pushes fluid into your hands.

SAFE PHYSICAL ACTIVITY

Here are the safest forms of physical activity to consider:

- **Swimming** combines muscle action on the inside with water pressure on the outside.
- **Walking** is probably the most convenient, least expensive form of exercise that involves little to no instruction (see arm positioning suggestions below).
- **Yoga** involves gentle, gradual, and symmetrical use of your body to increase balance, range of motion, strength, and relaxation.
- **Gradual strengthening** utilizes repetitive exercises of all muscle groups using light weights.
- **Arm stretches** increase flow in the lymphatic channels and help you maintain a wide range of motion.

Activities such as tennis, golf, bowling (using different types of equipment) can be done in moderation for women with slight to mild lymphedema, but it's best to ask your doctor or physical therapist whether it's okay for your particular situation. Some people do get into trouble when they engage in these sports.

YOGA. Gentle yoga movement can be a positive form of therapy for swelling, stiffness, discomfort, and range-of-motion issues. It teaches body awareness and posture combined with both energetic and restful breathing techniques. This can help you minimize any "guarding" (when you alter your body position to protect a tender area by rounding your shoulders), which adds to muscle and joint strain.

Gradual and *gentle* are the critical words to guide you. Be careful not to stress or put too much weight on your arms, shoulders, or chest muscles. Make sure you're ready before assuming positions like downward-facing dog and plank. No hand or shoulder stands or other fancy inversions.

Yoga is a noncompetitive way to improve your inner and outer strength: exercise with spiritual overtones, working within your own personal limits. Over time you can expect more from your body, protecting your affected limb as you go. Choose a class with an experienced yoga instructor who can help you figure out the safest way to work around or compensate for a problem area.

Gradual Strengthening and Arm Stretches

The use of weights to build up muscle is controversial in people who have lymphedema of the arm and breast areas. While everyone agrees that you want to enhance your body's natural lymph fluid pumping machinery—your muscles—you don't want to do anything to strain or injure your muscles because it will increase blood flow to the injured area and worsen the lymph fluid backup.

The most important thing is for you to use your arm, shoulder, and chest muscles in a safe and effective manner, with expert guidance, to slowly build up your strength, range of motion, flexibility, and overall conditioning. Everything in gentle moderation!

Start by moving just the weight of your arm—which is considerable when you figure that the average weight of an arm is 5 to 6 percent of your body weight. For example, if you weigh 150 pounds, your arm would weigh about 7 to 8 pounds, and it can weigh a lot more if it has lymphedema. Range-of-motion, mild stretching, and gentle strengthening exercises for your arm are best: moving your arms from by your side to above your head, and from back to front, while sitting or standing. The longer you can have your arms above the height of your shoulders, the better, as this allows for gravity to pull the fluid down your arm and back into circulation. (You will quickly see how heavy your arm is when you do these exercises.) If you already have lymphedema, while exercising, wear a custom sleeve or wrap your arm with a specialized bandage, prescribed by a physical therapist.

A great resource for these arm stretches is the book *Stretching* by Bob Anderson. Yoga arm and shoulder flow movements are excellent (but again, get clearance from doctor before doing positions like downward-facing dog or plank). Go to a gentle yoga class, visit online sites such as Yogabasics.com and ABC-of-yoga.com, or borrow or purchase a DVD or tape at your local library or Gaiam.com.

If you're working with weights, increase the amount of weights you're using in a gradual manner, beginning with a light weight. More repetitions with a low weight are better than fewer reps with a higher weight. Feeling strain is a signal to stop immediately.

Manual Lymphatic Drainage

Manual lymphatic drainage, also known as complex decongestive physiotherapy, consists of hands-on stimulation of all the soft tissues of the arm and shoulder, as well as the breast area tissues if they are affected by swelling and stiffness. More traditional massage concentrates mainly on muscle and can be quite vigorous. If that kind of massage makes you sore, it could potentially worsen lymphedema rather than making it better.

With manual lymphatic drainage, a professional therapist gently stimulates the affected arm, starting at your hand, using delicate rhythmic movements of her fingers on the surface of your skin, moving the skin slowly with a pumping motion directed toward your shoulder. This technique requires specific training and certification.

At the end of every session, the therapist applies a customized bandage or sleeve, which provides light compression of the arm without restricting the flow of lymph in order to minimize reaccumulation of fluid. You'll be prescribed exercises to perform with the bandage in place and given instructions on how to apply the bandage yourself (this can be tricky and requires practice to get it right). Arm elevation is also recommended.

Manual lymphatic drainage is usually one session a day, three to five days a week, for about three to nine weeks, depending on your situation. Sessions take about an hour to an hour and a half. Find out about the cost and coverage up front; the procedure can be expensive and may not be part of your medical insurance plan. The success of manual drainage is closely tied to the skill and enthusiasm of the therapist.

Air-Driven Pumps

Air-driven or pneumatic pumps can be a very effective treatment for lymphedema. Your arm is placed into a full-length plastic sleeve that fills with air, compressing your tissues, thereby moving the backed-up fluids out of the swollen arm into channels of normal lymph flow.

An effective pump must have two features. One is *gradient pressure,* meaning the pump exerts stronger pressure on the hand area than it does on the upper arm, to propel fluid in the proper, upward direction. (Less useful pumps exert equal pressure over the whole arm.) The second necessary feature is *sequential pressure.* The pump should exert pressure that moves from the hand up the arm with a sort of "milking" technique.

This treatment requires about a two-hour commitment each day to obtain temporary though significant relief. The therapy is done in your home while you are reading or watching TV, but it must be intermittently supervised by a qualified professional. When it works, it can work great and be a very sustainable long-term management solution, particularly if you have ongoing swelling and you can't continue—for practical or financial reasons—to get manual lymphatic drainage at a center several days a week, week after week, month after month.

Before buying or renting a pump to use at home, make sure this technique works for you. Start off with the pump in the physical or occupational therapist's office. If you make good progress, ask your therapist where to get a pump for home use. Good pumps are expensive to buy ($5,000 to $6,000), but most medical insurance plans cover part if not all of the cost. They can also be rented from some surgical supply stores. There has been a sudden surge of medical practices and independent companies promoting the pump; some of these companies lack trained physical therapists to supervise an individual's care. Watch out. Buy or rent a pump only from a rehabilitation center or through the recommendation of your physical therapist.

Weight Loss and Diet

Weight gain is common with chemotherapy, hormonal therapy, and the inactivity that tends to accompany treatment, compounding your arm edema problem. Losing weight can really help you reduce edema.

But weight loss is so hard to achieve (see Chapter 18). One suggestion that can help, especially with edema issues, is to restrict your salt and sugar intake. (Read the labels of any canned or prepared food you plan to eat, to avoid consumption of excess salt.) This will reduce the amount of fluid your body retains, thus helping you control your weight as well as reducing the fluid buildup in your arm. Another suggestion is to restrict the amount of protein you consume: high protein density in your tissues attracts more fluid to the area. See Chapter 17 for more on eating a balanced diet.

Diuretics

Diuretics or "water pills" are a type of medication that removes excess water from your whole body, including your arm, shoulder, armpit, and breast area. They may be able to ease your discomfort and reduce the swelling, but they do not eliminate these problems, and the relief is temporary. That's because the protein remains in the tissues, drawing fluid back to cause the arm to swell up once again.

Diuretics require a physician's supervision; regular blood tests must be taken to make sure your blood chemistry is not out of whack as a result of taking them. I tell my patients to avoid the use of diuretics unless no other therapy has worked for them, or they have a general underlying medical condition that warrants fluid restriction and the use of diuretics anyway (such as high blood pressure, congestive heart

WARNING!

Do *not* use unproven "medicines" or surgical procedures to treat lymphedema. In fact, they can make lymphedema and your overall health *much* worse.

One example is a group of medicines called benzopyrones. Coumarin is the most commonly used benzopyrone (not to be confused with Coumadin, the blood thinner). Its promoters claim that it removes proteins and the extra fluid that holds on to them. But be aware:

- Benzopyrones are unproven by clinical trials.
- They're not approved by the Food and Drug Administration (FDA).
- They're capable of causing liver damage.

Surgery is another example. Some claim it can create new avenues through which the fluid backup can escape from the arm, either by bypassing or opening up blocked channels or by bringing new tissue into the area. It's promoted as a last resort for cases of lymphedema that do not respond to the less invasive, less aggressive techniques described above. But be warned:

- It's unproven as a treatment for lymphedema.
- Surgery can cause problems with healing.
- It can seriously worsen your condition.

There are very few tissue reconstruction plastic and blood vessel surgeons who have the ability to perform surgery with a significant chance of benefits—and with an acceptable risk of complications.

When you're dealing with significant lymphedema that won't go away, these treatment claims can grab your interest and give you false hope—but they end up making matters worse. Be extremely careful.

failure, or general edema). Before trying diuretics, it's best to first try salt restriction in your diet, since salt makes your body hold on to water.

✣ Moving Forward

Managing lingering lymphedema and stiffness involves a lot of work, dedication, inconvenience, and expense. You can expect both real progress and frustrating setbacks. Over time, your goal is to take individual steps that will eventually become healthy habits that get integrated into the routine of your daily life. This is a long-term investment in the quality of your life—an insurance policy to keep you active, fully functioning, and feeling good about yourself.

CHAPTER ELEVEN

Hair Loss and Nail Changes: Terrible but Temporary

Nothing was as bad as losing my hair. My best friend called me when I was feeling so blue about it and told me, "We're going out to get you a wig." "I can't—it's a really bad day for me," I said. "Look, getting a wig is one of the worst things you can do—so why screw up a good day? I'm coming over, and we'll screw up the rest of a bad day!"

My fancy human hair wig is back in its box, where it will stay—too hot, tight, and scratchy. A silk scarf with bangs and a ponytail works so much better for me.

Within four weeks, I lost the best part of my figure—my breasts— and all my hair, including eyebrows and eyelashes. I was at my lowest. I know now just how important a beautiful wig can be.

I went bald and looked bold and beautiful—but it took really cool earrings to give me the guts to pull it off.

It wasn't until after chemo was all over that my nails started to lift up off my fingers and toes—ugly and painful. Months later my new nails grew in. Getting a manicure now is a celebration.

✣ First Things First

Hair Loss

One of the cruelest side effects of cancer treatment is hair loss. Some treatments lead to complete hair loss; others lead to all-over thinning or to partial or patchy hair loss. Hair loss is usually temporary, rarely permanent. But the amount and type of hair that you grow back after treatment is over can be different from what you had before.

If you check out "hair loss" on Google, you'll be slammed with a million ads, pop-ups that refuse to go away, and all kinds of medical sites speckled with confusing terms like "diffuse vs. patterned alopecia" (*alopecia* is the medical word for hair loss) and "telogen effluvium" (when the cells of the hair follicles go into a resting mode and the hair falls out a few months later).

The average person has about 100,000 hairs on her head, and they grow about one-half inch per month (six inches per year). Hair loss occurs from decreased growth and increased hair fallout, damage, or removal, and from side effects of certain chemo mixtures.

Cells that grow hair are alive and active, but the hair *crop* they produce is made of protein that has no living cells. Like all cells in your body, the hair-producing cells grow and rest; the usual ratio of growing to resting cells is ten to one. This ratio can shift quickly to less growing and more resting if there is any significant change in your health or your body's internal hormonal environment due to hormonal therapies. Chemotherapy also damages the hair-making cells themselves, which can halt all hair growth immediately.

Nail Changes

Onycholysis is the official term for the finger and toe nail changes that can occur as a side effect of some chemotherapies (Taxotere is the guiltiest, followed by Taxol, then Adriamycin). About 30 percent of patients who receive Taxotere will experience nail changes. All twenty nails are usually affected to a variable degree.

Apart from their obvious aesthetic value, hair and nails perform important functions: hair helps retain body heat, and nails protect the tender and sensitive tissue at the tips of your fingers and toes. It's no wonder that you can dearly miss and suffer from their absence or compromised condition.

Focus on the light at the end of the tunnel: when the health problem or medication insult is over, or when your body has adjusted to its new internal environment, your hair and nails will eventually grow back. This chapter will help you face the emotional and physical challenges in the interim, so that you're able to devote your energy to your recovery.

❧ Challenges

Hair Loss

Within a few weeks of starting chemotherapy, you may lose some or all of your hair. Some drugs affect only the hair on the top of your head; others cause the loss of eyebrows and eyelashes, pubic hair, hair on your legs, or hair on and under your arms. The extent and timing of hair loss depends on the type, amount, frequency, and duration of medicines used. Going into early menopause or going on or off hormonal therapies (tamoxifen, aromatase inhibitors) changes your internal hormone levels, making more of your hair cells stop growing and

---

COMMON CHEMOTHERAPY MEDICATIONS AND HAIR LOSS

- **Taxol and Taxotere** usually cause complete hair loss in all areas: head, brows, lashes, pubic area, legs, and arms.
- **Adriamycin** causes complete hair loss in all women, usually within the first few weeks after receiving the drug. Some women also lose lashes and eyebrows, which usually fall out long after the hair on your head.
- **Cytoxan, methotrexate, and 5-fluorouracil** (the ingredients of the CMF chemotherapy plan) can cause thinning of hair in many women, no hair loss in some— but rarely complete hair loss.
- **Xeloda (capecitabine), Gemzar (gemcitabine), and carboplatin** do not usually cause significant hair loss.

Note: When some of these same medications are given in more frequent, lower doses, such as once a week, there may be less hair loss (for example, regular-dose Taxol given once every two to three weeks causes complete hair loss, whereas weekly low-dose Taxol may just cause thinning).

Hair on your head goes first, eyebrows and lashes last.

start resting. Radiation therapy can cause hair loss limited to the area within the treatment field.

Hair loss from breast cancer treatment doesn't work in isolation. Many non-cancer-related factors can cause or contribute to the problem of hair loss, including emotional struggles (anxiety); poor nutrition; sleep deprivation; medical conditions (autoimmune conditions, chronic anemia); and hormonal shifts (over- or underactive thyroid, pregnancy and the postpartum period, stopping or starting postmenopausal hormone therapy or birth control pills); tendencies (obsessive-compulsive disorder with hair pulling); and medications. In addition, hair can be damaged by brushing and combing; heat (hair dryers, curlers, the sun); hair products (dyes, straighteners, shampoo, setting solutions); high wind; salt and chlorinated water; and air pollution. And don't forget family genetics.

All of these factors produce overall changes in the growth signals of your whole scalp and all its hair-growing cells. That's why these changes tend to produce loss of all hair (diffuse) rather than just a patch here or there (patterned). Sometimes, however, certain areas of hair-making cells are more sensitive than others—which can lead to patches of hair loss with or without thinning in other areas.

When Your Hair Grows Back

Bobbi was beside herself when she went bald. "What if it doesn't grow back?" she asked her doctor, who replied, "Then you'll be the first one." It took six months: first fuzz, then real lush hair—curly, too. Bobbi had always wanted curly hair, and here it was. "I was ecstatic. I figured this was my reward—but I felt like an impostor."

How quickly your hair grows back depends on the kind of treatments you're on and have had, and how fast your hair normally grows. Very, very rarely, permanent baldness occurs after many years of continuous or on-and-off chemotherapy: hair follicles get "burned out" and they shut down. Or, also rarely, an autoimmune disorder can occur that involves baldness and is unrelated to prior breast cancer treatment.

AFTER CHEMO AND HORMONAL THERAPY. Hair may be a little slower to grow back after hair-harsh chemo such as full-dose Taxol, compared to other regimens, like TC (Taxotere and Cytoxan). Here are some general guidelines to go by:

- A few weeks after chemotherapy is finished, you might feel a little peach fuzz.
- Around a month, you might feel the bristle of some nubs.
- By six weeks, your new hair should be visible.
- By a few months, you may have an inch or more.

Once your hair gets growing, it will probably continue to grow at its normal rate. Some women notice that their hair is thinner all over, particularly on the top and in the temple area (consistent with male-pattern hair loss). This is due to the change in your body's hormonal environment. It may or may not get better on its own, but there are things you can do. (See the "Solutions" section of this chapter.) If you are currently taking hormonal therapy, such as tamoxifen or one of the aromatase inhibitors (Arimidex, Femara, Aromasin), the thinning continues to a certain point—about a year—then it usually stabilizes, but in some women the tendency continues as long as they are taking the medicine.

Your hair may remain thinner after you stop taking hormonal therapy, or it may recover a little. It's unlikely to recover completely, however. You can try the products mentioned in this chapter to help it along the way.

AFTER RADIATION. If you have hair loss after radiation to the head area, it can take four to six months before you regrow an inch of hair. Your new hair will probably be thinner than it used to be, and you may have a small bald spot along the very top and/or back of your head. Letting the surrounding hair grow longer to cover the bald spots can solve the problem, particularly if you have a clever hairstylist. Hair extensions can be a good solution. You also might want to hold on to your wig or headgear to spruce up for special occasions.

Hair Loss Hits Home

No other side effect of breast cancer treatment seems to be more disturbing than hair loss. For many women, it's worse than losing a breast. Hair loss threatens your privacy because it is so visible. And hair is so much a part of your image that when it goes, you look so transformed. It's the final insult, on top of the gray skin, the look of exhaustion, and the weight gain. "It's hard enough to have cancer and feel bad, but to have to look bad, too?" It's so traumatic—but it's also temporary.

Nancy's two-year-old daughter had the hardest time. She always loved to sit on her mother's lap and play with her mother's hair, and she was terribly upset when it started to fall out. "I got a wig very quickly after that, and Nora was okay with that. But when she'd wake up in the middle of the night, I'd have to pull the wig on—half asleep and in the dark—before going in to see to her."

Cynthia's eight-year-old daughter had her own influence on her mother's use of a wig. "Hair is very important to an eight-year-old," said Cynthia, "so I hadn't told her about my hair loss. But one day when we were at the dinner table and I scratched my scalp, Skye said, 'Mom, your whole hair just moved when you itched it. Are you wearing a wig? Can I see it?' So I pulled the wig back a little bit and she said, 'Oh, Mom, that's not such a big deal. But I don't want you outside this apartment without your wig!' "

Deena, a bold and independent-minded person, was ready to skip the wigs and do-rags and just go bald. But her preteen daughter stopped her cold; she wanted her mother to look exactly as she had before the cancer therapy. The only way to come near accomplishing that was for Deena to buy a wig just like her natural hair. She gave in, got the wig, and calmed her daughter's distress.

Nail Changes

Early nail changes may not be visible at first. But over weeks to months, darkening, ridging, and pitting of the nails occur, followed by separation and lifting of the nails off the nail bed. There's also inflammation of the tissues that surround and hold on to your nails, and there may be oozing of small amounts of blood or other fluid. Sometimes the most significant nail side effects don't show up until *after* chemo is over.

Reddened and tender soft-tissue changes of the fingertips and toes, hands, and feet—with possible small blisters and fissures in the skin—can be side effects of another common chemotherapy called Xeloda. Treatment with both Taxotere and Xeloda can produce a double whammy.

TIMING OF HAIR AND NAIL CHANGES

Hair loss may be gradual or dramatic: clumps in your hairbrush, handfuls in the drain of your shower or on your pillow a few weeks into chemotherapy. The nail changes evolve more slowly midway through chemotherapy and when it's all over. No matter how forewarned you may be, it's always miserable. You see these changes even if no one else does. Luckily, there are things you can do about it.

Thin and brittle nails can occur while on antiestrogen hormonal therapies such as tamoxifen and the aromatase inhibitors.

Bad habits, including nail biting and smoking, can worsen these difficult nail problems.

These changes can be very painful—and for many women, they are unsightly and embarrassing. The small blood or fluid collections that can build up under the nail or in the surrounding tender tissues are at increased risk of infection (particularly when your immune cell counts are low). And using your hands and feet for everyday functions at home and work may be quite difficult. Making matters worse, loose fingernails can get caught on clothing and other stuff, causing further pain and separation of the nail.

Solutions

Covering Your Head—or Not

Until your hair returns—and it will—you have a choice of cover-ups, or you can decide to go bold and bald. One young woman I know went for the bare-head look, with great makeup and big, flashy earrings. She was stunning. Most women, however, want to find some way to disguise their bareness—and keep warm in the winter or protected from the sun in the summer. Then it's a matter of what you're most comfortable with: a wig, a scarf, a hat, or a baseball cap.

Preparing for the Fallout

If you have lead time, it's less troubling to select a wig before you lose all your hair, because you can get used to wearing the wig in short trial sessions before you need to wear it all the time. And if you still have your hair, it's easier to match your hair color and style. But if the wig is fitted while you still have a full head of hair, it can be too big once your hair falls out.

It's also a good idea to have your hair cut short before chemotherapy begins. It's a lot less traumatic to lose short clumps of hair than long ones, and it's easier to get fitted for a wig.

Wigs

You want a wig that looks natural, that looks like it belongs on your head. You can order a wig made of real hair, but it could cost you

---

YOU MAY HAVE TO TELL PEOPLE WHAT HAPPENED TO YOUR HAIR

Keeping your breast cancer diagnosis a secret is extremely taxing and difficult—and usually impossible. Losing your hair is the biggest tip-off. It's unrealistic to expect your wig or other solution to keep your secret from others; even the best wigs aren't good enough to fool everyone. You can assume that anyone close to you who matters already knows that you've been dealing with breast cancer.

The need to keep a secret is usually driven by your need to protect your privacy, avoid unwanted attention, make everything appear normal, and stay in control. My patients who own businesses or who are the lead adviser or consultant don't want their clients to lose confidence or worry about them, so they have an urgent drive to keep it secret. Secrets can also be a denial technique—a coping strategy we all use when we're trying to block out something that's disturbing.

My advice:

- Give up the secret. Most everyone knows people who've had breast cancer. After all, breast cancer is the most common cancer to affect women. There's nothing shameful about it; you should not be embarrassed.
- Avoid putting excess and unnecessary pressure on yourself. Don't try to look and be exactly as you were before your diagnosis. Do the most critical client functions with backup as needed.
- Go with your day-to-day flow and expend reasonable effort to look the best you can.

You want to save your precious personal energy for what's really important to you and within your control.

between $800 and $3,000 or more, and it requires more care than you give your own hair. After four to six months, real hair wigs may start to look dull because they lack the natural oils your scalp usually makes to protect your hair from damage due to brushing and styling, sunning, and using hair dryers. (Taking your wig to a hair stylist can help spruce it up.)

Most women choose synthetic hair: It looks and feels good, needs very little attention and care, and costs much less than real hair ($30 to $500). You may feel that a synthetic wig looks too shiny and perfect and may be noticeably out of character for you, particularly if you had a natural, wind-tossed pretreatment hairdo. A good compromise is a wig that combines real and synthetic hair: you save on cost and improve on maintenance.

As for wig length, a short wig is easier to wear and to care for, and if your hair is already short, you'll have an easier time living with temporary hair that's a similar length. (A great stylist can give your wig a haircut, but be careful—wig hair doesn't grow back.) Besides, if you get used to yourself in short hair, you can get rid of a short wig a lot faster since it takes much less time to regrow your hair to a short length without anyone noticing.

If you do get a long wig, you may want to ease the transition back to your short hair at the end of treatment (which would otherwise take years to regrow to the length of the wig's hair). Schedule serial haircuts for your wig, bringing its length up to the length of your new real hair. Then you'll be better prepared to toss the wig.

Shorter is also cooler, an important consideration, because wigs usually feel hot in any season—particularly if you're prone to hot flashes.

Here are some other important wig selection guidelines:

Color
- Go with a somewhat lighter color than your own hair because:
  - ~ Dark wigs harshly contrast with pale skin.
  - ~ Synthetic hair or real hair from Asian women is usually thicker than your own, which could make your normal shade appear much darker.
- Avoid yellow-blond wigs if you have yellow skin tones.
- Look for a wig with natural color variation.

Comfort and fit

- Fits your head without hair, but isn't too tight
- Isn't scratchy against your scalp
- Doesn't have an obvious part line
- Won't get matted or look like you're wearing a hat or helmet.

Most wigs are designed for women who have some hair, so don't assume it will be comfortable to wear against your scalp or that it's going to fit you once your hair comes out. Work with an expert, experienced wig fitter to pick the most comfortable and best-fitting wig. If the mesh stretches out and the wig becomes loose, small adjustments can fix the problem.

> **HAIR EXTENSIONS**
>
> Hair extensions and clip-on hair pieces (ponytails, bangs) can be a practical and glamorous solution to everyday thin hair, a way to get long hair quickly once your hair grows back in, or a fabulous way to create a fancy hairdo for a big occasion.
>
> You don't want to glue or sew in anything that's too heavy and pulls too hard on your newly regrown, sensitive hair. It's best to go to an experienced hair extension expert who knows how to attach many small pieces of hair (rather than a few big pieces) or who can recommend special pieces anchored by a hair comb or hair band.

Your satisfaction with a wig depends on much more than its cost. You can get a $50 wig that you end up wearing every day and a $5,000 wig that just sits in the back of your closet. To manage the costs, ask your doctor for a prescription for an "extracranial prosthesis" (aka wig) that you can submit to your health insurance company. Not every health insurance company will reimburse you, but try for partial if not complete coverage. It is, after all, a remedy for a cancer treatment side effect; antinausea medication is covered as a side effect remedy, so a wig should be handled in the same manner. Some hospital cancer centers and American Cancer Society branches offer free wigs. You can also Google "free wigs."

You might even find that wearing a wig is something that gives you a smile or two. Try a new color, a new length, a new style. You may as well find something upbeat in this experience. Mary Beth had always toyed with being a blonde, so she bought a high-styled blond wig, and she liked it so much she dyed her own hair blond after it grew back.

"When my hair started to go," Florrie said, "my husband shaved off all of his. Then he put on a Howard Stern wig and we horsed around and had a few laughs." Annamarie's husband cajoled her into shaving her head bald once she started to shed clumps of her hair, and then he did his, too—that sparked a lot of conehead jokes. Annamarie did get a wig, exactly like her own hair, and none of her friends realized the difference. "When my hair was about an inch long, my husband

FINDING THE RIGHT WIG

You can ask your oncologist's office, hairdresser, or local breast cancer organization for a list of wig specialists in your area. Some wig specialists will come to your home if you are concerned about privacy. One of the cheapest sources of synthetic wigs is the Paula Young catalog (800-343-9695, 800-472-4017). For a high-quality glamorous synthetic wig with va-va-voom, check out Henry Margu wigs (about $120–$300; www.henrymargu.com). On the other hand, if you're interested in a fabulous hand-woven, custom-made human hair wig, check out Bitz-n-Pieces in New York City (it can cost between $2,000 and $4,000 and requires an initial consultation and fitting). A full head of hair extensions starts at $500 and can easily go up to $1,000 or more.

No Guarantees

When your hair expectations hit reality, the crash may derail you. Don't panic when you're buying a wig. Take the time you need to find your best wig solution. Bring with you a trusted friend or family member who has great taste and will be totally honest with you.

Try on as many wigs as you can, go with the winner, and leave the rejects in the store. You can be more relaxed and take more risks with inexpensive synthetic wigs. For high-priced real hair wigs, be absolutely sure it's what you want before you shell out a few thousand green ones. Avoid special-order wigs that you're obligated to purchase. Only go with a custom order if it's pay-on-approval. Make sure you're totally satisfied before making your decision; wigs are generally not returnable.

Later, if you're dissatisfied or tired of your wig, you can give it to someone else who might need and enjoy it (or donate it to your hospital cancer center or a nonprofit wig bank and take the tax deduction).

told me, 'You look so much better with short hair,' so I kept it that way. It had been ash blond before and it grew back gray with blond streaks. I wanted it brown, so I dyed it, and it came out purple. I kept it purple for a while—life was kind of wild, so why not a wild hair color?"

"My friend Jane had begun to lose her hair long before she ever got breast cancer, so when she lost it all after chemotherapy, she felt she had a proper excuse for getting a really good wig. It was beautiful, she was beautiful—and she looked ten years younger."

Scarves

Head scarves suit some women better than a wig. "I knew my hair would be coming back, and I was just more comfortable in a scarf. I didn't let anyone see me bald, my husband in particular. I figured he'd had enough to deal with, and I guess I was worried he'd find me unappealing. I wore beautiful scarves and earrings and made myself up, something I never normally did. It made me feel much better about myself."

You can learn to tie scarves in clever, creative ways. Top the scarf with a dramatic hat and it needn't look anything like a disguise for lost hair.

WIG CARE

Taking good care of your wig will help it last as long as you need it—about a year or less. Human hair wigs require more care than synthetic wigs, and they tend to get dry and damaged over time. Mixing up your repertoire—wig, turban, scarf, hat—makes the wig solution last longer. Resting your wig on a stand each night will keep it looking fresh. (You can fashion your own wig stand with two 2-liter plastic soda bottles. Cut them in half, discard the tops, face the cut edges of the bottoms together, and force one inside another to get a football-shaped stand.)

Synthetic wigs wash easily using a shampoo for dry hair followed by conditioner (every two weeks is recommended). You can set them with warm curlers, sprays, or gels. The only thing you have to worry about is high heat—stay away from hair dryers, curling irons, and even hot ovens. "The front of my wig was all singed when I got too close taking a pizza out of the oven."

If you have the money in your budget, drop your wig at the hairdresser's for a few hours once a month while you work or run errands, and have them shampoo, condition, trim, and set the wig for you. What a relief to have someone else fuss with your hair—and you don't have to be there! (Use a turban, scarf, cap, or backup wig while your main "lady" is at the salon.)

FIND YOUR STYLE

Check out online resources for clever, useful, and fun ways to use scarves, turbans, and hats:

- Breastcancer.org discussion boards (www.breastcancer.org)
- Headcovers Unlimited (www.headcovers.com)
- Hats with Heart (www.heidesmastectomy.com; www.hatswithheart.com)
- Cover Your Hair (www.coveryourhair.com)
- American Cancer Society's TLC (www.tlcdirect.org)

Turbans

Turbans fit close to your entire head, unlike hats, which tend to sit on the upper part of your head. Unlike scarves, turbans don't need tying or adjusting—you just pull them on. Turbans may fit like a simple cloche or sport a twist, or they may have pleated folds of fabric. They come in terry cloth, jersey, or felt. They're easy to put on and take off, many are washable, and they're cheap (most cost between $5 to $15, with a few as high as $100). Elsie wore a turban alternately with a wig. "I wear the turban to sleep, for warmth. Apart from how it looks, a bald head gets cold at night." (The Paula Young catalog offers a full line of attractive, inexpensive turbans; see www.paulayoung.com or call 800-364-9060.)

You can also wear a hairpiece—designed to be worn with a turban or baseball cap—that looks like you have bangs or a ponytail. Some are already sewn into the turban or hat; others can be attached wherever you want them.

Hats

Deena went to work in hats (she was never comfortable with her wig), and her co-workers started wearing hats to work, too, to help make her feel better. When Jeannie lost her hair, she bought a supply of baseball caps, snug-fitting and funky, and wore one of them to work each day. After the first day, everyone in her office showed up in caps, and wore them every day after that, until Jeannie gave hers up when her hair grew back.

Makeup for Lost Brows and Lashes

If you lose your eyebrows and eyelashes, you may want to use makeup to restore the balance in your features. You may be surprised at what a pleasing effect this can create. (While I certainly don't recommend it, there are some women who normally shave off their natural eyebrows to paint on eyebrows they believe are more becoming in shape and color. If you compare early photos of Greta Garbo with later ones, you'll see how much more beautiful and dramatic she looked when Hollywood gave her those graceful arching eyebrows that became part of her personal signature.)

Thumb through a good fashion magazine to come up with possibilities. Then take a little time in front of a mirror and practice your technique with shapes you like. To get the most natural look, choose two different shades of a color that's a little lighter than your wig, and apply both, in alternation, with feathered strokes. (The Anastasia brand and application technique is my favorite; it's not cheap, but it works great and one pencil lasts a year. Go online for a large selection of places to buy this product.) It takes practice to get it right. You can even get a stencil to help you create the same shape on each side and from day to day. You can also get help at your local beauty parlor or a makeup store like Sephora.

As for eyelashes, you can try eye shadow to give the effect of contrast and drama around your eyes, or if you really miss your eyelashes, you can buy false ones. (Think of Liza Minnelli or Dolly Parton.) You can also ask your doctor about a directly applied medicated cream called Latisse that makes your eyelashes grow in fuller and darker.

Be careful not to overdo the makeup; wearing a lot of makeup when you're washed out can make you look clownlike. Do not get permanent tattooed makeup—not only are you likely to change your mind about how you like your brows and eyeliner to look, but the tattoo ink might contain metal molecules that react during an MRI scan, causing heat and discomfort.

Medical Solutions

For medical hair loss solutions, a dermatologist is best. He or she will do a full history and physical and try to identify any underlying disease or condition that might produce hair loss (for example, excess stress, overactive thyroid, autoimmune problem), as well as any medication that may be contributing to your problem (for example, steroids, stopping hormone replacement). Because any medication you're on may have a unique or uncommon side effect, it's best to run through the list of the medications and over-the-counter products (drugs, herbals, supplements) you're using to see if hair loss is a reported side effect. (This is your doctor's job, but it never hurts to keep on top of what's going on with your treatment. After all, who cares more about you than you?) A great resource for this is Litt's Drug Eruption Reference Manual (your dermatologist or primary care doctor will have this in the office, and you might find a copy in the library; online access to this and other resources may also be possible).

Rogaine or minoxidil (same thing, just different names) has been shown to stimulate hair growth and is a safe and effective approach to hormonal-therapy-related hair loss, but it's a messy daily chore and it's expensive. One of my patients followed the daily Rogaine ritual for years, but she finally got tired of it and stopped. Her hair loss has stabilized, and she still has a full head of hair, although she says it's not as thick and lush as it once was.

A hormonal imbalance consisting of a little too much testosterone can cause male-pattern hair loss (thinning at the top and temples and pulling back of your hairline) or excess body hair with not enough hair on the top of your head! Your dermatologist may suggest that you try a medication, spironolactone, which works by nudging your body's testosterone out of its receptor—the place where testosterone exerts its negative effect on hair growth on your head.

Just as for men, there are hair transplantation procedures that can work for women. Transferring tiny crops or "plugs" of hair from the back of the scalp to fill in thin

THINGS THAT DON'T WORK

Keep in mind that hair loss products are a multibillion-dollar international market. Do you remember the *Seinfeld* episode when George orders hair-growing cream from China? He spends a fortune on products and gets no results.

Don't expect extra vitamins to produce extra hair growth. Supplemental biotin (from the B-vitamin family) on top of a healthy diet has no proven hair-growing benefit despite grand claims.

Special shampoos may make your hair appear thicker by plumping up the hair shafts, but they don't stimulate hair growth. Watch out for sound-alike products (like Progaine shampoo) named after proven products, like Rogaine, in order to drive sales through name recognition. Save your money and avoid them.

areas at the top and around your hairline is a hair solution that works for many. Ask your dermatologist or primary care physician for a reputable hair transplantation practitioner.

To stimulate the regrowth of your eyelashes, there is the medicated cream Latisse, mentioned earlier. Ongoing studies are looking at the ability of Latisse to help with hair growth in other areas as well.

When Your Hair Grows Back

Once it grows in, your new hair may be just like your old hair. It may also be thicker, curlier, or straighter than your original hair, and it may be a different color. This new texture and color may stay the same or revert back to your original hair type. You may have persistent bald spots or areas of thinning. Get creative with your haircuts to cover these areas. Don't restart or begin bad habits like twirling and pulling your new hair; your hair may be more likely to come out.

Most women are surprised to see how gray their hair is when it regrows—mostly because they had been dyeing it for years and never really got a good look at its true color. You can keep it gray—which is actually a gentler contrast to your paler complexion—or you can hit the bottle again and zip it up with some color. Watch out, however, because the color might not take exactly as you'd expect. You might try some temporary dyes first until you find the color you want.

Gerry's hair used to be straight and wispy, but it grew back curly and thick. "Your hair looks so good! Where'd you have it done?" asked a friend. Gerry's reply: "Paoli Hospital." Dee's daughter started calling her "Mary," as in "Mary Had a Little Lamb," because Dee's hair grew back in as soft curly swirls that piled up on each other. "Mary" was just happy to have hair again.

Taking Care of Your Finger- and Toenails

There are a number of things you need to do (or not do) to take care of your finger- and toenails to keep them from getting worse, to avoid infection and bleeding, to reduce pain, and to maximize your ability to function properly and fully.

Dos

- Inspect regularly for healing progress as well as signs of trouble (like infection).
- Cut nails short, but not too short, using a clean, small pair of sharp curved scissors.
- Keep hands and feet extra clean.
- Moisturize hands, feet, and nails.
- Wear gloves to do household chores such as washing dishes, cutting onions, or using the oven.
- Wear open-toe shoes or ones with a big toe box so your toes aren't squooshed together.
- Avoid injury and excess heat.

Don'ts

- Use harsh chemicals and detergents
- Expose yourself to poison ivy
- Use hot paraffin hand treatment
- Bite your nails
- Smoke

You can use nail polish, but minimize your use of nail polish remover, leave your cuticles alone, and avoid artificial nails. To provide some protection or to conceal a lost or damaged nail, you can use a Band-Aid—put the gauze pad of the Band-Aid over the nail and the adhesive part over the flesh of the finger or toe.

Eventually this nasty side effect will go away. Healing is not immediate, however, and the problem can take up to six months to resolve.

✿ Moving Forward

As terrible as hair loss is and as unattractive and disabling as nail changes can be, these treatment side effects are temporary. The good news is that there are lots of products you can use to help you deal with these side effects. Finding the best solutions for your own situation will require resourcefulness, creativity, and an open mind to a new look.

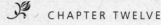

CHAPTER TWELVE

Bone Health: Weaknesses and Strengths

I started on an aromatase inhibitor, and I was on it about a year when my primary care doctor asked if I was taking bone-building medication. I wasn't, and he was upset. It seems my medication, which was great for fighting breast cancer, wasn't so great for my bones. I got on bone-building medication, and the last time I had a DEXA scan of my bones I was in pretty good shape. I'm just relieved that my regular doctor was on top of my care—but disappointed that my oncologist let it fall through the cracks.

After ten years on bone builders, the bone density in my spine was still not up to my doctor's expectations. I was almost six feet tall to start with, so my loss of height didn't bother me so much, but my doctor wanted me to improve my spine density. The common medicines didn't work. Eventually I went on Forteo for a year and had great results. At first I was squeamish about using that needle and stuff, but it was really easy. No pain at all, and no fuss.

First Things First

Your bones give your body its shape, help you move, and support your body. Bones also provide protection around your heart, lungs, and brain. Even though your bones feel hard and rigid, bones are living tissues that are constantly rebuilding themselves during your lifetime.

Bones come in two varieties: compact bone that forms the outer hard, dense, white part (about 80 percent of total bone) and trabecular bone, which fills the inside of the compact bones with a scaffolding of spongy bone like a honeycomb, filled with bone-making cells.

Bones are always in a sensitive, continuous process of resorption and growth with specialized bone cells: osteoclasts and osteoblasts. Old bone is dissolved and removed by osteoclasts; new bone is rebuilt by osteoblasts in a process called mineralization. During this process, osteoblasts apply a kind of spackle—made of the protein collagen fortified with calcium and phosphorus—to the walls that fill up the spaces inside your bones. Mineralization is stimulated by a cascade of hormones and by using your bones in various forms of activity.

Bones need calcium, vitamin D, and weight-bearing physical activity to stay healthy and strong. If you don't have a healthy diet full of bone-building nutrients and don't get enough of certain kinds of exercise, bones can start to weaken without your awareness. The higher your bone's density, measured with a DEXA scan, the stronger and healthier your bones are.

While some bone loss is natural as you age, along the way things can happen to upset or improve the balance between bone building and bone loss, including breast cancer treatment effects, diet and lifestyle choices, physical activity, medications, and other medical conditions. Some shifts in the balance between bone building and removal are beyond your control, but there are quite a few areas where you are in direct control.

This chapter will outline the challenges to bone health and identify solutions to tip your balance in favor of strong bones for an active life— standing tall and moving with strength, comfort, and ease.

❧ Challenges

Bones stay strong as long as there is an even balance between bone building and bone resorption. There are a full range of factors that can influence how your bone makes, remodels, and removes bone, including:

- Growing older
- Experiencing low estrogen levels

- Being postmenopausal (a combination of growing older and lower estrogen levels)
- Getting little or no exercise
- Being small and very thin (associated with low estrogen levels and less weight bearing on the bones)
- Having low bone mass to begin with
- Having a family history of osteoporosis or broken bones
- Smoking over an extended period of time
- Not getting enough calcium or vitamin D/sunlight
- Poor nutrition
- Having more than two alcoholic drinks per week
- Taking certain medications over a significant period of time, including steroids, thiazide diuretics, digoxin, some antibiotics (such as tetracycline), or regular use of mineral oil or antacids containing aluminum or magnesium
- Experiencing chronic stress

In addition, having one (or more) of the following medical conditions challenges your ability to rebuild bone or threatens to break down existing bone mass:

- Hyperthyroidism or hyperparathyroidism
- Kidney disease
- Arthritis
- Inability to absorb key vitamins, minerals, and other nutrients (due, for example, to inflammatory bowel disease)
- Cancer in the bones
- Chronic lung disease
- Cushing's disease
- Multiple sclerosis

Comparing Risk Factors

Having a risk factor for bone loss doesn't mean you're going to get bone loss—it just means that you're more likely to develop the problem than someone who doesn't have the same risk factor. And each risk factor can affect different people differently. Furthermore, not all risk factors are

SOME PEOPLE HAVE LOW VITAMIN D LEVELS

Some people with dark skin tend to have low vitamin D levels and have trouble getting enough calcium. The main reasons are:

- They are more likely to be lactose intolerant and thus consume little to no dairy products (a major source of dietary calcium)
- Pigments in dark skin absorb much of the UVB component of sunlight before it has a chance to activate vitamin D
- Low vitamin D levels make it harder to absorb calcium from the gastrointestinal tract

Other people at risk for bone loss because of minimal sunshine or from little to no consumption of dairy products include:

- Women of Islamic faith who cover nearly all of their skin with clothing
- Elderly people who spend most of their time indoors, often housebound or bedridden
- People who adhere to a vegan diet and usually consume no animal products

These obstacles can be overcome with the consumption of other foods rich in calcium and vitamin D, the use of supplements, and more time in the sun (privately, for religious and modest women).

created equal. For example, the overall aging process has a greater effect on bone loss than a shift of estrogen levels. Smoking is way worse than alcohol. A family history of osteoporosis can be outweighed by regular physical activity.

The amount of stuff you take or are exposed to and the length of time you take it, or the duration of the exposure all matter a great deal. Short-term exposure to steroids, smoking, or a high-protein diet has essentially no lasting effect, but long-term exposure to these factors can have a severe impact.

Your starting point matters, too. If your bones start out supersturdy, you can weather some hits and still come out strong and upright. If your bones are weak to begin with, even small insults can make a difference.

Changes in Bone Strength as You Age

During your childhood and teenage years, your body adds new bone faster than it gets rid of old bone. That's when you grow taller and broader. Then for years and years, your bones are in perfect balance: new bone is added at the same rate as old bone is removed. Your body structure is stable.

Your bones are strongest in your twenties and thirties. Beyond age thirty-five, bone removal gradually begins to outstrip bone formation, resulting in very slow loss of bone mass. After menopause, there is about a five-year period of accelerated bone loss, then the rate slows and returns to a regular age-related rate. Your bone strength can stay within normal range for a long time when everything is going well. But as bone mass diminishes with age, osteopenia becomes an issue—when bone mass is at the bottom of the normal range but is not yet critical. Most people lose some height as they age, although more than two inches can be a matter of concern.

Eventually, with the passage of many years or with a combination of risk factors, bone mass and strength can fall significantly—a condition called osteoporosis—putting you at increased risk for broken bones.

Breast Cancer Treatments That Decrease Bone Strength

When you experience a shift in your body's internal hormonal environment—from natural or breast cancer treatment–induced menopause, ongoing hormonal therapy, or other medical conditions— estrogen levels can drop sharply. And since estrogen helps maintain bone mass, such a drop can cause significant bone loss. Here are some breast cancer treatments that can weaken the bones:

- Chemotherapy, particularly if it brings on temporary or permanent menopause. Significant bone loss may result while you're still under treatment and continue until your menstrual periods resume or a bone protector is used. (If your periods cease, age-related bone loss will persist.)

CALL TO ACTION: OSTEOPENIA AND OSTEOPOROSIS

A diagnosis of osteopenia—low but not significantly low bone loss—is an opportunity to make changes in your life that will help you restore the bone strength you're missing.

Getting a diagnosis of osteoporosis—critically low bone mass and strength—calls for extra measures to get you back on the right track:

- Moderate osteoporosis, associated with an increased risk of fracture, calls for moderate steps.
- Severe osteoporosis, associated with actual fractures, usually requires immediate big steps.

Osteoporosis can lead to excessive loss of height and small fractures of the wrist and back bones. You're also more vulnerable to larger fractures of the hip that can have a significant effect on your quality of life, limiting your comfort and ability to perform many activities. Particularly if an elderly woman fractures a hip, forcing her to stay in bed, she is at significant risk for developing complications from the fracture and/or extended inactivity. Few of these women return to their prior lifestyle—and there is even a risk of death, usually due to a blood clot to the lung.

- Aromatase inhibitor hormonal therapy in postmenopausal women:
  ~Arimidex (anastrozole)
  ~Aromasin (exemestane)
  ~Femara (letrozole)
  All work by blocking the formation of estrogen. Lower estrogen levels during the five or more years on the medication can lead to bone loss.
- Ovarian shutdown in premenopausal women quickly lowers estrogen levels:
  ~Removal of the ovaries causes a sudden, permanent menopause resulting in an immediate increased rate of bone loss.
  ~Ovarian shutdown using medicine (such as Lupron or Zoladex) temporarily stops your ovaries from producing estrogen. It takes a few weeks to shut down your ovaries, and once they are defunct, the rate of bone loss increases. When the ovarian shutdown medication is discontinued, your ovaries

will get back to work if they still have premenopausal life left in them. Then the rate of bone loss will slow down.

The period of greatest bone loss occurs during the first few years after a significant change in your body's internal hormonal environment.

℘ Solutions

The best plan for making bones strong starts with an accurate understanding of your current situation: the strength of your bones right now, the medicines that you're currently on and those you expect to take, and other medical conditions. Once your situation is defined and mapped out, the solutions will become relatively clear.

Know Your Baseline

The main "window" used to see and measure the strength of your bones and predict your risk of fracture is a DEXA (dual-energy X-ray absorptiometry) scan. This X-ray scan measures the bone density

SOME HORMONAL THERAPIES PROTECT BONE

Not all hormonal treatments weaken bone. In fact, selective estrogen receptor modulator medicines (SERMs) can have an estrogen-like protective effect on your bones. The most commonly used SERMs are tamoxifen (available as a generic) and raloxifene (Evista). These two medicines have very similar chemical structures. Tamoxifen is an effective treatment against all stages of breast cancer as well as for breast cancer prevention. Raloxifene is primarily used as a bone protector in postmenopausal women. It also offers the secondary benefit of breast cancer prevention; however, once breast cancer is diagnosed, raloxifene is not used to treat the breast cancer.

(thickness or mass) throughout your body, giving particular attention to your lumbar spine and hips, since these areas are usually the first to experience loss of bone mass and have the highest risk for bone loss–related fractures. (A DEXA scan is different from a bone scan, which you may have had to check for evidence of cancer spread to the bone.)

The main purpose and value of DEXA scans is to provide a report card of how your bones are doing. This report will then be used to guide your medical management and lifestyle choices so that your bones can stay strong, aligned, and straight, and you can remain active and empowered. In the past, you only found out that you had critical bone loss *after* a fracture or after losing meaningful height each year (both signs of significant osteoporosis). With DEXA scans, it is now possible to diagnose osteopenia and osteoporosis from the start and begin treatment *prior* to any fracture.

DEXA scans recommendations are based on your risk for developing osteopenia or osteoporosis. It's advisable to get a baseline DEXA scan if you're:

- Over the age of 65
- On the cusp of or in the midst of menopause or you're postmenopausal and under 65, and you have significant risk for osteoporosis
- About to start treatment with an aromatase inhibitor
- Likely to go into early menopause with chemotherapy or hormonal therapy that shuts down or removes the ovaries and your doctor is concerned about your bone strength to begin with because of other risk factors (being a smoker, or being thin with a family history of osteoporosis)

You need a baseline study to assess your starting bone density. Any future scan can then be compared to this early one to chart your progress.

The frequency of repeat DEXA scans over time depends on what your baseline DEXA scan shows, the likelihood of significant bone loss from your past and ongoing treatments, and your other risks for osteoporosis. For example, DEXA scanning every two years is the usual approach for women without significant risk factors for bone loss, whereas yearly DEXA scans may be recommended for women on aromatase inhibitors to help decide if and when bone-protecting medications are needed and if they are working.

More frequent DEXA scans are unlikely to detect significant bone loss unless you're in a unique situation with a predicted high rate of bone loss moving forward. This kind of rapid bone loss might occur if you have combined risk factors such as:

- You already have osteopenia or osteoporosis.
- You're about to go through or you recently went through an early menopause.

- You're on an aromatase inhibitor.
- You have significant pain or a physical limitation and you expect to be inactive.
- You have a personal history of heavy smoking.
- You have a family history of osteoporosis.
- You are on regular steroids for a medical condition.
- You have abnormal thyroid, parathyroid, or kidney function.

Under such circumstances, it's best to have expert care by a doctor who specializes in osteoporosis. For some women, rather than have more frequent DEXA scans (and their associated exposure to radiation), a specialist may obtain other tests to measure your bone metabolism, such as urine N-telopeptide.

DEXA scans should *not* be done if you are or think you might be pregnant.

For more information about the DEXA scan technique and the location of a scanner near you, as well as general information on osteoporosis and the various medications used to treat it, call the National Osteoporosis Foundation (800-231-4222) or go to their website (www .nof.org).

Keeping Your Bones Strong

The full menu of bone-strengthening solutions—lifestyle changes, supplements, and medications—divides into three basic categories:

- Supply necessary bone-building blocks
- Stop bone weakening
- Increase bone building

For each category, let's go over the practical considerations and review the choices you can make together with your doctor.

Supply Necessary Bone-Building Blocks

Giving your bones the materials they need to stay strong is an essential first step. This includes getting enough calcium.

CALCIUM FROM FOOD. About 1,000 to 1,500 milligrams of daily calcium is recommended, depending on your age and medical situation. (First check with your doctor to be sure your calcium level is not too high to begin with and to clarify your recommended intake.) The best way to get the calcium you need is from a combination of foods and supplements. Foods that are high in calcium include dairy products, calcium-fortified drinks, dark green leafy vegetables, beans, almonds, vitamin-fortified cereal, and canned salmon with bones. See Table 12.1 for the amount of calcium in various foods.

CALCIUM BY SUPPLEMENT. Consider your calcium intake from all sources before taking calcium supplements. Keep in mind that you can only absorb 500 mg of calcium at a time, so you have to spread your total daily dose throughout the day (for example, 500 mg in the morning, at noon, and at night) if you're depending mainly on your supplements. If you are consuming significant amounts of calcium in your diet, you should not take supplements, as very high doses of calcium are unhealthy and can lead to high blood calcium, kidney stones, and interference with absorption of other important minerals.

If you don't get enough calcium in your diet and require supplements, two of the most common and effective options include calcium citrate and calcium carbonate.

Most people buy the supplement that appeals to them based on the container and rarely notice the difference between preparations. If the differences are important to you, based on advice from your doctor, take time to pick out the best option for your situation.

GETTING ENOUGH VITAMIN D. Vitamin D helps your body absorb calcium from your gastrointestinal tract. The recommended daily dose varies, mostly between 200 to 600 IU daily (IU stands for "international units") depending on your age:

- 200 IU if you're under 50
- 400 IU if you're between 50 and 70
- 600 IU if you're over 70

TABLE 12.1 Selected Food Sources of Calcium

Food	Calcium (mg)	% DV*
Yogurt, plain, low-fat, 8 oz.	415	42%
Yogurt, fruit, low-fat, 8 oz.	245–384	25–38%
Sardines, canned in oil, with bones, 3 oz.	324	32%
Cheddar cheese, shredded, 1½ oz.	306	31%
Milk, nonfat, 8 fl. oz.	302	30%
Milk, reduced-fat (2% milkfat), no solids, 8 fl. oz.	297	30%
Mlik, whole (3.25% milkfat), 8 fl. oz.	291	29%
Milk, buttermilk, 8 fl. oz.	285	29%
Milk, lactose-reduced, 8 fl. oz.**	285–302	29–30%
Mozzarella, part-skim, 1½ oz.	275	28%
Tofu, firm, made w/calcium sulfate, ½ cup***	204	20%
Orange juice, calcium-fortified, 6 fl. oz.	200–260	20–26%
Salmon, pink, canned, solids with bone, 3 oz.	181	18%
Pudding, chocolate, instant, made with 2% milk, ½ cup	153	15%
Cottage cheese, 1% milkfat, 1 cup, unpacked	138	14%
Tofu, soft, made w/calcium sulfate, ½ cup***	138	14%
Spinach, cooked, ½ cup	120	12%
Instant breakfast drink, various flavors and brands, powder prepared with water, 8 fl. oz.	105–250	10–25%
Frozen yogurt, vanilla, soft-serve, ½ cup	103	10%
Ready-to-eat cereal, calcium-fortified, 1 cup	100–1,000	10–100%
Turnip greens, boiled, ½ cup	99	10%
Kale, cooked, 1 cup	94	9%

Kale, raw, 1 cup	90	9%
Ice cream, vanilla, ½ cup	85	8.5%
Soy beverage, calcium-fortified, 8 fl. oz.	80–500	8–50%
Chinese cabbage, raw, 1 cup	74	7%
Tortilla, corn, ready to bake/fry, 1 medium	42	4%
Tortilla, flour, ready to bake/fry, one 6" diameter	37	4%
Sour cream, reduced-fat, cultured, 2 tbsp.	32	3%
Bread, white, 1 oz.	31	3%
Broccoli, raw, ½ cup	21	2%
Bread, whole-wheat, 1 slice	20	2%
Cream cheese, regular, 1 tbsp	12	1%

*DV = Daily value, based on 1,000 mg calcium.
**Content varies slightly according to fat content; average = 300 mg calcium.
***Calcium values only for tofu processed with a calcium salt; tofu processed with a noncalcium salt will not contain significant amounts of calcium.
Table courtesy of the National Institutes of Health, Office of Dietary Supplements.

(Your doctor may recommend higher doses of vitamin D for other reasons, such as if you are vitamin D–deficient, you're hoping to cool off hot flashes, etc.)

The three main sources of vitamin D are sunlight (sunshine converts inactive vitamin D in your skin to its active form; the sun is responsible for about 90 percent of our active vitamin D); dietary sources; and supplements. (Most calcium supplements are packaged with vitamin D in varying doses.)

If you're indoors most of the time or live in an area where sunlight is limited, you will have to add foods rich in vitamin D to your diet (see Table 12.2), and you may need to include vitamin supplements as well (but even the supplements require sun to activate them).

GETTING ENOUGH SUNSHINE. Too much sun causes skin cancer; not enough causes low vitamin D levels. So how much sun is safe and necessary for your body to make the vitamin D that it needs?

TABLE 12.2 Selected Food Sources of Vitamin D

Food	IU per serving*	Percent DV**
Cod liver oil, 1 tbsp.	1,360	340
Salmon, cooked, 3½ oz.	360	90
Mackerel, cooked, 3½ oz.	345	90
Tuna fish, canned in oil, 3 oz.	200	50
Sardines, canned in oil, drained, 1¾ oz.	250	70
Milk, nonfat, reduced-fat, and whole, vitamin D fortified, 1 cup	98	25
Margarine, fortified, 1 tbsp.	60	15
Ready-to-eat cereal, fortified with 10% of the DV for vitamin D, ¾–1 cup (more heavily fortified cereals might provide more of the DV)	40	10
Egg, 1 whole (vitamin D is found in yolk)	20	6
Liver, beef, cooked, 3½ oz.	15	4
Cheese, Swiss, 1 oz.	12	4

*IU = international units.
**DV = Daily value, based on 400 IU for adults.
Table courtesy of the National Institutes of Health, Office of Dietary Supplements.

Between 10:00 a.m. and 3:00 p.m., you need five to thirty minutes of unblocked sun exposure to the face, arms, hands, or back at least twice a week. But if you live in a very sunny place, it's best to avoid the skin-damaging effect of the midday sun and get your sun exposure before 10:00 or after 3:00. Recommendations for this time frame include about ten to fifteen minutes of unprotected sun exposure of the face, arms, and hands three or four times a week.

Stop Bone Weakening

Even as you're supplying your bones with the building materials they need, you need to take immediate steps to stop bone deterioration:

• Stop smoking.
• Limit your alcohol use.

HERE COMES THE SUN: RECOMMENDATIONS CAN VARY

Ask the question "How much sun do I need?" and you can get a bunch of complicated answers. That's because the amount of sun that actually hits your skin depends on:

- Where you live relative to the equator
- Season of the year and time of day
- Air considerations: ozone layer thickness, air quality (smog), cloud cover, and altitude
- Lightness or darkness of your skin: the darker the skin, the more sun exposure is necessary to make vitamin D (dark-skinned people need around six times more exposure to UV radiation to produce as much vitamin D as someone with fair skin; the good news is that the extra skin pigment protects them against sun damage to their skin)
- SPF of any sunscreen you might be wearing (an SPF of 8 will block the sun conversion of vitamin D—but it's unusual for people to apply enough to all surfaces to effectively block the sun's effect)
- Type of surface you're on (reflective or absorbent: boat, beach, backyard)
- Whether you're outdoors or indoors (UVB doesn't penetrate glass, so if you're enjoying a little sunshine through a window, it's not going to turn on the vitamin D you need)

According to the National Institutes of Health's Office of Dietary Supplements, if you live north of Chicago you're unlikely to make enough vitamin D from November to February. And while Los Angeles has direct sun through much of the year, its poor air quality can limit the sun's access to your skin.

- Avoid high-protein diets; balance your proteins with fruits and vegetables.
- Manage chronic stress.
- Get enough rest.

You also want to work with your doctor to manage any medical problems or medications that rob your bones of their strength, including:

- Reducing or eliminating your need for steroid medications if possible

- Treating any thyroid, parathyroid, or kidney disease
- Managing conditions that shift calcium from the bone to the bloodstream, which can sometimes accompany advanced breast cancer
- Treating bowel problems that limit your ability to absorb necessary nutrients
- Relieving pain and stiffness from arthritis so you are comfortable enough to move around, stay active, and keep your bones strong

You know how much longer it takes you to fill up the sink if the plug isn't tightly in the drain. Same thing is true for your bones: you have to stop the leakage of bone mass if you want to fortify your bones.

SERMs (SELECTIVE ESTROGEN RECEPTOR MODULATORS). The selective estrogen receptor modulator (SERM) raloxifene (Evista) helps keep bones strong by reducing bone resorption and decreasing overall bone remodeling. As noted earlier in this chapter, raloxifene does have another benefit: to lower risk of hormone receptor–positive invasive breast cancer.

The SERM tarnoxifen, designed as an anticancer hormonal medicine, also has a secondary benefit: like raloxifene, it helps keep bones strong. The SERMs' protective effect on bone strength is mild to moderate, less potent than bisphosphonate medications (discussed in the next section). SERMs should not be taken along with aromatase inhibitors or chemotherapy because they can add extra side effects without any added benefit. SERMS may in fact interfere with chemotherapy's effectiveness—that's why hormonal therapy is not given during chemotherapy.

BISPHOSPHONATES. The group of medicines commonly used to keep bones strong and reduce the risk of fracture is the bisphosphonates. Here are some of the names they go by:

Taken by pill
- Fosamax (alendronate sodium)
- Actonel (risedronate)
- Boniva (ibandronate)
- Didronel (etidronate)
- Skelid (tiludronate)

ORAL BISPHOSPHONATES: STANDING UP ON EMPTY

All of the oral bisphosphonates (taken by pill) are supposed to be taken on an empty stomach with a glass of water. After taking the medication, no other medications, foods, or beverages should be ingested for at least thirty minutes; an hour is probably better. This is because bisphosphonates are poorly absorbed by your gastrointestinal tract, though once in your system, the medication doesn't require any fancy enzymes to make it work. It lasts a long time in the body—some of it stored in your bones and released every time old bone "spackle" is removed.

Oral bisphosphonates can irritate your esophagus (the food tube between your mouth and stomach), causing heartburn—that's why you have to stand or sit up for a half hour after taking the medication. Intravenous bisphosphonates avoid the esophageal irritation and the poor-absorption issues.

Given by injection:
- Reclast or Zometa (zoledronate)
- Aredia (pamidronate)

Most share a similar chemical structure but differ in various ways, including the method by which they're administered (by pill or injection), the frequency of delivery (daily, once a week or month, once or twice a year, etc.), side effects, and effectiveness. Each medication has different official FDA-approved indications. All require your doctor's prescription.

Bisphosphonates all work by inactivating the osteoclast cells responsible for removing old bone material, thus:

- Halting or slowing bone loss
- Reducing the number and severity of bone fractures
- Restoring some of the bone mass you have lost

There is also evidence that bisphosphonates may have antitumor action—perhaps directly on the cancer, or indirectly, by making the bones' internal environment hostile to any cancer cell activity. Studies of women taking this type of medicine showed a reduced risk of cancer spread to the bone and other organs.

CALCITONIN. The hormone calcitonin, naturally made by your thyroid gland, is an active player on the bone scene. It stops the osteoclasts from removing bone, and it juggles calcium and other mineral levels in the body.

SERIOUS BUT RARE SIDE EFFECT OF BISPHOSPHONATES: OSTEONECROSIS OF THE JAW

Bisphosphonates given in significant doses over a long period of time can cause a rare but serious side effect, osteonecrosis of the jaw, in which the bone cells in a compromised part of the jawbone start to die. Tissue repair fails to occur properly, blood flow to the area is limited, and eventually the affected area of the jaw bone weakens, teeth loosen, infection can occur, and the tissues may stay open—unable to heal and come together.

This rare condition is usually triggered by a dental procedure like a tooth extraction that involves a manipulation and requires a lot of extra healing—but it can also happen without any clear precipitating event. It's still not clear what causes it and why this happens in some people and not in others.

Current recommendations include a careful dental examination and preventative tooth and gum care before you start a bisphosphonate. Dental extractions should be avoided at all costs. If any signs of dental decay or other form of compromise occur, the bisphosphonate medication should be discontinued and expert dental evaluation should be sought immediately. If you're already taking a bisphosphonate and you haven't seen your dentist, contact your dentist and make an appointment right away. Together, you and your dentist can work out a regular maintenance schedule that keeps your teeth healthy and minimizes your risk of osteonecrosis of the jaw.

The medication form of calcitonin is Miacalcin, which is taken once a day by nasal spray. Its main use is for the treatment of osteoporosis in postmenopausal women. Generally it's well tolerated; the most common side effects include irritation of the lining of the nose.

Increase Bone Building

From the stairs to the gym to the medicine cabinet, there are a number of changes you can make in your life now to build up your bone strength.

REGULAR PHYSICAL ACTIVITY. You have to let your bones know how much you need them in order to get them to work harder at getting stronger. It's easier than you think to get this important message across: anything you do to consistently exert weight and repetitive balanced tension on your bones helps stimulate new bone mineralization. An exercise routine that includes a variety of activities is the best way to give all of your bones a good workout, avoid boredom, and get you to stick to your program. Here are a number of effective ways to show your bones how much you need them:

- Walking
- Jogging
- Jumping rope
- Stair climbing
- Playing tennis, racquetball, or squash
- Dancing
- Kick boxing, spinning, aerobics
- Rowing, sculling
- Lifting weights (women who've had breast surgery should check with their doctors before doing any weight lifting)

Weight-bearing exercise is the most effective bone-building workout and should ideally be performed thirty minutes a day, three or more days a week. (You can do your thirty minutes of exercise ten minutes at a time during the day to make it easier to squeeze in.)

FORTEO (TERIPARATIDE). For people who continue to have significant bone loss despite other medications, Forteo (teriparatide) may be an option. It is injected just under the skin every day with a tiny needle; people very quickly get used to this procedure. Forteo works by increasing the activity of the bone-making cells (the osteoblasts), whereas most of other bone medicines work by stopping the bone-dissolving cells (the osteoclasts). Over time, Forteo increases bone density and strength and decreases the risk of fracture. Although it's more effective than the bisphosphonates, this medicine is only used for people with severe or unresponsive osteoporosis because of cost, route of delivery, and side effects.

Forteo's side effects (besides the unpleasantness of a daily injection) may include dizziness (particularly when first standing up), muscle spasm, nausea, vomiting, constipation, sluggishness, slowed reaction time, and irregular heartbeats. During laboratory testing in rats, high doses of Forteo given over an extended period of time were associated with a rare risk of bone cancer (osteosarcoma). Although this serious complication hasn't been seen in humans, to be extra careful, the FDA's label says that it shouldn't be given to anyone with a history of bone cancer, a history of Paget's disease (a bone condition, unrelated to Paget's of the breast), or radiation therapy to a bone. Generally it is given for a limited period of time. (Another drawback is that the medication must be kept refrigerated at all times, so if you are traveling, you must arrange for cold packs to keep the stuff cool.)

FLUORIDE AND CALCIUM. Another option your doctor might discuss with you is slow-release fluoride taken with ongoing calcium citrate supplementation. Some studies indicate that taking this combination over several years can stimulate new bone formation and reduce the risk of spinal fractures, but not all studies show consistent benefit. If you are dealing with significant osteoporosis and other options haven't worked, it's worth discussing this option with a bone metabolism doctor.

EXTRA-SPECIAL CARE REQUIRED: CURVATURE OF THE SPINE

Bone health is particularly important if you have a curvature of the spine. Your back may be crooked in one or more different ways:

- Kyphosis (humplike curved spine)
- Scoliosis (side-to-side curved spine)
- Another type of significant spinal deformity

When the bones of your back (called vertebrae) are not neatly stacked right on top of each other, your weight is unevenly distributed over each vertebra. The result: extra pressure is placed on only part of the backbone (the pressure is greatest on the inside of the curve of your back). Weak bones can give out under this extra pressure, causing compression of the bone and further curvature of the spine. Any nerves in the area can get pinched, stretched, or twisted, producing pain, numbness, and possible weakness in another part of the body.

Your situation will determine the best approach to take. If you have a curvature of the spine and your bones are nice and strong, fabulous! You still need to preserve your current bone strength, prevent any bone loss, and closely monitor your bone health well into the future.

If you already have or are at high risk of developing osteopenia, osteoporosis, or complications from these conditions, aggressive medical management is necessary. Under these circumstances, you need to immediately address the role of lifestyle changes, supplements, improved nutrition, and medications, as well as possible orthopedic intervention. Compression fractures can be partly reexpanded with the injection of cementlike material to fill in the compressed vertebral body. Another special surgical procedure involves the use of metal rods to correct or stabilize significant curvature of the spine (following surgery, a full-torso body cast is required for several months).

Working with a team of doctors who specialize in bone health is critical if you have a significant curvature of the spine and you're dealing with breast cancer treatments and their effects. Besides your primary care physician, your team may include a:

- Bone endocrinologist—a doctor with expertise in the hormones that control bone health
- Rheumatologist—a doctor who specializes in the joints between bones and the tissues that connect them
- Orthopedic surgeon—a surgeon who specializes in the health, conditions, and diseases of the bone.
- Physical and occupational therapists—to maximize your range of motion, strength, comfort, and function

Communication and persistence are essential to getting the most benefit from working with your team.

Posture

How you hold your body and carry yourself affects the alignment and wear and tear on your bones. Regardless of your bone health, good posture is critical to positive maintenance of your bones. You want to be able to stand as tall and symmetrical as possible so you function optimally, are physically comfortable, look good, and have a strong presence. (If you are slumped or curved over, it's hard to breathe fully, back pain can develop, and you may appear vulnerable and diminished.)

Practical steps are crucial. If you're not looking where you're going, you're likely to fall; preventing accidents is critical (see Chapter 13). The chair you use and the position of your computer monitor can have a significant impact on your posture. Discreet reminders to stand up straight with shoulders back can be helpful: a special bracelet, a ribbon on your finger—whatever works!

Yoga has a major focus on posture, called *asana*. With beginner or gentle yoga classes near your home, or with a DVD, TV, or online program, you can quickly learn a lot about how to stand and move straight up without stiffness.

Special posture braces can make a big difference, too. These are available from medical supply stores and online vendors. Most have adjustable straps; just make sure the brace fits properly and doesn't dig in and cause yet another problem.

✣ Moving Forward

Great strides in recent years have yielded effective new medications to halt bone loss and facilitate bone building. I'm hopeful that more options will continue to emerge with ongoing research. Get together with your doctor for a focused conversation about your bone health. Pull in additional expertise if you already have significant osteopenia or osteoporosis and your situation calls for an anti-breast-cancer treatment that is likely to produce significant bone loss. A bone metabolism doctor or bone endocrinologist (hormone doctor) usually has the appropriate skill set. Your goal should be to prevent additional bone loss and to try to build back the bone that you may be missing. Ask about available new treatments even as you monitor your progress on your existing treatment plan.

If current therapies have fallen short, consider a clinical trial to get access to promising new agents that are otherwise out of reach. Clinical trials are the only way to advance science—your participation makes an important contribution. Stay tuned as well to Breastcancer.org's Research News and special programs for new information about fortifying your bone health in the years to come.

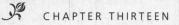

CHAPTER THIRTEEN

Thinking and Remembering: Clearing the Fog and Sharpening Your Mind

What is happening to my mind? I'm forgetting everything, names don't come, I miss appointments, screw up all over the place! Can it be this treatment—or am I getting old faster than I think?

It feels like I'm in a fog, I just can't think as clearly as I used to, can't find the right words like I used to.

I forget what I've just been told—the details just escape me.

I forget the names of my own children—and I'm only forty-four years old!

✿ First Things First

Many people treated for cancer notice significant problems with their ability to manage everyday mental functions such as memory, the expression of thoughts and feelings, and the collecting, sorting, organizing, storing, retrieving, and processing of information. Technically a form of cognitive dysfunction, these symptoms are often described collectively as "chemo-brain." The condition is poorly understood, lacking a formal medical name and definition, and it can occur with no connection to chemotherapy. So I prefer to use the term "mind fog"—it's more descriptive, and it can be associated with causes other than chemo.

The more treatments you have, the larger and faster the changes in your body and your life, the higher your risk of mind fog. About 20 percent of individuals can be expected to experience this challenging condition after breast cancer diagnosis and treatment. While the changes in your ability to think, remember, and juggle tasks may be obvious to you, they are often invisible to others, so it's up to you to inform your doctor and seek treatment. How you perform your everyday tasks is probably the most practical test of how well you're functioning—a true reality check, helping you measure how you're doing now compared to the past.

MIND FOG TARGETS YOUR FRONTAL LOBES

The front of your brain, the frontal lobes, makes up about one-third of your brain and serves as the headquarters for controlling and coordinating your thinking, feeling, remembering, and action, including these important functions:

- **Executive function.** Involves your ability to manage yourself and get your act together. Includes high-level decision making, problem solving, and processing new information.
- **Short-term memory.** Holds simple information in your mind for a moment, like remembering a phone number just long enough to dial it, or repeating back something you were just told.
- **Working memory.** Retains information until you accomplish a given task, like remembering where you put your car in the parking lot just long enough to find your car and leave the lot.
- **Episodic memory.** Describes information and experiences that stick with you as long as you're motivated to remember them (for example, math tables or names of people at a family reunion).
- **Psychomotor speed.** The rate at which you can control, process, and coordinate your thoughts, memory, and actions (using the computer for instance, requires rapid attention as you scan and hit the right keys).

These frontal lobe functions are the most vulnerable to the effects of mind fog.

There are relatively reliable specialized questionnaire tests that assess learning issues, memory challenges, and mood problems such as stress, anxiety, and depression. These tests are usually conducted by a neuropsychologist. "For most people, chemo-related effects tend to be mild—although they may be troubling on a day-to-day basis. But when a person goes through a detailed battery of tests, we may see that performance is slightly less than what we'd expect for persons of that age, education, achievements, etc.," says Dr. Andrew Saykin, director of the Indiana University Center for Neuroimaging.

Tests that show what the brain physically *looks like* (such as CAT scans and regular MRIs) usually don't reveal any obvious changes. Any detectable changes are generally pretty subtle and difficult to hang any diagnosis on.

Tests that show how the brain *works* may show more specific changes. The pattern of brain activity on a PET scan or functional MRI (active parts of the brain take up a special contrast or tracer agent that shows up on the study) may reveal a weak area that partly explains your loss of function.

Causes of Mind Fog

Chemotherapy

There are a lot of important questions about the connection between chemotherapy and mind fog that we don't yet know the answers to. For starters:

- Is chemo the main cause of mind fog?
- Are specific chemotherapies—alone or in combination—more or less likely to contribute to the problem?
- Does the dose of chemo matter?
- Does the length of chemo matter?
- Is the foggy effect due in part to non-chemo-related factors: other treatments, other ongoing circumstances, or both?

In women who do seem to have mind fog due to chemotherapy, it's often hard to tell how much of chemotherapy's insult is due to a direct chemical effect on the brain versus an indirect effect such as plummeting hormone levels from early menopause (caused by the chemo shutting down the ovaries).

Researchers at the University of Texas M.D. Anderson Cancer Center have confirmed the presence of mind fog after chemotherapy treatment. But they also discovered that a significant number of patients (22 percent) had less than expected cognitive ability even before chemotherapy was started. So the trauma of the breast cancer experience alone can cause or greatly contribute to this condition.

The absence of solid answers to these important questions about the impact of chemo on your mental functioning is very frustrating. But at least this area is finally the focus of research by a number of talented investigators. (Breastcancer.org will have updates on the latest research information.)

Hormonal Changes

Decreasing estrogen levels inside your body is one of the most effective ways to stop the progression of breast cancer cells that depend upon estrogen for their growth—but it does a helluva job on your head.

As your body scrambles to adjust to the low estrogen levels, you may experience a wide range of symptoms that can contribute to mind fog: hot flashes, night sweats, insomnia, mood shifts, concentration and memory problems, and difficulty with smooth speaking (finding the right word when you want it).

In addition, if you're age forty or older, there is a significant risk that chemo will put you into early menopause, causing even more major and rapid hormonal changes. What might have happened naturally over five to ten years gets condensed into a few months. Wham! Mind fog can really get you in its grip.

Radiation Changes

Radiation to the brain to treat cancer cells there can cause mind fog—fatigue in particular, and loss of short-term memory. Radiation to the breast has no impact on mind fog, but the disruption of your routine required with six to seven weeks of daily radiation can tire you out and cause you to function less well overall.

Emotional Strain

The emotional chaos and disruption of your life upon diagnosis bear a good share of responsibility for mind fog.

Stress is a major trigger. A diagnosis brings on a wave of new information in what can seem like a foreign language, causing even a full professor of English to feel overwhelmed, confused, and "stupid." (I hate using that word, but it is so commonly used by the people I take care of to describe how they feel.)

Anxiety, depression, and self-doubt further pollute your feelings and thoughts. Given how complex your life can be and how finely tuned, highly coordinated, and overstretched you are, you quickly notice any change in how you function. So many of you, like the women I take care of, are working extra jobs on top of managing your primary job, home, and community responsibilities.

Adding to the list of emotional stressors are problems such as pain, sleep disturbance, and insomnia that can make mind fog worse, last longer, and leave you feeling even more disheartened. "I was stupid for a whole year. Slowly my smarts crept back over the following year. I'm finally pretty much back to normal."

One study found that a third of women experiencing chemo-brain had similar problems with cognitive function prior to treatment. In the M.D. Anderson study mentioned earlier, 22 percent of patients were found to have lower than expected cognitive abilities after diagnosis (and prior to treatment) but had no prediagnosis testing on record to determine if this low cognitive level was present before the whole breast cancer situation began.

You may have had a learning disability such as dyslexia or an attention deficit disorder all your life, which produced some of the same symptoms as mind fog, and then with the diagnosis and treatment of breast cancer, your symptoms got worse. Distinguishing old from new symptoms is difficult—often it's mostly the same symptoms, only amplified. This leads some people to have a previously undiagnosed cognitive disorder identified for the first time after being diagnosed with breast cancer.

Most if not all of the costs of your mind-fog evaluation and management should be covered by your health care insurance. But when insurance carriers see the term *psych* they may categorize the claim as a mental health benefit and deny the claim if you don't have that type of coverage. A letter of appeal, written by your neuropsychologist, primary care doctor, or medical oncologist, can help get the costs covered.

✣ Challenges

Wrapping Your Head Around Chemo-Brain

Many of my patients say they feel like they're losing their mind. I've heard some people describe it as a drought condition of the brain, like a plant that hasn't been watered. The leaves and buds of their words and memory have wilted and there's little sign of vitality. Mental activities that once were automatic as a young person and may have taken additional effort as a mature adult are now missing, flickering, or at half strength. Here are some of the common symptoms that people report:

- Missing and forgetting things, like a doctor's appointment, invitation to an event, kid's car pool, kettle on the stove, grocery items, the thing you ran upstairs to fetch
- Regularly losing things like your keys, glasses, and cell phone, or forgetting where you put your car in the parking lot
- Dropping, breaking, and bumping into things; slipping and falling: your cell phone falls into the toilet, the water glass drops out of your hand, you slip off the last step of stairs you've come down for years
- Less capable of multitasking; doing two or more things at once—like driving while talking on your cell phone—becomes even more dangerous (don't do it!)
- Trouble learning new things, like a new task at work, new financial forms and rules, or how a new electronic gadget works
- Being easily distracted, with trouble keeping your attention focused through completion of a task: you load the washing machine but forget to turn it on; you do the assignment but forget to pass it in; you can't remember the plot from one book chapter to the next

• Thinking slowly (in contrast to past speed), in figuring out how to get from here to there, coordinating your calendar, planning a trip, keeping up the pace at work, getting out the door in the morning

• Trouble managing your emotions and responding appropriately: feeling weepy, saying the wrong thing, lashing out

Many of these signs and symptoms relate to thought processing and memory, as well as coordinating these thoughts and feelings with physical actions. And all of these issues are worsened by emotional distress and any preexisting conditions or tendencies, such as attention deficit disorder or being accident prone. As with fatigue, you'll have to set realistic expectations for yourself and seek help if and when you need it.

Worst Nightmares: Alzheimer's, Dementia, Recurrence

The full range of mind fog symptoms can make you worry that you're on the verge of Alzheimer's disease or another type of dementia, or fearful that the cancer has gone to your brain.

Mind fog from breast cancer treatment can be distinguished

UNREALISTIC EXPECTATIONS AND SELF-DOUBT

The expectations you have for yourself are often greater than what others expect from you. With any change of your cognitive ability, you become hyperaware, compare yourself to others, and often feel worse about yourself. And since you're the one living with yourself twenty-four hours a day, seven days a week, you're likely to notice changes in yourself before most other people do. This can play out in a variety of ways. For example, you may:

• Become acutely aware and worry about your shortcomings—and amplify them

• Feel embarrassed or ashamed

• Experience a sense of failure

• Revert back to childhood patterns of behavior

• Lose touch and miss cues

• Find yourself in denial

These self-destructive tendencies can snowball, throwing you into the middle of a vicious cycle: self-doubt leads to loss of confidence, which leads to disappointing performance, and on and on. If you believe that others think you are slipping, ask a close friend or relative for honest feedback. Most important is to set realistic expectations for yourself and reach out for help. Getting better is your first priority.

from Alzheimer's and dementia relatively easily. Alzheimer's involves very significant defects in very specific areas: reasoning or problem solving, and loss of episodic memory (the kind of memory that sets, stores, and retrieves a record of your experiences). Confusion and trouble talking are also symptoms of dementia, including Alzheimer's. In contrast, mind fog involves minimal or very subtle nonspecific changes: inefficient thinking and acting, muddled memory. These are detectable by various tests. If you've developed relatively sudden onset of any of these symptoms and they've persisted or are getting worse, contact your doctor for an evaluation.

Brain involvement with cancer generally shows up with other types of specific symptoms, such as headache, nausea, or loss of a particular function, like weakness on one side of your body, trouble with balance, falling, or a change in vision. New onset of confusion and trouble talking can occur and get worse over time. (In contrast, mind fog tends to be mild and nonprogressive.) Testing for cancer involvement of the brain is straightforward, using an MRI or CAT scan together with an IV contrast agent.

Test Results Get Tricky and Muddy

To better understand the reasons for or causes of your symptoms, you'd ideally need a full and careful set of assessments:

- Recent, before-diagnosis assessment
- After-diagnosis, before-treatment assessment
- After-treatment evaluations and repeated studies at appropriate intervals

If you missed the before-diagnosis test, by the time you take the after-diagnosis/before-treatment assessment, you may already be struggling to think straight and control your emotions. If your first official evaluation occurs after treatment is over, you have no valid baseline because the test results may have been already "polluted" by the effects of your breast cancer diagnosis and treatments. Working with your doctor, however, you can figure out a rough starting point. Says Dr. Saykin, "If someone comes in for whom I have no pre-chemo data, but they have significant complaints, we can figure out what their baseline would be (based on age, education, etc.) and then we figure out what we'd expect their function to be. Then we can work on a comparison."

Emotional distress during test taking—especially anxiety—interferes with your ability to perform executive functioning, and can result in a misleading interpretation of your cognitive test results. That's why it's so important to address your emotional concerns, to free up your mind to do the work of thinking, feeling, remembering, speaking, and acting.

✿ Solutions

O f one thing you can be absolutely sure: there is no single simple solution for mind fog because there is no single cause of its symptoms. The first step is to obtain an evaluation of your situation. From there, a combination and/or sequence of simple and small solutions can add up to results that can make you feel much better and carry you along till mind fog recedes. In the meantime, try not to be discouraged.

"We want our patients to know that we are trying to understand what happens and that there are a wide variety of therapies available to help them," says Christina Meyers, professor of neuropsychology at the M.D. Anderson Cancer Center in Houston, Texas. "We have a whole platter of treatments to choose from that can help patients, from medications to accepted alternative therapies."

Find the Right Health Care Professionals to Guide You

No one doctor or specialist can handle this kind of challenge. Start with your primary care physician. She or he can consult with the appropriate members of your cancer treatment team and bring in other experts, depending on your situation. Here are your possible team members:

- A medical oncologist, if you've had chemo or are on hormonal therapy
- A neuropsychologist, who is a health care professional (typically

based in a neurology or psychiatry practice) specializing in how your mind learns, thinks, remembers, and coordinates thoughts with actions
- A neurologist, who is a doctor specializing in the brain and nervous system, including how your mind and body thinks, moves, and feels
- A physiatrist (rehabilitation specialist), who focuses on rehabilitation and recovery after a devastating event or illness such as a stroke or head trauma
- A psychiatrist, a doctor who specializes in your behavior, emotional well-being, and distress, including anxiety, depression, and post-traumatic stress disorder.

The complex causes of mind fog can go well beyond breast cancer–related issues. It is essential that you and your doctor rule out any other manageable causes of these symptoms: depression, weakening of the heart, thyroid problems, sleep disorders, Lyme disease, chronic fatigue syndrome, previously undiagnosed learning disability, major loss or stress (death of a child, spouse, or parent; divorce; loss of a job and health insurance; foreclosure of your house; struggles with teenage children).

Despite the negative impact of these illnesses and unfortunate circumstances, many of these issues and situations can be treated and/or significantly improved.

Safety First

When you are not feeling and functioning at your best, you must be extra careful. Safety is a major concern. Fatigue, anxiety, discomfort, stiffness, numbness, and more can throw off your balance, equilibrium, and spatial perception, making you more likely to stumble, fall, bump into things, cut or burn yourself, or get into a motor vehicle accident—even burn your house down.

To put safety first, you have to get practical and take some immediate steps in each arena of your life—home, work, and community. Here are some dos and don'ts to follow:

Decrease trippers, slippers, and bumpers

- Do anchor area rugs with a pad or heavy furniture.
- Do widen the walkways between furniture.
- Do put bumpers around corners of pointed furniture.
- Don't wear very high heels or platform shoes.
- Don't wear wide-legged pants.
- Don't store stuff on the stairs.
- Don't lift heavy objects or work with heavy machinery.

Accident-proof your house

- Do check your hot water heater setting so you don't burn yourself.
- Do install a gate at the top of any stairs that you tend to slip on; it will force you to stop and slow down.
- Don't put poisons or other harsh chemicals in high places where they can fall off and spill.
- Don't overload upper cabinets, to avoid a potential avalanche when opening the cabinet door.

Slow down

- Do pace yourself: break down jobs into smaller units and attack them in order one at a time.
- Do eat and drink slowly, particularly with foods you could easily choke on, such as meat, apples, and carrots.
- Do make sure to catch important conversations: ask people to repeat what they've just said, take notes, or use a tape recorder.
- Do drive at no more than the speed limit.
- Don't drive aggressively.
- Don't enter situations or accept tasks that require quick thinking (let someone else accept the crossing-guard job at a busy corner).
- Don't hesitate to ask for help.

Avoid multitasking disasters

- Do fasten your safety belt before you turn on the car engine.
- Do focus on the task at hand and minimize distractions.
- Don't eat and talk at the same time, to reduce your risk of choking.
- Don't pick a fight or argue when you're very upset. Wait until you're more clearheaded and able to construct a thoughtful

discussion, obtaining the results you're seeking. (Unless it's really worth it, save your personal energy for more important issues.)

• Don't do anything potentially dangerous (like chopping onions with a sharp knife) while experiencing distressing thoughts (after an argument with an unruly teenager or a fuming husband).

Push Back

Like many of the high-powered women I take care of, you, too, are probably trying to do way too much and are stretched beyond your limits. This is particularly true if you're dealing with mind fog, because you're even more limited and are in unfamiliar territory. It's time to cut back on some of your daily responsibilities and demands, and to develop reasonable expectations for yourself. But hold on to the activities, routines, and rituals that give your life meaning and joy.

If you keep pushing to "do it all," you may reach your breaking point—if you haven't done so already. On occasion, I'll have a patient who doesn't take my warning seriously enough, who keeps pressing way past her limit, and I've had to step in to make her slow down or stop. To make things easier for her to cut back, I can help with communications: a doctor's phone call or note to her employer to explain necessary time off from work or to family members to excuse her from day-to-day responsibilities. This might mean moving from full-time to part-time work or even taking short-term disability. (There is a reason why these benefits exist.) See Chapter 2, on support, and Chapter 8, on fatigue, to learn how to conserve your precious personal energy reserves.

Emotional Care and Support

If emotional challenges such as depression and anxiety are intruding into your life, look at how you might seek help and better manage these problems. "It's vital to be able to reassure patients that mind fog can be a normal consequence of the breast cancer experience and its treatment," says Dr. Christina Meyers.

Your cancer center may be the place to go for your emotional care. Ask your primary care physician for guidance on best next steps: individual counselor (psychologist, psychiatrist, social worker); executive or life coach; group therapy, support groups; yoga, meditation, acupuncture/acupressure, massage, or other complementary therapies.

Many people turn to Breastcancer.org's online community chat rooms and discussion boards for support and practical advice. You can participate in support groups through the Wellness Community, Gilda's Club, or SHARE, or at your local hospital. Or you can pick up the phone and call a trained breast cancer survivor at the Network of Strength's YourShoes 24/7 Hotline (previously called Y-me, 800-221-2141) or at the Living Beyond Breast Cancer Helpline (888-753-5222).

GET ORGANIZED

Here are some suggested tools to help you supplement and reinforce your executive functioning, memory, and thinking.

- **Calendar system** (pocket-size, desktop, or computer-, phone-, or Blackberry-based) to provide you with regular organizational structure and an up-to-date daily schedule. Make appointments only when your reminder system is open in front of you, and record the full names and contact information of people from whom you've accepted invitations, as well as the start and end of any meeting.
- **Lists** to assist in your ability to gather, track and prioritize all of your must-dos—from grocery lists to call lists.
- **Menus** to help you plan, cook, and serve your meals each day. Use a favorite cookbook or online recipe site for assistance.
- **Directions** to help you get to your destination faster and safer without getting lost. MapQuest, Google Maps, GPS, and AAA maps are all great options.
- **Instructions** to provide clear steps on how to execute tasks or operate a device. Owner's manuals and the like remove the guesswork and frustration when you encounter a new task.

On a daily basis, each of these aids can help you feel more capable, effective, organized, confident, and in control of your life. And rather than depend on your memory and organizational skills for the mundane everyday tasks, list making and other prompts can help you conserve your precious mental energy for more important responsibilities.

Memory Aids and Organizing Systems

Given the negative impact that mind fog has on your executive functioning, you will need tools and tricks to help you remember and organize your tasks and responsibilities, document progress at work and home, establish a daily routine, and build your confidence. "My day starts with a three-by-five card that tells me what I must get done. I depend on this easy reminder system, even though my brain is working pretty well at the moment. Anything I wear must have pockets, to hold these cards and a pen, so I can add items and cross others off."

Build Brainpower

Your brain is your most powerful organ even when it's running a deficit. It can still do amazing things—and once it recovers, it will perform even better for you. But it's going to take a long time to bounce back; patience and persistence are necessary. You really do have to believe.

You can do a lot to offset the severity of your symptoms by sharpening your skills, practicing your routine, removing self-doubt, building your confidence, protecting your rest, and nourishing your mind.

Dr. Martha Denckla, a widely acclaimed developmental neurologist, prescribes practical ways to reinforce your ability to learn new information. Combine mental activity with a physical activity—like taking notes when you're listening to a lecture. Social interaction can turn a dry, boring learning experience into one that's memorable. Getting a tutor to help learn the material or taking a class with a buddy might work well for you. Rather than read a book on your own, join a book club. Finally, great learning can come from teaching. Showing someone else how to do something reinforces your knowledge and stimulates your thinking.

Exercise Your Mind

Working your brain can significantly improve mind fog. Here are a bunch of different mental exercises that you can do:

- Hum, sing, or belt out your favorite songs. Try a karaoke bar.
- Read out loud: rhymes and joke books (comes with the side

benefit of a good laugh), poetry, treasured books from your childhood, storybooks, newspapers, magazines.

- Say your prayers, chant your mantras.
- Expand your vocabulary—carry a small dictionary or thesaurus around with you.
- Learn a new language a few words, and phrases at a time.
- Listen to books on tape.
- Memorize poems and great short speeches.
- Have fun with word games, crossword puzzles, Boggle, Scrabble, etc.
- Practice math tables; solve math word problems.
- Play card games such as Concentration and solitaire.
- Enjoy relaxing and comforting activities such as quilting or knitting.
- Mix up your exercise routine to get variety and avoid boredom—it will invigorate your mind.

You can perform these functions better by consuming a balanced diet with quality foods, plenty of liquids, and rest.

Rest Your Mind

During the day, take regular mental time-outs. Try setting aside five minutes every half hour to stop what you're doing, turn off the worries and thoughts, and focus inward on your energy and breathing. Meditation, visualization, yoga, or regular prayer can also help you handle the stress of mind fog and make you more awake to experiencing life.

It's impossible to overestimate the importance of regular restful sleep for anyone recovering from breast cancer—particularly if you are dealing with mind fog. Sleep tucks in your feelings, organizes your thoughts, and cleans up your concerns, making you fresh and ready for action the following day. An occasional short nap can refresh you (but too much napping can steal from your higher-quality nighttime sleep). To learn much more about how to practice sleep hygiene and get the rest that you need, turn to Chapter 15.

Medications

If you didn't get enough improvement from the other measures described in this chapter, talk to your doctor about medications that might help. Because mind fog can be due to one or more causes across a broad spectrum, there is no one medication specifically designed to help people with mind fog. The best approach is to work with your doctor to identify the best treatment for the specific symptoms that are bothering you the most. Here are some examples:

- *Caffeine.* If your speech is loosey-goosey, your thoughts are unfocused, and your energy drags each morning, something as simple as caffeine (from tea, coffee, Coke, Mountain Dew, Yoo-Hoo—whatever) might improve your ability to function. (But be aware of its possible negative effect on your nighttime sleep.)
- *Antianxiety and depression medication.* Mind fog can be made much worse by panic attacks, anxiety, and depression. Individual counseling and medication can make a very big difference in the way you feel and function. Consult with your primary care doctor or a psychiatrist to find the right medication and dosage. (Watch out for interactions between these types of medications and tamoxifen; see Chapter 7.)
- *Attention-focusing medicines.* If you have mind fog and everything takes you much longer and requires more effort than ever before, then you might run out of energy and focus before completing your everyday tasks and responsibilities. If nothing else you've tried has made a big enough difference, ask your doctor if you might benefit from a medication such as Provigil (modafinil), a stimulant that's sometimes used for people dealing with mind fog (although this use is without official FDA approval). If you were already on medication for an attention deficit problem (for example, with Adderall or Ritalin) and now you're experiencing mind fog, your doctor may need to reevaluate your treatment plan, including the choice of medicine and the dose.
- *Other medications.* You doctor might suggest other medications if you still have significant symptoms despite trying other measures and medications described in this section. While most forms of mind fog are distinct from Alzheimer's, some people might have

an overlap of symptoms and may respond to medication that tends to be helpful to people struggling with this form of dementia. For example, a patient who was very forgetful before breast cancer and whose symptoms get worse after breast cancer may respond to the medication Aricept (only approved for the treatment of people with Alzheimer's-type dementia; untested in people with mind fog). This medication should only be prescribed by a neurologist or psychiatrist who specializes in this area of medicine.

Whenever someone takes a medication, there can be side effects. Sometimes those side effects become a real problem and may require treatment. For example, mental stimulant medications such as Ritalin can worsen anxiety; successful anxiety treatment with Paxil can leave you feeling disorganized.

Make sure any medication you take is prescribed for *you* by your doctor and does not interfere with the effectiveness of your other medicines (for example, Paxil can decrease tamoxifen's effectiveness). Do not take anybody else's medicines—it's much too risky.

✣ Moving Forward

With or without medications, the good news is that most mind fog symptoms improve over time. Many people are able to remember and think more clearly six months to a year after completion of treatment—with further improvement to follow.

More good news is the publication of two significant books on mind fog: *Chemobrain* by Ellen Clegg (Prometheus Books) and *Your Brain After Chemo* by Dr. Daniel Silverman and Idelle Davidson (DaCapo Press).

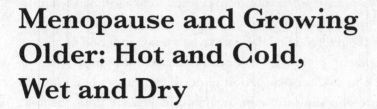

CHAPTER FOURTEEN

Menopause and Growing Older: Hot and Cold, Wet and Dry

I'm thirty-five going on seventy after that chemo, starting out each day stiff and poky. My kids fly around me, even my mother moves faster than I do. I finally pick up speed by midday, then I'm okay till 7:00 p.m., crash by 9:00, and it starts all over again the next morning.

When I look in the mirror there's an old woman, but the spirit inside me isn't yet fifty. Why is "old" such a dirty word?

I had a lumpectomy, radiation, and then a hysterectomy. The hardest part was I couldn't produce estrogen and I couldn't take it. It was devastating to my sex life. But I started on alternatives, Catapres and an occasional Bellergal, and I began to use Astroglide, and they all helped. The bottom line: my husband's been great and we're good.

My thermostat is completely broken. One minute I'm hot and dripping with sweat, the next minute I'm freezing and shaking cold. There's no way I can predict when the floodgates or the ice age will come on—or how to stop them. I'm stuck feeling exhausted, miserable, and sorry for myself.

✣ First Things First

Your hormones set you on a lifelong roller-coaster ride: on and off, up and down. Estrogen, progesterone, and testosterone launch you into adolescence, when your ovaries respond to age-timed brain signals. Ovulation and menstruation follow, leading into your most fertile years, until about forty. Then there's maybe a ten-year period of gradual decline in ovarian production of hormones, called the climacteric, followed by a one- to three-year period of perimenopause, when estrogen and progesterone levels dip even further and become unpredictable. Your periods become irregular; hot flashes flare; moods get edgy. Eventually hormone production drops below the level sufficient to keep your periods going, menstruation stops, your ability to reproduce ends, and there you are: menopause.

Menopause officially starts twelve consecutive months after your last period. Natural menopause occurs at a median age of about fifty-one, and for many women menopause comes on gently, after a long, smooth, and easy hormonal slide. But breast cancer treatment can bring on an early and abrupt menopause, with your production of hormones coming to a screeching stop.

Treatment-Induced Menopause

Menopause can be brought on early and quickly by various medical and surgical interventions. Certain chemotherapy medicines (depending on the agent, dose, and frequency) and hormonal therapies (Zoladex and Lupron) can push your ovaries into early retirement. The older you are, the higher the risk of early menopause.

Menopausal symptoms occur from hormonal therapies' direct and indirect effects on your body's hormone receptors. Aromatase inhibitors (Arimidex, Femara, Aromasin) and ovarian removal and shutdown measures all decrease the amount of estrogen that makes it to the estrogen receptors. Although aromatase inhibitors are only given to postmenopausal women, they can bring on or worsen menopausal symptoms in this way. While the effect of low estrogen on the breast is desirable, the deprivation of estrogen can have profound negative effects on bone and muscle, cholesterol metabolism, energy, hair and nail growth, and cognitive abilities.

The group of medications called selective estrogen receptor modulators (SERMs; tamoxifen and raloxifene) do not bring on early menopause unless you're on the threshold of menopause, in which case they may tip you in somewhat earlier. But they do often cause other menopause-related symptoms, as they directly target the estrogen receptor with both antiestrogen and estrogenic activity, which may be desirable or undesirable:

- Desired antiestrogen activity: inhibits breast cell growth
- Desired estrogenlike effects: reduces cholesterol, keeps bones strong

ESTROGEN RECEPTORS: WHERE HORMONES EXERT THEIR POWER

All female hormones interact with your cells through estrogen receptors, which are like little locks that can only be unlocked by an estrogen key. Once the estrogen key is in its receptor lock, the cells' activities are turned on and growth occurs. There are various estrogen receptors in your body, each with unique "assignments."

- Brain estrogen receptors control your body's thermostat (hot flashes), memory, sleep, and concentration.
- Breast estrogen receptors are responsible for breast cell growth.
- Uterine estrogen receptors stimulate uterine lining and wall cells.
- Bone estrogen receptors determine bone mass and strength.
- Liver estrogen receptors process both sex hormones and cholesterol.

How these receptors function differs widely, depending on the following:

- The number of receptors available for interaction with the hormone (measured as hormone receptor positivity) and the condition and configuration of the receptors (whether they're in the mood for action)
- The various types and amounts of estrogen and estrogenlike substances that are in the vicinity of the receptor
- The presence or absence of co-activators—other proteins and complex molecules that interact with estrogen and the estrogen receptor

- Unwanted estrogenlike effects: overstimulates the lining of the uterus and is associated with an increased risk of endometrial cancer (with long-term use in postmenopausal women)
- Unwanted antiestrogen side effects: causes hot flashes, vaginal dryness, hair thinning

It would be great to find the perfect molecular compound to turn on all the right receptors throughout your body (in cholesterol and

HORMONAL THERAPY VERSUS HORMONE REPLACEMENT THERAPY

The terms used to describe various hormone treatments can be confusing. Here are the different terms and what they mean:

- **Hormone replacement therapy (HRT)** is the most common term used to describe the use of estrogen (with or without progesterone) to ease the signs and symptoms of menopause. HRT increases the estrogen blood level between the usual premenopausal and postmenopausal values. For women who have undergone a medical or surgical menopause while in their thirties or forties, the concept of hormone *replacement* therapy remains appropriate (you're restoring estrogen levels to where they're supposed to be). But the term *replacement* is not accurate for women who go through natural menopause because nothing is missing (it's normal to have low estrogen levels during and after menopause).
- **Menopausal hormone therapy (MHT)** is a more appropriate term to describe the use of estrogen to treat menopausal symptoms in women who have gone through menopause.
- **Hormonal therapy** and **antiestrogen therapy** are the terms used to describe medicines that decrease estrogen levels or block the effects of estrogen on breast cells (normal cells and cancer cells).

I took care of an eighty-four-year-old woman who had just been diagnosed with serious breast cancer. More important to her, however, she had just been taken off the menopausal estrogen replacement treatment that she had been using for forty years. "Menopause at eighty-four stinks," she announced. Still a very healthy woman, her next step was antiestrogen hormonal therapy to combat her breast cancer.

TEST FOR MENOPAUSE

You may not know whether you have actually gone into menopause. You may have been finished with chemotherapy for six months, had your last period ten months ago, and be wondering now if your periods will ever return. Or you might have had a hysterectomy, so your periods have stopped, but you still have your ovaries, and you're not sure if they're still working. Special blood hormone tests can help you and your doctors figure out your menopausal status. These blood tests measure follicle-stimulating hormone (FSH) and luteinizing hormone (LH). Both hormones are made by the brain to stimulate each month's ovulation by the ovaries. If your ovaries are beyond menopause, they cease to respond to FSH and LH, and your brain reacts by sending out even more of these hormones. Persistent elevated levels of FSH (13 to 90 milli–international units per milliliter) and LH (15 to 50 mIU/mL) are consistent with being in menopause.

Another blood test that can help assess your internal hormonal environment is your estradiol level, although levels can vary significantly from one woman to another. Normal estrogen levels before menopause peak at 150 to 300 picograms per milliliter each month (depending on where you are in your menstrual cycle), falling to less than 20 pg/mL after ovarian function declines.

These blood tests are not the final answer to whether or not you are in menopause, however. Temporary ovarian shutdown can produce postmenopausal levels of FSH, LH, and estrogen. If someday in the future your ovaries decide to wake up and get back to work, FSH and LH levels will drop and estrogen levels will rise. Your periods can return even after a long break (see Chapter 20 on fertility).

Other factors that help sort out the answer are timing and repeat testing. The longer your menstrual periods have been stopped, the less likely that they will return. If you have serial blood hormone test results over twelve to eighteen months that are consistent with menopause, without any inching back toward premenopause, you are most likely in permanent menopause. That said, I have one patient who resumed her periods after three and a half years and several others who had their periods return between eighteen months and three years. Keep this in mind if you are sexually active: use birth control if you do not want to become pregnant—or until you're sure that you're in menopause for good.

mental processing, bone, vagina, and brain) and to shut off the "wrong" receptors in the breast and the uterus. (Many scientists are working on it.)

Stopping postmenopausal hormone replacement therapy (HRT) upon a diagnosis of breast cancer can bring on a flood of recurrent menopausal symptoms. These may be the very symptoms you were taking HRT to get rid of. This combination of natural and medical menopause—characterized by a significant drop in estrogen when discontinuing HRT—can feel like "cold turkey" menopause.

Severity of Menopausal Symptoms

How mild or severe your menopausal symptoms are depends on how fast your transition to menopause occurs and how much back-up estrogen your body has from other sources, such as adrenal gland androgens (which are converted to estrogens by fat and muscle cells—the more fat you have, the higher the level of non-ovarian-produced estrogen). My patients say natural menopause is like a fender bender, whereas medical or surgical menopause can be like hitting a brick wall at sixty miles an hour.

A major sustained drop in hormone levels can make you feel much older than you are or than your menopausal symptoms would suggest. If you are thirty-five and caught in medical menopause, your ovaries may have gone into early retirement, but the rest of your body is still that of a thirty-five-year-old woman. Thus it's a challenge to bring how you are feeling closer to what your actual age is. Your hormones are playing the notes, but your age is the keyboard—probably the most important factor in how you respond to what life is throwing at you at any particular moment.

Regardless of the shifts in your hormone levels and no matter what your age is, relieving troublesome symptoms and feeling well as you grow older deserve your highest priority and require a strong ongoing commitment. Support, expert advice, and guidance from your doctors, nurses, family, friends, and co-workers are also essential. This chapter gives you a solid place to start.

❧ Challenges

Your experience of menopause may have been uneventful up until this point, maybe even gratifying: you've reached your late forties or fifties, your family is on its way to independence, you're looking ahead instead of back, and you're not sad to see the end of monthly blood flow and emotional ups and downs.

But for many of you, menopause on top of a breast cancer diagnosis is more than a major disruption. It can wreck your sex life, dash hopes of having a baby, trigger mood swings, produce debilitating hot flashes, cause weight gain, drain your energy, worsen aches and pains, bring on jealousy or anger or resentment, and leave you feeling bad about yourself.

"Isn't breast cancer enough? I need this insult, too?" You may find it's these menopausal changes, not the breast cancer or the immediate effects of treatment, that may interfere most with your day-to-day quality of life.

Physical Effects of Menopause

As you approach menopause (or you're propelled into it), the immediate issues are usually the in-your-face symptoms: hot flashes, weight gain, dry vagina, mood swings and depression, loss of energy, memory loss, skin and hair changes, and muscle and joint aches. Long-range issues are osteoporosis, heart and vascular disease, and how to live a full and reasonably happy life. This chapter will focus primarily on hot flashes; other chapters go into depth on weight (Chapter 18), fatigue (Chapter 8), thinking and remembering (Chapter 13), bone health (Chapter 12), and sleep (Chapter 15).

Hot Flashes

Most women experience mild hot flashes, but if you are taking hormonal therapy on top of early menopause you can experience severe and debilitating hot flashes. They can hit hard, bringing on a sudden, intense hot sensation on your face and upper body, preceded and perhaps accompanied by rapid heartbeat and sweating; sometimes they are accompanied by nausea, dizziness, anxiety, headache, weakness, or a suffocating haze. "It's not like being hot, it's like being on fire!" Some women have an "aura," an uneasy feeling just before the hot flash that lets them know what's coming.

Hot flashes are primarily caused by a drop in estrogen levels that confuses the brain's thermostat (the hypothalamus) and make it read "too hot." The brain responds to this wildcat report by broadcasting an all-out chemical alert to the heart, blood vessels, and nervous system: *Get rid of the heat!* In response, your heart pumps faster, the blood vessels in your skin dilate to circulate more blood to radiate off the heat, and your sweat glands release sweat to cool you off even more. (Skin temperature can rise 10 degrees Fahrenheit during a hot flash.) The excess sweat cools you down quickly—making you feel cold. Blood vessels clamp down to conserve heat. You may end up shivering to warm yourself back up again.

Eighty-five percent of the women in the United States experience hot flashes as they approach menopause and for the first year or two after their periods stop. Twenty to 50 percent of women continue to have them for many more years. As time goes on, the intensity does decrease.

If you've had breast cancer, hot flashes can follow the same pattern as for women in general, or they can be more intense and last longer, particularly if:

- You went through early menopause.
- You are taking hormonal therapy and your body is still having trouble adjusting to it.

There is considerable variation in time of onset, duration, frequency, and the nature of hot flashes, whether a woman has had breast cancer or not. An episode can last a few seconds or a few minutes, occasionally even an hour, and it can take another half hour for you to feel yourself again. The most common time of onset is between six and eight in the morning and six and ten at night.

Vaginal and Vulva Dryness, Irritation, and Pain

During chemotherapy, sores of the vulva and vagina can appear. On top of that downer, chemotherapy and/or antiestrogen hormonal therapies can lead to a drop in estrogen level and early menopause. Gone is your sex life. Even without the direct effects of breast cancer therapy, the drop in estrogen after a natural menopause can lead to vaginal thinning, loss of elasticity, and decreased lubrication. Sexual intercourse may be uncomfortable or painful. Your libido can disappear.

Other tissues right around the vagina may also be affected. Your vulva can become so sensitive that it may be hard to sit, walk long distances, or have intercourse. Itching can also be a problem. In addition, you may experience burning on urination, involving your urethra (the opening through which your urine comes out) and the sensitive tissues right around it (inside the vulva, your clitoris, and the bottom of your vagina). (See Chapter 19 for more information about intimacy.)

BOILING OVER

About 10 to 15 percent of women in the general population experience severe hot flashes for which they seek medical attention. The tendency to suffer debilitating hot flashes is higher for women who have had breast cancer.

The faster you go through the transition from regular periods to no periods, the more significant your hot flashes will be. Hot flashes are severe after surgical menopause, and they can also be quite difficult after a chemotherapy-induced medical menopause. If you haven't been warned about hot flashes, a sudden severe episode can be frightening; you might even confuse the flash with a heart attack.

In a study randomizing women with breast cancer to tamoxifen or placebo, 13 percent of women on tamoxifen for a year experienced severe hot flashes, compared with 3 percent of women taking a placebo. The intensity of hot flashes accompanying treatment with tamoxifen eventually improves for most women (but not all) after the first three to six months.

Heavy or muscular women tend to experience fewer and less severe hot flashes than thin women because of the conversion of androstenedione into a type of estrogen, estrone, by fat and muscle cells. But if these women are taking an aromatase inhibitor that blocks estrone production, hot flashes can become significant. Smokers may have prolonged hot flashes: their blood vessels don't expand well enough to accommodate the increased blood flow that helps release the extra heat.

Wrinkles and Sun Damage

Okay, so wrinkles and other skin changes are not much of an issue compared to breast cancer, but they still may be important to you. They are to many women—how else would all those cosmetic specialists and manufacturers rake in billions for collagen, Botox, and Restylane injections and moisturizing creams if we didn't care about how our skin looks?

Wrinkles are often attributed to menopause, but they are more properly attributed to aging and lifestyle factors. That's because natural menopause comes at a time when the cumulative effects of sun exposure, smoking, aging, gravity, and genetic predisposition produce wrinkles—especially wrinkles on the face. There is no evidence that chemotherapy or tamoxifen causes wrinkles, and the hormonal flux of menopause contribute relatively little to the development of wrinkles. Instead, it's believed that aged skin has less supportive tissue beneath it, so it loses some of its fullness; add in ever-present gravity and sun exposure and you've got little sags and bags as well as wrinkles.

Your genetic makeup contributes to how resilient your skin is. If your mother went wrinkle-free into her seventies, you can probably skip the skin care creams; if your mother had weathered creases and lines by her sixties without heavy sun exposure or smoking to blame for the effects, expect similar evidence of aging, and save up for sunscreen and anti-wrinkle products like Retin-A. Although exposure to the sun is probably the most significant lifestyle cause of wrinkles, smoking runs a close second. Smoking constricts the little blood vessels that nourish the skin and results in three times as many wrinkles as in women who don't smoke.

Heart Health

One out of eight or nine women gets breast cancer, and one out of two or three women gets heart disease, but more women fear breast cancer than heart disease. This thinking is backward because 30 percent of all women die of heart disease, compared to the much smaller percentage who die of breast cancer.

Women who have had breast cancer are as much at risk of heart disease as all other women, and that risk increases most significantly with age. However, some of the treatments for breast cancer can further increase the risk of heart disease, including adriamycin chemotherapy, Herceptin, and radiation to the heart (although side effects to the heart are rare today with improved radiation techniques). If your doctor treats the internal mammary lymph nodes that are located just beneath the chest wall on each side of the breastbone, the risk of heart side effects increases. Radiation to the left breast that excludes the heart (located on the left) should have no risk of heart disease. You have a 10 percent risk of developing heart muscle weakness, or cardiomyopathy, if you take adriamycin in doses of more than 450 mg per square meter. (Most women receive only about 350 mg with a six-cycle treatment course.) Herceptin can cause weakening of the heart muscle that's usually reversible when caught early and the medicine is stopped.

Other risk factors in your life have a major effect on heart disease: high blood pressure, high cholesterol, diabetes, or a family history of early heart disease. Smoking, obesity, a sedentary lifestyle, and diet are also very important factors.

Psychological Effects of Menopause

Sadness and Depression

While studies show that natural menopause is not associated with a greater risk of depression, an abrupt onset of early menopause together with its rapid decline in hormone levels can throw you into a depression similar to postpartum depression. Sadness can combine with depression to drain the color from your world. Sadness is a natural part of your breast cancer experience, something you need to express and move through. If you don't allow yourself to feel sad and grieve, the unresolved grief gets in the way of feeling better, getting better, and moving on. Besides a feeling of sadness, depression can include:

- An inability to cope
- An overwhelming feeling of helplessness and hopelessness
- Inertia and lack of motivation
- Inability to concentrate
- Memory problems
- Panic attacks
- Loss of pleasure in what used to make you happy

- Lack of interest in sex or food
- Sleep problems

These are all possible signs of clinical depression, and all of these stresses, strains, and losses affect your well-being.

✣ Solutions

Y ou may have only a few menopausal symptoms, or you may have every one in the book. If they began because of a medical or surgical menopause, and if a particular symptom is especially debilitating for you, you may be highly motivated and anxious to get help.

Treatment recommendations involve a range of suggestions covering lifestyle choices, complementary therapies, and conventional medications. Most effective therapies and remedies carry some risks; they're worth taking only if the potential benefits clearly outweigh the side effects. Start with the simplest, mildest step with the broadest benefit and the smallest sacrifice or least number of side effects. If step one doesn't do the trick, then gradually move on to more significant shifts in lifestyle and/or stronger forms or amounts of treatment.

Managing Hot Flashes

The most effective way to treat hot flashes is through prevention, and figuring out the various factors that send your temperature soaring is your first step to finding the best solutions. To identify your hot flash triggers and patterns of onset, keep a record of the where, what, when, and how:

- When did they occur (day or night, work or home, weekdays or weekends)?
- What were you doing at the time?
- How were you feeling at the time?
- What other symptoms did you have at the time?
- How long did they last?
- How often do they occur?
- What makes them go away?

Any patterns should lead you to an examination of the small and big choices you make throughout each day and night, so you can avoid the triggers and utilize the coolers of your hot flashes.

Avoid triggers

- Stop smoking.
- Limit use of caffeine and alcohol.
- Avoid spicy foods and hot (temperature) foods.
- Limit weight gain.
- Don't wear wool or nonbreathable synthetics, and be wary of silk. (Look at the bright side: You'll save on cleaning and you can stop worrying about moths.)
- Avoid turtlenecks and bulky clothes.
- Stay away from hot tubs, saunas, hot showers, hot rooms, and hot weather.
- Reduce stress and anxiety. Allow more time to plan your work, rehearse your presentations, make deadlines, commute between meetings and arrive on time (or early). Avoid medications that can make you anxious (like diet and performance meds).
- Control expectations: don't set yourself up to fall short or fail.

Use coolers

- Dress in thin layers, so you can peel them off to cool down or put them back on to warm up once the hot flash ends.
- Pick clothing that allows you to release the extra heat quickly. Stick with open-neck and button-front shirts in natural fabrics (cotton, rayon, hemp, linen, etc.).
- Experiment with quick-drying fabrics that won't retain heat and don't stay wet (like athletic garments made by Under Armour and Nike).
- Wear pajamas or a nightgown—if you perspire a lot at night, nightclothes are easier to change than the sheets. Use cotton sheets only, not synthetics.
- Keep ice water at hand throughout the day in an insulated cup so you can sip to cool down your insides and stay well hydrated.

- Lower the house or room or workplace thermostat where possible.
- Use a room air conditioner, ceiling fan, or desk fan.
- On the go, try a little handheld battery-operated fan or the old-fashioned foldable kind you flutter in front of your face.
- Get the coolest seat at work meetings and in your home (near an open window, a fan, or the air conditioner).
- Try poking your head in the freezer at home (or in the market) when a hot flash hits.
- Try a cool nighttime shower just before going to bed.
- Get a bigger bed if you and your partner are on different heat planets but you still want to stay in close orbit. Getting a good night's sleep is also very important.
- Keep up regular physical activity and exercise.
- Use relaxation techniques: meditation, yoga, visualization, chanting, prayer, breathing exercises, biofeedback techniques, or hypnosis to avoid stress and shorten the hot flash or lessen its severity.
- Consider acupuncture or acupressure.

Use your symptom journal to chart your progress. If your hot flashes are still interfering with your quality of life, additional steps beyond prevention are in order.

Your first approach to treatment should be the most practical, useful, gentle, natural, and least invasive. Instead of estrogen therapy, consider less drastic, non-pharmaceutical measures first, partly because estrogen therapy is not believed safe for women with a history of breast cancer. Careful exercise is an example of a solution that involves a lot of work and an investment of time (and sometimes money), but it comes with a big payoff and nearly no side effects. It strengthens your bones and heart, controls weight, lessens hot flashes, improves your sleep, boosts your energy, revs up your sex drive, and makes your skin glow.

Diet Changes

Making changes in your diet to maximize your energy, manage your weight, and control hot flashes usually involves sticking to small, light, regular meals with relatively few calories, less fat, and more vegetables

and fruit, without heavy sauces or spices, served cold, room temperature, or warmed (not hot). Think of it as being more like bird food than
bear food.

EXERCISE, EXERCISE, EXERCISE

Increasing your level of activity and integrating exercise into your life can
reduce hot flashes and have a positive impact on just about every other symptom attributed to menopause and growing older. Regular exercise increases
endorphin levels, resulting in:

- Higher pain threshold
- Fewer mood swings
- Perkier libido
- Better sleep

Healthy muscle tissue helps:

- Provide a natural low level of estrogens for maintenance of basic
  function
- Push and pull against bones to keep them strong
- Keep your metabolism up, which slims you down

Exercise maximizes the health of your heart and blood vessels, which
helps you:

- Stay alert and energized
- Release excess heat from hot flashes
- Lower the risk of heart disease

Exercise increases metabolism and facilitates even distribution of weight,
helping you:

- Lose weight and keep it off
- Retain your curves and minimize weight buildup in your middle
- Enhance your self-image

Plus, regular exercise is associated with a lower risk of breast cancer. There
is no pill big enough or strong enough to give you all the lifesaving and life-
enhancing benefits of regular exercise. Shoot for a goal of three to four hours
of exercise per week (thirty minutes a day) in order to capture all these big
benefits.

Traditional Chinese Medicine for Menopausal Symptoms

Chinese medicine has a long tradition of evaluating and treating menopausal symptoms. The tradition distinguishes between a "hot" menopause and a "cold" menopause as well as between various kinds of hot flashes.

Chinese medical practitioners start by taking a full history and performing a complete physical examination, with particular attention to your tongue and pulse. Treatment usually involves a combination of acupuncture and Chinese herbs.

To find a practitioner of traditional Chinese medicine, ask your regular doctor or local hospital or medical school for a recommendation, or consult professional societies or the National Certification Commission for Acupuncture and Oriental Medicine (NCCAOM) online.

HERBS. Many different herbs are prepared together to make a tea (the recipe is customized to your particular symptoms). Common to all Chinese herbal mixes for menopausal symptoms is dong quai, a very weak plant estrogenlike substance. Some of the other herbs in the mix may include ginseng, licorice root, red raspberry leaves, sarsaparilla, spearmint, damiana, motherwort, chasteberry (aka vitex), black cohosh, red clover, wild yam, and evening primrose oil. (Ayurvedic medicine, originating in India, utilizes some of these herbal products in addition to other methods such as massage and yoga.)

Caution is necessary because the relative safety of these herbs in women who have had breast cancer is not known. It's critical for your traditional Chinese medicine practitioner to work with your conventional cancer doctors to select a safe and effective herbal combination.

ACUPUNCTURE. Acupuncture, which activates your *chi* (your inner wind, energy, or spirit) is a popular treatment, performed by doctors skilled in Western as well as Chinese medicine. Very thin needles are inserted in special points along lines of energy flow throughout your body. Acupuncture can help ease symptoms such as hot flashes, pain, stress, fatigue, and more.

COMBINED PLAN. The choice and sequence of Chinese medicine therapies—and the chance for success—depend on the type, nature, and severity of your symptoms along with your ability to make essential lifestyle changes described in this chapter. For example, all the herbs in the world won't take your hot flashes away if you're still smoking a pack a day and stuck on the couch. And even if you do everything perfectly, Chinese medicine may not be strong enough to eliminate severe hot flashes—but they can help. Even a small benefit can significantly improve your quality of life; acupuncture and herbal tea have minimal side effects, after all.

A CAVEAT OR TWO

As you shop for foods and supplements, don't be lured in by labels reading "natural," "pure," "wholesome," "home-grown," "local," "green"— these words sound good but carry no official meaning nor guarantee any health benefits. Concentrated supplements conform to no fixed standard. Natural doesn't mean harmless—and can even prove harmful.

Herbal remedies may depend on their plant estrogenlike substance, but just because it comes from a plant doesn't mean it's okay. For example, DHEA in wild yam from the natural food store can convert into active estrogens with just a few chemical reactions inside you. A concentrated pill can deliver a strong dose of unwelcome estrogenlike substances.

Hot Flash Medications

If you still have uncomfortable hot flashes despite lifestyle and dietary changes and alternative medicine therapies, you may be ready to try over-the-counter medicines or stronger prescription medications.

Tylenol (acetaminophen) is one of your over-the-counter options with antifever properties. Some women may have a good response to vitamin E (800 IU/day) even though studies show no benefit over placebo.

Here are some stronger medications requiring your doctor's prescription:

- Bellergal-S (contains phenobarbital and ergotamine), one pill twice a day
- Catapres TTS (clonidine patch), 0.1 mg/24 hrs, applied once a week

- Aldomet (methyldopa), 250–500 mg by pill twice a day
- Effexor (venlafaxine), 12.5–75 mg by pill each day
- Neurontin (gabapentin), 900 mg by pill daily
- Paxil (paroxetine), 20 mg by pill each day
- Prozac (fluoxetine), 20 mg by pill each day

These medicines intercept the faulty chemical messengers sent by your brain, forestalling hot flashes altogether or lessening your body's response to your brain's hot flash signal. (Note that Paxil and Prozac should not be taken with tamoxifen. See Chapter 7.)

SPECIAL CONSIDERATIONS: HOT FLASHES ON HORMONAL THERAPIES

Here are two important things to consider if you're experiencing significant hot flashes while on hormonal therapy:

- Avoid using Prozac and Paxil (also Wellbutrin) if you are on tamoxifen because these medicines can interfere with tamoxifen's effectiveness (read more in Chapter 7).
- Talk to your doctor about other hormonal breast cancer therapy options if you are still having severe hot flashes on hormonal therapy despite various remedies. Don't stop your hormonal therapy without a plan. There may be another form of hormonal therapy with equal benefits and more tolerable side effects.

Estrogen Therapy for Hot Flashes

If you have had breast cancer, you may be automatically told you *cannot* have estrogen therapy, as a matter of inflexible policy, without regard to your individual case. That's not to say that any estrogen therapy in all women is absolutely forbidden. Each person deserves her own individualized evaluation and management plan that's responsive to her needs, and that will work. If you are suffering from severe hot flashes despite nonestrogen remedies, some oncologists may give women with hormone-receptor-negative breast cancer a little more leeway to use estrogen therapy, and may even offer some wiggle room for low-dose estrogen in women with noninvasive breast cancer (like DCIS). But doctors are likely to be stubbornly resistant to prescribing estrogen therapy to women with significant-stage hormone receptor–positive disease.

You first need to try the full range of nonestrogen therapies and solutions that might serve your particular needs. If severe hot flashes are driving you absolutely crazy on the heels of a big shift in your body's natural hormone levels (say, after removal of the ovaries), a short period of decreasing estrogen therapy might be necessary to restore a decent quality of life and get you back into your groove. To find out more about the possible role estrogen therapy might have in your situation, work with your doctor and consult with a menopause specialist as needed.

Vagina and Vulva Care

Treatment of dryness, pain, and itching of the vagina and nearby tissues requires an open mind, creativity, resourcefulness, and extra-careful attention to your most sensitive tissues.

Goal number one is comfort and absence of pain. Next is recovery of basic function: peeing without burning, walking without discomfort and itching, and sexual intercourse that's not just tolerable but enjoyable.

First, avoid any unnecessary trauma when your tissues are raw or sensitive:

- Wait for sores on your vulva and in your vagina to heal before having sex.
- Stay away from harsh products on the vagina (Ivory, Irish Spring, and Dial soaps; wet wipes that contain alcohol; douching, etc.).
- Avoid using any products with fragrance near this area.
- Avoid activities, such as spinning, that put excess pressure or friction on your crotch.
- Wear wide-crotch soft cotton underpants without lace in the crotch area (you might even try men's underpants); stay away from thongs.
- Stay out of hot tubs or swimming pools, as the hot water temperature and chlorine can burn and dry you out further.
- Use a barrier cream such as Aquaphor or Eucerin on the vulva area when you take a bath or if you must swim in a chlorinated pool.

CURVE BALL: VAGINAL YEAST INFECTIONS

A vaginal yeast infection is a common side effect of antibiotics, steroids, and some chemotherapies. It can produce its own unpleasant symptoms (thick white vaginal discharge, soreness, itching, and a funky smell) on top of underlying vaginal and vulva discomfort.

The good news is that yeast infections usually respond quickly to various treatments, such as:

- Antiyeast medications by pill or creams
- *Lactobacillus acidophilus* capsules or a spoonful of live-culture *plain* yogurt inserted in the vagina to counterbalance the yeast overgrowth
- Vinegar/water douche to make the vagina more acidic (but only if you're sure that you have a yeast infection and you have no sores on the walls of your vagina)

If you think you have a yeast infection, contact your doctor to confirm the diagnosis and start the treatment you need.

Any treatable condition that's complicating the underlying menopause-related changes needs to be taken care of, such as:

- Yeast infection
- Bacterial overgrowth
- Herpes outbreak
- Urinary tract infection

Work with your doctor to resolve these problems right away. Once they've been taken care of, you're ready to take additional steps.

Lubricants

For vaginal and vulvar dryness, you can use lubricants that provide wetness and decrease friction. Water-based, fragrance-free lubricants are best, such as Astroglide, Sylk, K-Y, Motion Lotion, Surgilube, etc. (go to www.goodvibes.com for numerous options). Which one works best for you depends on your personal preference. Some women I take care of swear by natural oil-based lubricants such as olive oil (but this option can't be used with a diaphragm or a latex condom, as the oil will degrade the rubber).

You can try Replens alone or together with a lubricant, depending on what you need. Replens is designed to moisturize and stick to the walls of the vagina—sort of like hanging pads on the walls of an elevator to protect them from bumps, rubs, and bruises while moving furniture. It works well for many women, but for some, the "drip-out" is annoying (but can be handled with a panty liner). If Replens helps but you still need more wetness, add a lubricant.

The best lubricant is made by your own vagina—stimulated by arousal, desire, and good foreplay (with or without a partner). When you're ready for sexual activity, turn to Chapter 19, on intimacy.

Vaginal Estrogen Preparations

If you've taken all the steps above and you're still suffering from significant dryness and pain of the vagina and vulva, talk to your doctor about the possible role of adding a vaginal estrogen preparation to your treatment plan. You only want to use vaginal estrogen for its greatest benefit: to make the walls of the vagina thicker, more elastic, and less painful. (If you need more wetness and less friction, use a lubricant.)

Vaginal estrogens come in various types and in different forms. Here are some examples:

- Premarin estrogen cream can be applied inside the vagina (use just a small dab) each day for up to three weeks, then cut back to once or twice a week.
- Vagifem is a pill in a preloaded applicator, placed at the top of the vagina once a day for two weeks, then two times a week.
- Estring is a soft rubber ring that slowly releases estrogen and is replaced every 90 days.

With any of these preparations, a little goes a long way. If you and your doctor decide that vaginal estrogen is a reasonable option for you, you'll want to select the preparation that's most likely to relieve your symptoms and concentrate its effect on the vagina and nearby tissues.

There is still a concern about the possible increased risk of breast cancer from absorption of estrogen into the rest of your body through the vagina. Some preparations may remain in the vagina better than others. Ask your doctor about the results of ongoing studies comparing whole-body uptake of vaginal estrogen preparations.

Vaginal Discharge

Troubling vaginal discharge and wetness can also occur with menopause and antiestrogen hormonal therapies. Of the women taking tamoxifen, 80 percent will have no change in vaginal symptoms, 10 percent will have vaginal dryness, and 10 percent will have vaginal discharge.

Your doctor can evaluate you and figure out if the extra wetness is fluid coming from the vagina or leakage of urine from the bladder. If an infection is the cause of the new leak, immediate treatment is necessary. If you have minimal discharge from tamoxifen or a little urine leaking regularly after a cough or big laugh, a panty liner or thin diaper can usually take care of the problem. A bigger leak may require a urologist to solve the problem.

Skin Care

Protect Your Skin

It's never too late to protect your skin against additional wear and tear from growing older and the effects of the outside environment. Basic prescription: stop smoking and avoid the sun.

If you're not prepared to give up sunbathing, at least protect your skin from the sun. This is especially important if you're receiving:

- Certain chemotherapies such as 5-FU, Xeloda, or Adriamycin
- Radiation therapy to an area that gets sun exposure
- Certain antibiotics such as tetracycline
- Skin medications such as Retin-A

Sunscreen only works if you wear it, apply it before sun exposure, and reapply it periodically. It also needs to be strong enough to block the intensity of the sun you're going to be exposed to. Here are a few tips:

- Apply sunscreen a half hour before going outside.
- Wear a moisturizer or makeup base with a sun protection factor (SPF) of at least 15 in the spring and fall.
- Use an SPF of at least 30 during the summer, during or immediately after cancer treatment, or when you spend a lot of time outside.
- Go for a waterproof lotion with an SPF of at least 30 if you tend to sweat, go in the water, or are at the beach more than a few hours.

If you hate to apply and wear sunscreen lotion (or even moisturizing lotion), as I do, you can purchase special protective clothing with an SPF of 30, or find a long-sleeved, tightly woven cotton coverall. (A regular T-shirt alone will not provide complete protection—it has an SPF of only 8.)

You'll also need a tightly woven hat with a brim of four inches or more. When I go to the beach, I have to be particularly careful because I have a bunch of atypical moles (funky cancer-prone spots). So I stay away from the beach between 10:00 a.m. and 4:00 p.m., and when I do go I wear a tightly woven oversized men's button-down cotton shirt (the cuffs cover my hands, the collar covers my neck) and long yoga pants. Another option is special clothing from Sun Precautions (sunprecautions.com or 800-882-7860) or Solartex (solartex.com or 877-476-5789), which are designed to keep you cool and covered (not necessarily stylish).

Despite all the health risks of too much sun exposure, I have a number of patients who are addicted to the sun and to getting tanned. This calls for a serious conversation about the dangers of sun exposure, the reality that your skin is more sensitive and less able to heal from sun damage, and the variety of suntan alternatives. If you want to look tan, it's safe to use tinted makeup or self-tanning lotions that affect only the uppermost layer of your skin. Tanning salons are dangerous and should be avoided altogether.

Moisturize

It's important to keep your skin moist and supple with a moisturizer of your choice. The best moisturizers have both a humectant (a substance that holds on to the water you apply to your skin) and a sealer (a substance that keeps the moisture in the skin). These combinations may be cut with alcohol to make the products more spreadable and appealing; however, too much alcohol can cause dry skin (any ingredient that ends with *-ol* means it's a form of alcohol, and if it's one of the first few ingredients listed on the label, a significant amount may be present; cetyl alcohol is less drying). Also, don't dry out your skin with strong soaps such as Ivory, Dial, Irish Spring, and Noxzema. To find environmentally friendly skin products without unhealthy additives, go to the Environmental Working Group's website (www.ewg.org) and check out their section on consumer products.

To prepare your skin for moisturizing, many women like to use the Clarisonic handheld electric skin brush (available in drugstores and online). It removes old skin cells, stimulates the growth of new skin, and can be used to apply moisturizers.

Smoothing the Wrinkles

If you have wrinkles and you are unhappy with them, you do have options. Fine wrinkles can be smoothed in a number of ways that provide short-term results. Renova cream, containing the vitamin A derivative tretinoin, increases skin cell growth and turnover, increases collagen production, and reduces keratoses (those raised, scaly, brown-black spots that tend to appear as we age). A 25 percent alpha-hydroxy lotion and Retin-A are also effective and work the same way. All three require a prescription.

Less effective but still worth trying for fine wrinkles are potions from nature's medicine cupboard: fruit and milk acids that cause a mild skin reaction, resulting in increased firmness of the skin. These acids are the active ingredients in a range of wrinkle creams on the shelf of your drugstore, and include:

- Glycolic acid (from sugar cane)
- Citric acid (from citrus fruits)
- Lactic acid (from soured milk)
- Malic acid (from apples)
- Tartaric acid (from grapes)
- Tannic acid (from wine)

For moderate to more pronounced wrinkles, there are options such as:

- Chemical peels
- Injections with fillers or smoothers, such as collagen, fat, Restylane, Botox
- Laser therapy
- Face tucks, snips, and lifts

Taking any of the above steps makes no sense unless you also make a commitment to protect your skin from the sun and stop smoking, because these two negative influences will keep making more wrinkles and loosen your skin further. They'll also increase your risk of skin cancer.

Boosting Your Heart Health

The best way to keep your heart and blood vessels happy and healthy is through a combination of lifestyle modifications:

- Stop smoking
- Exercise
- Lose excess weight and stick to a healthy weight
- Control blood pressure
- Reduce the "bad" cholesterol (low-density lipoproteins, LDL) and increase the "good" cholesterol (high-density lipoproteins, HDL)
- Keep blood flowing to minimize risk of blood clots

Each item on the list helps with most of the others. For example, a low-fat diet helps with both weight loss and cholesterol; exercise helps with blood pressure, weight management, blood circulation, and cholesterol. Stopping smoking helps with everything on the list, and it also provides some additional health benefits. Add in relaxation techniques and you'll see major progress on all fronts. Lifestyle changes can also go a long way to improve your sense of self and well-being.

Beyond changes in your lifestyle, there are powerful medications that your doctor might recommend to manage the health of your heart and circulatory system, including medicines to keep the blood moving (a daily baby aspirin), lower blood pressure, decrease cholesterol, get rid of extra fluid (diuretics), and bolster your heart strength.

Check with your doctor about an exercise program, cholesterol and blood pressure levels, and medications. It's a big burden to deal with both heart health challenges and breast cancer issues—and you must attend to both. Luckily, you can address both issues with many of the same steps. For example, stopping smoking, exercise, weight management, and eating well all promote heart health and breast health, and decrease the risks of heart disease and breast cancer.

Treating Sadness and Depression

Getting the support you need from family, friends, co-workers, and support groups can help with the blues—but when depression and stubborn

TAKE EXTRA CARE

Reducing stress and injury is more important now than ever before as you go through menopause and grow older. Starting at about age thirty to thirty-five, your body begins to experience a very slow and subtle decline in function and activity:

- Your tissues are stiffer and more vulnerable to stress and injury.
- Muscle mass and strength slowly decrease.
- Your reaction time is slower.
- Healing and repair take longer and may be incomplete.

But it's not too late to make changes in your life to protect your body. In fact, the changes you make now will make a bigger difference because:

- You're more mature and more likely to follow your health resolutions, such as eating better and stopping smoking.
- Your body is less forgiving of what you may be doing, such as smoking or drinking too much.

So now is the time to take extra care to avoid injury, insults, and other damage to your body.

sadness hits, you need to take it seriously and reach out for professional attention and care.

Counseling and Lifestyle Changes

A psychiatrist, psychologist, or trained counselor will meet with you, listen to your concerns, and outline a plan of action. A series of regular counseling sessions is the backbone of your care—pulling in other resources to help work out your problems and help you build a support network or fortify the one you already have. Social workers can work with you to identify practical solutions for any logistical or financial hurdles you might be facing. Parallel to counseling, you have to make critical lifestyle changes. Regular exercise becomes absolutely mandatory, and extra physical and mindfulness activities such as yoga can go a long way toward making you feel so much better.

Medications Can Make a Big Difference

Counseling and lifestyle changes may combine to make you feel better. But for many women, more therapy may be needed. Your health care practitioner may also recommend the use of antidepressant medication, alone or in combination. Although another round of medication may worry you, these medications represent a major medical breakthrough. They help rebalance chemical levels in your brain that are in charge of moods, feelings, energy, motivation, and interest in living.

To most quickly identify the medication that will provide the greatest benefits with the least side effects, it's important to go to a psychiatrist who specializes in antidepressant medications. (Your oncologist is trained in cancer treatment, not depression medication.) But make sure that the prescribed antidepressant is compatible with your anti-cancer treatment plan (see Chapter 7 regarding antidepressant medications that can interfere with tamoxifen). Seek help early to forestall serious trouble and to avoid unnecessary side effects. Check your insurance plan's mental health benefits; insists on your rights to coverage if you need it.

Medication can take up to six weeks before you know if it's even working, and any adjustments in dose, or additions or subtractions of new medications, will take even longer. But all this time, effort, and energy are worth it. Past is past: you're investing in your future and your chance to feel better again.

✄ Moving Forward

Some of the hardest challenges to your quality of life are addressed in this chapter, and accepting a less vital self-image and quenching hot flashes top the charts. You may still be suffering these symptoms, even after doing everything that your doctor recommended and then some. Your frustration can deepen further if:

- Conventional medical solutions for these challenges come up short.
- Estrogen, the medication that may solve some of these tough problems, is considered off-limits.
- Your doctors are unwilling to endorse alternative and complementary medicine treatments that promise to make you feel better.

The conflict between what may improve your quality of life and what may threaten your survival is an unpleasant reminder of having had or living with breast cancer. No one wants to make these sacrifices and compromises. So what do you do? You can't just sit back and hope that you'll do okay. This is your life, and you've got to work on keeping it at its best.

Menopause is a wake-up call to a new phase of your life—and so is breast cancer. So decide what you'll be doing today and in the years ahead. It's time to set new priorities and confirm or toss past commitments, making sure to put your health and well-being at the top of the list.

You can make any number of risk-free lifestyle changes that will reduce your daily stresses and improve your health and quality of life. Whenever you can, find a practical way to integrate these lifestyle changes into regular patterns and habits you will stick with. Test-drive appropriate medication suggestions with your doctor's supervision and care. Check out alternative effective anticancer treatments that you might tolerate better. Don't use symptomatic treatments that are not fully approved until their risks are better understood.

Soon there will be more effective breast cancer treatment options with fewer side effects and more effective and safe symptomatic solutions in your future. Stay tuned to Breastcancer.org for immediate reports on these anticipated advances.

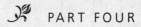

PART FOUR

Caring for Your New Self

CHAPTER FIFTEEN

Sleep: Restoration and Renewal

I used to be called the "Queen of Sleepa." Within two seconds of hitting the pillow I'd be off in lullaby land. No more! One o'clock, two o'clock, three o'clock in the morning, I'm wide awake—hit with a hot flash, a worry, a list of must-dos. I'm tired all night, tired all day— tired of being tired. Please help me.

I have no trouble falling asleep. My problem is waking up at three or four in the morning and being unable to fall back to sleep. It's lonely, frustrating, and exhausting.

The littlest things now wake me up: my husband's snoring, the birds outside my window, the wind in the trees, a noisy truck driving by. While I'm able to fall back to sleep, I never get a good solid stretch of time without interruption.

The sleep medicine works pretty well, but I'm afraid that I'm going to get hooked on it.

First Things First

Sleep is life's essential; there is no compromise on the real thing. It is tonic, balm, medicine, therapy. Restorative. Sleep is a mystery—a fall into the unconscious, a magical transformation. What makes it happen? If only we could flip that switch at our command!

You need adequate sleep to perform basic everyday functions plus anything above and beyond. Need to recover from the anxiety and intensity of the breast cancer experience? Stressed to meet major deadlines at work? Dizzy from the merry-go-round of demands at home? Want to think clearly, speak well, be one of the living? Need to revive your flattened spirit? Sleep is your first priority. Not snoozing, napping, daydreaming, resting, relaxing— we're talking about good, high-quality, solid sleep to revive your energy, focus, resources, motivation, and will to live your life fully.

What Happens During Sleep

Sleep cycles through various stages during the passage of a night. Normally, a person experiences about five sleep cycles during a night, with each cycle lasting about ninety minutes. Each cycle goes through these four stages:

1. *Light sleep* is a relatively short stretch (2 to 5 percent of the sleep cycle) when eye movement and muscle and brainwave activity begin a slowdown process. Light sleep can be easily interrupted.
2. *Middle sleep* lasts for 45 to 55 percent of the cycle. Eye movement ceases and brain waves continue their slowdown.

MELATONIN, THE SLEEP HORMONE

What helps flip your sleep switch to the on position? When lights are out and it's time for bed, a little gland in your brain (the pineal gland) makes a special hormone called melatonin, which slows down the cells of your body so you can get your ZZZs.

There have been some intriguing studies showing that too much light or work at night may be associated with a higher risk of breast cancer. While it's hard to make any solid conclusions without gold-standard studies, there is some evidence that melatonin can influence how breast cells grow. Here is one possible explanation for how melatonin might play a role in breast health: Each night melatonin helps to slow down cell growth and activity. When enough melatonin is present to do its job, your body's cells are more likely to stay well behaved. Over time, however, if there's too much light and too little melatonin is produced, there may not be enough melatonin to slow down cell growth, keep the misbehaving cells under control, and possibly protect you against breast cancer. This possible explanation has yet to be fully proved.

3. ***Deep sleep*** ranges from 13 to 23 percent of the total cycle. No eye movement or muscle activity occurs; metabolism has slowed and brainwave activity (called delta waves) is at a minimum.
4. ***REM (rapid eye movement) sleep*** lasts for 20 to 25 percent of the total sleep cycle. Active dreaming, brainwave activity, heart rate, and blood pressure are gradually ramped up and your arms and legs are temporarily paralyzed.

The reason you're paralyzed during REM sleep is probably so you don't act out your dreams. All that running and flying and whatever else you're dreaming about not only would exhaust you but also could prove quite dangerous. Waking from REM sleep is no big deal, but if you're dreaming about falling and then you wake up, you might find yourself flailing your way out of bed as the paralysis lifts.

As the night rolls through, deep sleep gets progressively less time in each cycle, while REM sleep takes up more time. Growing older can change the quality of your sleep: you tend to get less deep sleep and relatively more REM sleep.

The Main Purpose of Sleep

You depend on sleep for rest and restoration: while you're out for the count, a ton of work gets done. Sleep allows your mind to automatically:

• Consolidate your day's mental activities
• Organize what you've learned
• Add new data to your memory bank
• Edit the day's happenings into an orderly history
• Process the emotional experiences of your day
• Sort through your social encounters and settle them in context and perspective

Dreaming also helps achieve this consolidation.

Sleep allows your body to:

• Cleanse its internal self, keeping all your fluids flowing
• Reduce swelling in your legs (where gravity sends extra fluid

during the day when you're standing and sitting)—and possible
swelling in the breast region and arms—by moving fluids back
into circulation

- Flush out chemicals built up in your muscles
- Bolster your immune system
- Promote normal cell growth and development

Knowing how many critical jobs are accomplished during a good
night's sleep, you can better understand why you feel and function poorly
the day after a bad night's sleep—and why it's so important to learn how
you can improve this necessary and restorative part of your life.

❧ Challenges

Getting Enough Sleep

Nearly all of us say we don't get enough sleep. The crazy demands of modern life do steal precious sleep, and drain our energy reserves. On the
other hand, some people who feel like they have sleepless nights may be
getting more sleep than they think. Said one expert: "We have eight hours
of recorded sleep for one patient in our sleep lab who insisted she didn't
sleep a wink." Despite what may be an inaccurate sense of sleep quantity
and quality for some, true insomnia is a troublesome problem for many,
many women—and a good reason to seek evaluation. If you are sleep-
deficient on a regular basis, physical and emotional exhaustion can hit
hard:

- Things that ordinarily gave you pleasure no longer interest you.
- Routine problems can feel like emergencies; you may unravel
  and become a danger to yourself and those around you.
- Accidents and falls are more likely to happen.
- Hurtful words can slip out of your mouth before you can think.
- Judgment suffers and you overreact and underperform, much as
  if you'd had too much to drink.

There's no universal magic number when it comes to sleep. A
few individuals claim they can function well on only four to five hours a

night, but these people are unusual. (Naturally short sleepers may, in fact, have a genetic mutation that sets them up for fewer hours of sleep.) Most of us need from seven to nine hours a night. Some of us need even more. The myth of needing less sleep as you age is just that: a myth.

Interrupted and Irregular Sleep

The quality of your sleep is just as important as the amount of sleep that you get—and continuous sleep is essential in order to progress through the stages and get enough deep sleep. Because the brain has a hard time snapping to sudden wakefulness from deep sleep, interrupted deep sleep will likely cause confusion and irritation. Getting back to sleep soon after you've been awakened is critical to the overall restorative quality of that night's rest.

The regularity of your sleep routine is also very important. Do you have to catch sleep whenever you can—in between major family, community, and work demands? In my practice, I see a considerable number of women who work several jobs around the clock, meaning shifting work hours and erratic sleep schedules. Other women are worn down, mixed up, and strung out by the predictably unpredictable demands of managing the home base, stretching the finances, and taking care of everyone in the family—often including teenagers (and their friends).

Without a regular routine of work, play, eating, relaxation, and sleep, it is hard to train your body to get good-quality rest. Because your body knows the difference between night and day and between dark and light, when these outside cues are out of sync with your schedule your body gets confused and sleep suffers. Until you establish (or reestablish) a regular, consistent rhythm to your life, you'll feel disordered and vulnerable to stress and breakdown.

Sleep Anxiety

Both worry and anxiety can keep you from falling asleep and keep you awake in the middle of the night. You may even lose sleep over losing sleep—and if it takes a long time to fall to sleep, you may worry you'll oversleep in the morning.

Because anxiety about breast cancer often hits at night, your bed can become haunted by your fears about your health.

Medicines, Ingredients, Foods, and Beverages

You probably already know many of the things you should limit or avoid if you want to get a good night's sleep. Here are a few that need to be at the top of your list:

- Caffeine
- Heavy meals close to bedtime
- Spicy or rich foods
- Alcohol (although it may help you fall asleep, it ultimately makes you more tired because it interferes with deep sleep)
- Ritalin, Adderall, and other such medications taken for attention issues
- Antiestrogen medications
- Steroids (discussed in Chapter 8 on fatigue), which in moderate to high doses can affect the deep, restful part of your sleep that's most restorative
- Nicotine, from a patch or from cigarettes

Hot Flashes

Debilitating hot flashes that seriously interfere with sleep are often a side effect of chemotherapy, antiestrogen therapy, and natural menopause. There are various ways to minimize these hot flashes, and new methods are constantly being explored (see Chapter 14).

Noise and Discomfort

Pain will wake you at night. So will noise. You may find certain noises almost soothing (like lulling constant traffic sounds), while other noises, such as slamming doors and intermittent barking, can drive you up the wall.

Snoring

Snoring happens when air moving through a partially blocked airway makes the back of your throat vibrate. Lips can also rattle. Are you the snorer, or is it your partner? If you are the snorer, you may not be troubled by your own snores. But if it's your partner who snores, it can wake you and keep you up.

Sleep Apnea

Apnea is when breathing stops during sleep because the tissues in the back of your mouth block airflow. When breathing stops, your brain may be slow to get breathing going again, and your heart can be stressed. Apnea may continue on and off throughout the night. Each episode usually lasts for no more than ten seconds—occasionally a minute or more. You wake up tired, unaware perhaps of being troubled by this condition.

Hypopnea, or shallow breathing, is another form of sleep apnea. The shallow breathing diminishes the supply of oxygen needed by the cells of the body, resulting in less efficient sleep and more tiredness.

Apnea often affects very overweight people and can be a serious condition. If neglected, sleep apnea can even be life threatening.

✒ Solutions

The best gauge for whether you're getting enough sleep is how you fall asleep at night and how you feel when you wake up in the morning. A gentle falling off to sleep in a number of minutes is a good sign. If you wake up refreshed and energized, you've had a proper amount of sleep. If the morning finds you grumpy, groggy, and hard to rouse, you probably missed out on the sleep you needed.

If you fall asleep the moment your head hits the pillow, you may actually be sleep deprived. Aim to inch up the time you sleep, maybe an hour a night, till you've caught up on your sleep deficit, or treat yourself to an extra-long sleep on the weekend to make up for missed ZZZs.

Our sleep expert, Dr. Helena Schotland of Bryn Mawr Hospital, advises a general three-pronged approach to getting the sleep you need:

1. Attend to sleep hygiene—the conditions and habits that add up to your sleep environment.
2. Accept cognitive behavioral therapy—methods used to treat patients whose ideas, beliefs, or behaviors are causing them discomfort or unhappiness. Options include relaxation and distraction techniques and/or limited-time psychotherapy.

3. Consider sleep medication—preferably Rozerem, which has no tolerance issue, no problem with long-term use, and no dependence, and which is not a controlled substance (thus prescriptions are easier to obtain).

We'll start the "Solutions" section by first focusing on the essential elements of good sleep hygiene, which, when practiced together, will help you create the best setting, conditions, and practices to give you a solid, uninterrupted night's sleep.

Stick to a Regular Routine

Getting your body on a regular day-and-night schedule helps you form good sleep habits. Here are some important tips:

- Exercise on a regular basis during the day.
- Manage your hot flashes by avoiding the triggers and using the coolers described in Chapter 14.
- Try to get to bed at a regular time each night and get up at a regular time each morning.
- Eat your evening meal as early as possible before you go to sleep.
- Keep any later-night snacks light, and don't eat in bed.
- Avoid late-night phone calls unless there's an absolute emergency.
- Avoid late-night work that causes anxiety.
- Make sure the dog has been walked and is inside and settled before you go to sleep so that barking doesn't wake you up. Politely ask your neighbors to do the same. If your pets don't get it, put them in a distant room or the basement. They'll manage better than you think—and they'll probably get a better night's sleep, too.
- Don't stay in bed once you wake up.
- Make sure the alarm clock is set properly (not for yesterday's early-morning run to the airport).

These are some of the same steps you would use to train a baby. Setting up sleep limits gives your body a structure to work with and expect.

Avoid Caffeine and Other Stimulants

Caffeine from any of a variety of sources can compromise your sleep, particularly when taken after two o'clock in the afternoon (or even after noon if you're especially sensitive). Take extra care to limit or avoid using:

- Coffee and tea. Even decaffeinated versions of coffee and tea have more caffeine than you'd suspect.
- Sodas—Coke, Pepsi, Mountain Dew, Jolt, Surge, and even some orange sodas all have a lot of caffeine along with the bubbles (look at the ingredients).
- Chocolate, especially dark chocolate, keeps a lot of people up.
- Diet pills and nicotine (tobacco or patch) will keep you up at night. Neither is healthy, but if either is part of your life, avoid using it in the evening.
- Other medications can disrupt your sleep—for example, steroids. If a required medicine keeps you awake, ask your doctor if the amount or timing of the medicine can be changed, or if there is a more sleep-friendly, effective alternative.

It's best to stick to herbal teas, cold or hot lemonade, apple cider, or warm milk with a touch of honey. Seek beverages that soothe you, relax you, and make you sleepy. Avoid or limit alcohol consumption.

Set the Stage for Sleep

Just like anything else you do, you do it best when you're in the mood for it: eating, talking, listening, having sex, doing sports, reading—and sleeping. Here are some things you can do to get you in the mood for sleep:

- Massage your neck or legs.
- Take a warm bath.
- Daydream.
- Meditate.
- Try a light snack to satisfy late night hunger. Avoid anything heavy, spicy, or very sweet.

KEEP YOUR BEDROOM WORRY-FREE

To disassociate cancer-related anxieties from your bedroom and nighttime routine, establish your bed, and night, as a worry-free zone.

- Leave your bedroom when anxiety hits. If you wake up with lists of things to do or worry about and can't get back to sleep, get out of bed and go to another room if necessary.
- Write down your chores, tasks, and problems. Park your fears and worries on paper, and commit yourself to dealing with them the next day. Daytime is always much better than nighttime to deal with these issues.
- Make an appointment with yourself, a daily date with your worries. Take this task seriously—go over that list in the daytime, manage the worries that you can, and postpone those you need to work on further.
- Let someone else take over your worries for you. (My niece makes little worry dolls: you whisper your worries to the doll and let the doll work on your problems.)
- Return to your bed only after you've parked your fears somewhere else.

- Don't indulge in overstimulating experiences just before bedtime, like television news or action shows, or late-night exercise. (Sex, however, may help you get to sleep.)
- Avoid fluids near bedtime so you don't have to go to the bathroom in the middle of the night. Once up, you may have trouble getting back to sleep.
- Try cooling down your bedroom at night.
- Keep your room dark, soothing, and quiet. Curtains, blinds, a face mask, and silicone earplugs all may help. Darkness increases your brain's production of melatonin, the "sleep hormone."
- Be sure to have a comfortable, suitable mattress, adequate covers, and good pillows.
- Treat yourself to a new nightgown or pajamas.
- Turn your clock to the wall. Too much attention to how much time you're awake may only reinforce sleeplessness.
- Try a pillow over your eyes and ears to help block out noise and light (an old thin down pillow works great).

- Get your family to cooperate with your need for quiet, for sleep. Your motto can be "I'll protect your sleep if you guard mine."
- Try white noise—that's the kind of sound that makes your mind relax while it drowns out other noise. A whirring fan can work well, soothing you to sleep.

If your bedroom has become polluted by troublesome nighttime fears, change the scene. Rearrange the furniture, paint the walls another color, or cheer things up with a new quilt and sheets. You might even want to choose a different bedroom if possible.

Manage In-Bed Activities

When you have trouble sleeping, only use your bed for sleep or sex. If you're trying to sleep and you can't, you should leave your bed for a while. Try doing something relaxing or boring for thirty minutes, and then try again to fall asleep.

- Don't toss and turn for more than twenty minutes.
- Read a soothing or dull book or watch TV somewhere else.
- Count backward from 100. Count sheep, horses, or dogs if that works for you.
- Sing a familiar song to yourself, over and over.
- Concentrate on thinking the words *in* and *out* with every breath that comes in and goes out.

When it comes to sex, avoid nights when you have to get up early for work. I've told more than one patient who really needed her rest to hang a Do Not Disturb or Not Tonight sign over the bed. (That deal works as long as there is another side to the sign that says Tonight's the Night.)

Snore Stoppers

Snoring—your own, your partner's, or both—can be a huge problem that must be worked out.

- Experiment with earplugs until you find a kind that works for you.
- Find the sleep position that stops the snore. Sleeping on one's back usually makes snoring worse; sleeping on one's side often resolves the snoring.
- Consider wearing a belt with a big buckle turned onto your back to keep you from rolling onto your back.
- Consider one of those much-advertised snore stoppers: strips, straps, pillows. They may help; they can't hurt. But stay away from sprays—they can be harmful.
- Take charge of your partner's chin if he/she is a lip rattler (like mine ☹). Reach over and pull the chin down, and pray that it doesn't start up again.
- Move you or your partner to a couch if the snoring won't stop or it keeps restarting. Or it might be easier for you to find or set up a spare bedroom.

If the snoring persists as a significant issue, check with a doctor for a more serious medical approach. Your local hospital probably has a sleep specialist—usually in the pulmonary department (that's lung medicine).

Apnea Management

Sleep apnea can be a critical problem. Its proper diagnosis is usually established by an overnight sleep study, where the subject comes in to sleep at least one night under observation. Treatments are customized based on the specific type of apnea, and usually involve one or more of the following solutions:

- Weight loss—a major way of dealing with this problem.
- CPAP—a machine that provides continuous positive airway pressure through a specialized face mask. This is the gold standard of sleep apnea treatment. The machine may be rented or purchased, depending on your insurance. But it only works if you use it on a regular basis.
- Position therapy, similar to that recommended for snoring; techniques to keep the sleeper on her side and off her back.

• Oral appliance applied to the teeth, to pull the lower jaw forward. As devices go, the CPAP is more effective, but an appliance seems to work for some mild or average cases.

Surgery is kind of a last resort. There are various procedures to keep the airway unblocked, but we don't have positive proof of long-lasting results.

Sleep Medicine

By following the sleep hygiene suggestions outlined in this section, most sleep challenges can be improved or resolved. If you are still experiencing sleep challenges despite all your efforts, you might find yourself headed to the medicine cabinet.

Over-the-counter drugs for sleep usually contain diphenhydramine (benadryl)—bad news! This medicine may make you sleepy at first, but it disrupts sleep stages and you may wake up feeling hungover. Read labels, especially for heavily advertised sleep aids such as Tylenol PM. Also, diphenhydramine can interfere with tamoxifen's effectiveness (see Chapter 7).

It's better to ask your doctor for a prescription. Our expert recommends a medication that functions like the sleep hormone melatonin: Rozerem. Over-the-counter melatonin products should be avoided.

NAPS

If you are tired during the day, try a cat-nap, but beware of long naps—you'll pay for them later. You'll be wide awake in the middle of the night, wondering why you can't sleep. Most sleep experts advise against napping unless it's absolutely necessary because it can compete with your nighttime sleep. But, if you must have a nap in the daytime:

• Limit the nap to no more than thirty minutes, so you'll get some rest without falling into deep sleep, which could interfere with deep sleep at night. (If you wake up groggy from your nap, you are waking from deep sleep: you've napped too long.)
• Have the nap before two in the afternoon, to avoid spoiling your nighttime sleep.
• Schedule the nap for the same time each day if you need them on a regular basis.

Rest needs to be balanced with activity. Too much rest can undermine your resolve to keep moving. It's too easy to fall into a comfortable pattern of sitting back with a book or TV instead of braving the outdoors or getting on a treadmill.

If mild discomfort or hot flashes are keeping you up or waking you up, acetaminophen (Tylenol) or ibuprofen (Advil) might be enough to help you get to sleep. If transient anxiety is responsible for your sleeping problems, ask your doctor about a suitable solution—including medication if appropriate.

If your insomnia is nonspecific (not due to any particular cause or reason) and Rozerem doesn't do it for you, occasional use of something like short-acting Ambien or Lunesta can be helpful. Follow doctor's orders and don't take it more than two times a week or your body will get used to it and it may lose its effectiveness.

Most effective sleep medications can be obtained only with your doctor's prescription and should only be taken with your doctor's approval. Never borrow pills from a family member or friend. Stay away from alternative medications for sleep. Herbals and supplements are not regulated by the FDA, so you can never be sure of what's inside that bottle.

When to Seek a Sleep Consultation

If nothing in what you have read in this chapter helps you, if your sleep is still troubled and inadequate, it's probably time for you to seek help from a professional accredited sleep therapist or clinic. Many hospitals now have such resources available to the community. If you have no such local facility, contact the nonprofit National Sleep Foundation on the Web for help (www.sleepfoundation.org). If you are suffering from insomnia and can't find a specialized therapist or clinic near you, a good physician may be able to help you address the issue.

Moving Forward

Your sleep may never end up as perfect as you might hope. Our expert, Dr. Helena Schotland, says, "Don't shoot for perfection; shoot for improvement. Decrease the pressure on yourself about not being able to fall sleep. Ask yourself, what's the worst thing that can happen? So what if you don't get enough sleep on one particular night? Tell yourself that you can always make it up. We look for small steps that add up to something helpful."

CHAPTER SIXTEEN

Your Immune System: Blows and Boosts

I got an awful response to my second bout of chemo—fever, aches, chills, throat ulcers—and I had to go to the hospital. They did a blood count and the doctor came back in a panic: "You have no platelets and as for your white count—there's nothing lower on the scale!" But then my oncologist came in and told me not to worry. "General doctors don't see this reaction, so they get scared. I see it all the time. You're going to be fine, but we need to keep you in the hospital and give you some growth factor." I had a transfusion and I was on IV. After taking time off and taking care of myself, I got back my old strength.

I'm so conflicted. My breast cancer treatment is weakening the very part of my body—my immune system—that I'm counting on to get me out of this mess and keep me safe from cancer in the future.

It took a full year after all my treatments were over before my immune cells and energy level returned to normal.

I got my medicine from the hospital, my organic food nutrients from the grocery store, my vitamins from the health food store, my rest in my home—and somehow, with the support of my family and friends, I was able to pull it all together and ride through the storm.

First Things First

The human body is composed of many organs and systems that are vulnerable to attack, not only from outside, but also from inside the body: injury and disease, aging, cell damage, and mutations (genetic changes in gene structure or organization, including those that result in cancer). Vulnerable as it is, the body has amazing strength and defenses. The immune system reaches almost every tissue, alert and ready to help protect us against danger.

The immune system can distinguish between substances in the body that are foreign (or nonself) from those that are native (or self). It attacks these foreign substances, called antigens, trying to eliminate them, and then stops the attack before the body itself is damaged.

Women dealing with breast cancer inevitably wonder: "Can my immune system fight breast cancer? Do the surgery, chemo, and radiation therapy reduce my body's ability to fight breast cancer and infections? Did I get breast cancer because my immune system was weakened by stress, or by the wrong food? How can I fortify my immune system to help me become as healthy as possible?"

Over the course of this chapter, we'll discuss how your immune system works to protect you, and how scientists are looking for ways to reinforce the immune system's ability to fight cancer—and even to "invent" new immune system defense mechanisms.

Generalized Immune Response

The immune system responds immediately to danger with an innate, generalized, nonspecific reaction (such as inflammation) to fight any threat—for example, a virus or an injury. This response is like an army artillery attack, with shells bursting all over. It indiscriminately damages and kills all varieties of bacteria, viruses, and any other microorganisms that happen to be in range, as well as some of the body's own cells.

The crudest of your body's generalized defense forces are free radicals, highly reactive and unstable "warrior" molecules released to take quick action against the enemy or insult. These free radicals are produced by white blood cells, which are quickly mobilized by the presence of

THE IMMUNE SYSTEM'S DEFENSE TEAM

The major organs of the immune system are the thymus, spleen, bone marrow, and lymph nodes. The white cells of the blood are also part of the immune system, including:

- Lymphocytes—T and B cells—are central to the immune system because they carry out immune responses against antigens.
- Macrophages are necessary helper cells derived from white cells (monocytes).
- Neutrophils, eosinophils, and basophils are cells that contribute to inflammation, which is the initial, involuntary immune response.

These immune cells circulate through and between several immune system structures and organs:

- The thymus gland acts like a nursery for the development of T cells.
- The spleen accumulates macrophages (large cells that engulf and digest microorganisms and other antigens), which it filters from the blood.
- Lymph nodes filter lymph fluid, removing antigens, bacteria, and cancer cells that get trapped in their weblike structure, where macrophages, antibodies, and B and T cells can destroy them.
- The bone marrow generates T cells, B cells, and macrophages; these cells travel throughout the body in the blood and tissue fluids.

Treatment for breast cancer can have a negative effect on how your immune system's defense team functions. Chemotherapy affects bone marrow production of all immune cells, radiation can lower immune cell counts within the area treated, and surgery removes lymph nodes, which can compromise the local immune response. But because you have hundreds of lymph nodes located throughout your body, your overall lymph node protection remains intact.

cancer or the invasion of a dangerous microorganism. Free radicals are nonspecific—they react in the same way to bacteria as they do to a bruise, and even to the cells of normal tissue, if they get beyond their target area. Free radicals and other elements in the generalized defensive response induce the swelling, redness, heat, and pain of inflammation.

After the free radicals have finished their work, they are "turned off," converted into nonreactive, harmless molecules. Antioxidant vitamins are essential to this conversion process. You hear a lot about free radicals and oxidation being brought down by antioxidant vitamins A, C, D, and E. (See Chapter 17, on nutrition.)

This benefit of vitamins actually produces a dilemma. Because radiation therapy works in part by producing free radicals that attack cancer cells, some scientists wonder if vitamins might reduce this radiation effect and therefore should be avoided during radiation therapy.

Specific Immune Defenses

As the immune response continues, it becomes adaptive and more specific. The white cells of the blood and immune tissues produce special fighter proteins called antibodies that selectively kill the invading organism or foreign agent, called an antigen. Antigen and antibody link, and the immune response progresses, with the generation of huge numbers of antibodies to react with matching antigens. Other cells of the body are left undamaged by this specific response. It's as if the army's Rangers have zeroed in and are taking careful aim.

The B lymphocytes or B cells, the immune cells that produce antibodies, have a long memory for their enemies—those specific antigens. These B cells may remain in the body for years, ready to wage war quickly and powerfully by the explosive production of antibodies whenever that particular antigen shows up in the body again. This process is how your body acquires and sustains immunity after vaccination with the specific antigen of a particular infection, such as polio, measles, or the flu. If your B cells have never met up with that particular antigen before, however, there will be no antibody response.

There are a number of different ways in which antibodies destroy antigens. Antibodies cause the antigens to clump together, immobilizing them, so that they can be swallowed up by macrophages. Or antigen-covered cells are perforated by antibodies, their insides leak out, and they die. Or antibodies interlock with the antigen-covered cells, attracting immune cells (macrophages, in particular) like flies to honey, and the harmful cells are gobbled up.

It takes a while for the body to develop and implement the specific immune response. In contrast, the generalized immunity process responds immediately to a threat to your health.

✣ Challenges

Battling Cancer

Breast cancer cells start out as normal body cells that begin to grow out of control because of mutation or other damage. The immune system plays a major role in limiting the development of these mutations—often before cancer has a chance to develop beyond a very preliminary stage. As a result, many cancerous cells are eliminated before they do harm.

Scientists believe that there is a continuous process of cell overgrowth and genetic change, followed by growth arrest, destruction, and "mopping up." Damaged, premalignant cells may be a constant presence in the body, but an ever-alert immune system takes them out and protects us from many assaults of cancer that never get beyond the very earliest stage.

Occasionally, however, cells change from normal to abnormal without any changes to their surface markers. These changing cells manage to elude attack by the immune system in this way, and they grow and multiply into abnormal cells without triggering an immune response. Eventually, the resulting tumor becomes abnormal on the outside and can no longer hide its malignant character. That's when the immune system finally launches its attack.

The attack may succeed, or it may be too late: the tumor may be beyond the power of the immune system alone. Bold measures such as immune growth factors (drugs that stimulate the production of new immune cells) or vaccines may be able to turn the tide and arrest the disease, or non-immune-system intervention such as chemotherapy, radiation, or the surgical removal of the harmful growth may be necessary. Other promising approaches include anti-angiogenesis (the drying up of the blood supply to the tumor) or new medicines that make the cancer cells self-destruct.

Relying on a Compromised Immune System

You may worry, "What happens if I lose lymph nodes to surgery or my white count drops dramatically because of chemotherapy? Isn't my immune system weakened, and don't I again become vulnerable to cancer and infection?"

Fortunately, your immune system is very resilient and flexible. Various parts and cells can switch roles and fill in for one another, and there is a considerable reserve or surplus of immune cells and tissues. If some lymph nodes are removed, others take up the load, handling the circulation of lymph and the filtering of cancer cells, bacteria, and other unwanted elements. Key cells of the immune system move readily from place to place in the body, traveling through the tissues and circulating in the blood. Alerted by signals from cancer cells or inflammation, they quickly arrive at the site where they are needed. Since there is such a large reserve of blood cells and because immune cell growth factors are often given prophylactically together with chemo, cancer treatment can reduce your immune cells without putting you in serious danger.

Still, blood counts are used to assess the possible damage to your immune system and your associated risk of infection during treatment. The amount that the white blood cell count declines depends on the individual, the treatment given, the dose and the interval between dosage cycles, and the accumulated total dose given. Blood counts are most profoundly affected by chemotherapy, because the chemicals travel to all sites of immune cell production. There's a very small drop with radiation to the breast alone. When the lymph nodes are also irradiated, the decline is somewhat steeper. Radiation to bones for metastatic disease can cause low counts, especially if the vertebrae, pelvic bones, and leg bones are treated, because the marrow of these bones is where most new blood cells are produced.

The bone marrow, thymus gland, spleen, and lymph nodes respond to low blood counts by calling on their reserves and revving up the production of more white cells. When counts fall below a critical level, the risk of infection increases and your doctor will quickly initiate immune support treatment. Your chemotherapist will probably give you growth factors to speed up your immune cell production; antibiotics may also be given. Only occasionally are donated white blood cells used to boost your immune system and your ability to fight infection. Once your immune cell counts rise above this critical level (between 500 and 1,000 "frontline" cells, or neutrophils), your system is sufficiently intact to fight most infections. If you are in the middle of chemotherapy, it can usually resume when the count reaches between 2,000 and 2,500, and the dose given will depend on what your immune system can tolerate. But even with growth factors and other supportive measures, there can be some depression of immune cell counts that persists for weeks, months, or, in an occasional patient, a year or more.

✣ Solutions

Traditional Methods to Boost the Immune System

A vaccine can help build up the immune system. In this case, a solution made of weakened or dead breast cancer cells taken from the tumor that caused the disease serves as the antigen that stimulates an antibody response, resulting in antibodies primed to attack and destroy cancer cells. If any new cancer cells appear, the circulating antibodies of the vaccine-educated immune system should destroy them.

Although this approach is traditional for infectious diseases, it is very much in the experimental stage for cancer, and it is significantly handicapped by the nature of cancer progression. Cancer starts with a few abnormal cells that keep multiplying, generation after generation. Each generation produces variations, called mutations, so that eventually the cancer has countless faces, with a very mixed antigen profile. One vaccine, however, yields one or a limited number of different antibodies that were developed against the specific kinds of cancer cells in the vaccine preparation. As a result, they may not be effective against the full range of newly developing cancer cells.

In addition, an effective vaccine must produce antibodies that target the bad cells and leave normal cells alone. The trick is to catch or tag the cancer cells as they change from normal to abnormal, and direct a vaccine against the cells just after they've become newly malignant.

Researchers are investigating chemical markers that would identify cancer cells at a very early stage. These markers would tag the problem cells and alter them enough to make the immune system perceive them as abnormal. It's just a matter of time before scientists find ways to pinpoint and tag these markers and develop antibodies against the identified cancer cells.

Another traditional therapeutic approach is to produce antibodies against oncogenes, such as HER2 *neu* (Herceptin is an antibody therapy targeting HER2), and the gene for epidermal growth factor receptor (EGFR) (these medicines are under development). Oncogenes are genes that in normal form keep cell growth under control and suppress cancer formation. They carry out this function by directing the production of special proteins. If these oncogenes are abnormal and malfunction, they fail to regulate growth, and cancer—uncontrolled growth—can result.

By targeting cancer cell genes, or their receptors or proteins, these antibodies can more precisely recognize cancer cells, destroy them, and spare surrounding normal tissue. An elaboration of this approach delivers antibodies with attached poisons, such as nitrogen mustard or a radioactive agent, that will help kill the cancer cells. Animal studies in this area have been encouraging, and clinical trials are ongoing.

A serious obstacle to the success of these immune therapies is that the antibodies manufactured in response to the vaccine may not be able to get into the cells. To do their job, antibody molecules must be able to penetrate the cells' outer (and sometimes inner) barriers to truly destroy these cells.

Other research is looking for ways to boost T-cell activity against antigens, to encourage T cells and other fighting cells to work even harder and longer to find and destroy cancer.

The goal of current immune system research is to determine the ways to prevent cancer from ever starting, or, if it has started, to track and eliminate any potentially dangerous cells without damaging healthy cells—a less toxic result than the chemo or radiation therapies now in use.

Nontraditional Methods to Boost the Immune System

Nutrition, stress reduction, support groups, exercise—there is intriguing literature evolving that demonstrates the ability of these fundamental but nontraditional interventions to strengthen your immune system. For example, Dr. Fawzy Fawzy, a psychiatrist at UCLA, showed enhanced immune cell function after regular support group meetings for people with melanoma, a serious form of skin cancer.

Dr. Keith Block, of the University of Illinois and the Block Medical Center, makes nutrition central to his overall treatment plan to reduce cancer risk and increase quality of life. His work emphasizes low-fat veg-etarian diets coupled with stress reduction and other complementary medicine therapies, all of which he believes combine to strengthen the immune system.

Many experts believe that consuming high levels of cholesterol and unhealthy fats (see Chapter 17) depresses the immune system and increases the risk of cancer. They claim that fat appears to reduce white cell production, slows and dulls T-cell and macrophage activity, and compromises the lymphatic system, making the body more vulnerable to infection and disease. Ongoing studies are evaluating these claims.

There is wide consensus that whole foods are the best source of vita-mins and their "posse" of important co-factors (rather than processed supplements). Fresh fruits and vegetables, grains, mushrooms, herbs, teas, omega-3 fatty acids, complex carbohydrates, yogurt with active cul-tures, and seaweed are believed to increase the activity of T cells and their escort cells, and to promote the proliferation of antibodies and fighting cells. These claims—currently under study—continue to be strong beliefs rather than established facts that call for immediate action.

Keep in mind that any process your body performs is crippled by poor nutrition. This is true for healing a wound, building immune cell blood counts, and even managing stress. Attention to good nutrition makes sense whether it specifically benefits the immune system or not. (See Chapter 17, on nutrition.) Likewise, exercise, stress management, and taking care of your emotional and health needs are all important to your overall health.

✄ Moving Forward

Although your immune system may have been battered by the effects of breast cancer treatment, with the support of medica-tions, good nutrition, mindfulness, quality rest, and the healing effects of time, your immune system will recover and once again perform its critical functions: protecting normal cell growth and guarding you against infection.

CHAPTER SEVENTEEN

Sustenance: Nutrition and Supplements

My mom told me that a healthy diet was one way to minimize the risk of breast cancer. I wonder if she's right or if it's just in the hands of fate.

I'm totally confused. One day they say that all beans are good. The next day chocolate, coffee, and soybeans are out. A few months later, dark chocolate is voted back in. Why can't they agree on this stuff? It's not like these foods are new. When my sister and I were kids, my aunt Jean used to push a murky concoction of celery and carrot juice on us, the only guinea pigs within reach to carry out the prescription for good health she was reading about at the time. She also tried to get us to swallow huge pills of vitamin C and E and B complex. We rejected all her efforts, our jaws clamped shut. We thought she was a little nuts, not realizing she was actually ahead of her time by at least sixty years.

First Things First

Eat this. Eat that. Every year there seems to be new instructions, new studies, new warnings on diet and nutrition. Food, fad, fat, fuss, fraud, fear, fact? What do you do with the information that bombards you? Whom and what can you believe? And how do you make sense of all this information and figure out what's really good for you and what you should be doing?

After breast cancer, you want to do whatever you can to become as healthy as possible. Your doctors have guided you through treatment—surgery, anticancer medicines, antibiotics for infection, advice on anxiety—but who tells you what you should be eating? You know that the foods you eat and the vitamins and supplements you take influence your body's ability to fight disease and maintain good health. You've probably heard that at least one-third of all cancers can be attributed in some part to diet, and that's one of the breast cancer risk factors you have the most control over—so common sense demands that you pay attention to what you eat.

But when you hear that nutrition can influence your cancer risk and that you supposedly had control over what you put in your mouth, you can get hit by a major case of guilt and the "woulda, coulda, shouldas." So let's make a deal before you read another word in this chapter or in this book: Past is past. This is the point to start fresh, to take the opportunities and make the best nutritional decisions to help you recover from breast cancer treatment, enhance your immune system, provide energy, build strength, manage your weight, lessen the effects of aging, and keep the cells of your body growing normally.

ℐ Challenges

Pesticides and Other Chemicals

Every time you take a bite, you bring the external environment into your internal environment, where it can lead to health or havoc. According to the Environmental Protection Agency, about seventy pesticides currently in use are suspected carcinogens. For example, DDT and its breakdown products may increase the risk of breast cancer because they act a little like estrogen and build up in fat tissue over years. And while DDT is now illegal in the United States, it may be on foods we import from countries without DDT restrictions. (Ironically, pesticides banned in the United States may come back to us on fruits and vegetables we import from countries that buy these chemicals from us.)

Farmers are more likely to use pesticides to protect crops from bugs and rot if these crops:

- Bruise or fall apart easily
- Ripen quickly (chemicals are used to slow the ripening process)
- Have a short growing season (chemicals are used to help them last beyond their season)
- Come from far away (need to last longer, during transportation)
- Are grown in countries without laws restricting pesticide use or without enforcement of organic guidelines

The pesticide levels of commonly used nonorganic fruits and vegetables (as well as the juices that come from them) are listed in Table 17.1. These test results don't apply to all sources of each fruit. For example, some sources of bananas could be higher on the "guilty" list. And of course, things change and repeated test results over time may yield different results. The information in the chart below was prepared by the nonprofit organization Environmental Working Group (www.food news.org).

TABLE 17.1 Pesticide Levels: Fruits and Veggies

Rank	Fruit or Veggie	Score
1 (worst)	Peaches	100 (highest pesticide load)
2	Apples	96
3	Sweet bell peppers	86
4	Celery	85
5	Nectarines	84
6	Strawberries	83
7	Cherries	75
8	Lettuce	69
9	Grapes, imported	68
10	Pears	65
11	Spinach	60
12	Potatoes	58
13	Carrots	57
14	Green beans	55

15	Hot peppers	53
16	Cucumbers	52
17	Raspberries	47
18	Plums	46
19	Oranges	46
20	Grapes, domestic	46
21	Cauliflower	39
22	Tangerines	38
23	Mushrooms	37
24	Cantaloupe	34
25	Lemons	31
26	Honeydew melon	31
27	Grapefruit	31
28	Winter squash	31
29	Tomatoes	30
30	Sweet potatoes	30
31	Watermelon	25
32	Blueberries	24
33	Papaya	21
34	Eggplant	19
35	Broccoli	18
36	Cabbage	17
37	Bananas	16
38	Kiwi	14
39	Asparagus	11
40	Green peas, frozen	11
41	Mango	9
42	Pineapples	7
43	Sweet corn, frozen	2
44	Avocado	1
45 (best)	Onions	1 (lowest pesticide load)

Testing was done on washed (apples) or peeled (bananas) fruit by the U.S. Department of Agriculture and the U.S. Food and Drug Administration.

Chemicals used to kill weeds are frequently used to grow the most common food crops: Atrazine with corn and Roundup with soybeans. (Often seeds used to grow these crops have been genetically modified to withstand the effects of these herbicides.) These chemicals can remain on or in corn and soy, ingredients in many foods for people, and nearly all farm animals. Chemical runoff into rivers, streams, and drinking water is an additional potential health threat to all life, for both plants and animals. For example, Atrazine has been shown to increase aromatase activity in fish, thereby increasing their estrogen levels (believe it or not, biological processes in humans and fish are very similar).

Soybeans: The Controversy over Isoflavones

The nutritional benefits of soy are the main value, particularly to a vegetarian who needs nonanimal sources of protein. Soy is inexpensive, high in protein, and low in fat, with no cholesterol. Many soy foods are also high in calcium. But soy is somewhat controversial, as it contains weak estrogenlike substances called isoflavones, with a potential upside and downside for people who've had breast cancer.

The upside is a possible drop of blood cholesterol levels when daily soy replaces animal protein in your diet. The possible downside: soy's weak estrogenlike activity may stimulate breast cancer cell growth. This worry, however, is partly relieved by a few basic soy facts:

- Soy foods contain only a small amount of isoflavones.
- Isoflavones' estrogenlike power is much weaker than your own body's estrogen.
- Women in Asia consume a hundred times more isoflavones than women in the United States, yet they're much less likely to develop breast cancer.

To explain why this might be the case in Asian women, consider that the weaker estrogenlike compounds in soy may actually be blocking normal estrogen from your body's estrogen receptors, so stimulation of breast cell and breast cancer cell growth may be reduced. In this way, isoflavones may act like a relative antiestrogen.

But concern about the possible cancer-promoting effects of soy remains for someone who:

- Has an estrogen receptor–positive breast cancer
- Is on antiestrogen therapy and wants to reduce or avoid any other kind of estrogenlike substances, weak or strong
- Consumes large amounts of concentrated soy and isoflavone products (such as isoflavone supplements or soy protein powder)

Red Meat, Poultry and Dairy: Opportunities for Contamination

Just as you should watch the food you eat, you should also watch what your food eats and what enters its system. So if you consume meat, poultry, and dairy, the quality of the food these animals are fed and the medicines and chemicals they're given all matter. Here are some examples:

- Cows fed on grass are exposed to less pesticide than when they're given a diet of processed grains (such as corn and soy

exposed to Atrazine and Roundup, as previously discussed).

WORLD LIFESTYLE AND BREAST CANCER RATES

The incidence of breast cancer varies significantly around the world. Women living in China and Japan have much lower rates than women in the United States and England. There are several potential explanations for this phenomenon. Asian women living in Asia are more likely to:

- Follow a low-fat, low-calorie diet that is mostly vegetarian, high in soy, and low in animal protein and fat (little meat and barely any dairy products)
- Be at a healthy weight
- Smoke less tobacco and consume less alcohol
- Be more physically active
- Practice regular mind and body disciplines (like tai chi)

But these statistics are changing. When Asian women adopt more habits of Western culture, their risk of breast cancer goes up. Asian women who move to the United States and live the American lifestyle eventually encounter cancer rates that are similar to American women. The reverse is also true: when women from a high-risk country move to a low-risk area, their cancer levels go down as they adapt to the new culture.

- Antibiotics routinely used in animals raised in close quarters—to protect them from infection—get into their milk, meat, eggs.
- Hormones given to dairy cows to increase their milk production (the growth hormone rBGH or rBST) go into the cows' milk supply.
- Hormones given to beef cows to make them bigger also get into their meat and fat. (Hormones are not allowed to be given to poultry and non-beef red meat.)
- Preservatives put in processed and packaged meats, such as nitrites in hot dogs, bacon, and bologna, are not good for you.

A little of these foods from nonorganic sources, on occasion, is probably harmless. But a significant amount of these products over time may prove harmful.

Fish: Pay Attention to Quality

Fish is generally a healthful food, but some fish are more healthful than others. Just as for meat, poultry, and dairy products, the healthfulness of fish depends on what it eats, the water it swims in, and the life span of the fish.

Cold-water fish, such as salmon, haddock, and mackerel, contain omega-3 fats (considered health-promoting), as do smaller fish such as sardines, anchovies, and herring. Bigger fish have bigger issues. They live longer, have more fat, and accumulate more unhealthy chemicals in their fatty tissue. Large fish high on the food chain, such as tuna or swordfish, may contain high levels of mercury or other pollutants, including polychlorinated biphenyls (PCBs, from machine fluids, solvents, etc.) and polyvinylchloride (PVC, a chemical used in making plastic). Fish live in water 24 hours a day 365 days per year. If they live in polluted water, they will accumulate toxic substances. The reverse is also true: clean water, healthy fish.

The source of fish—wild (caught in their natural habitat) or farmed (raised in tanks, pens, or nets)—can make a difference in their quality and safety. But don't assume that wild is automatically better than farmed. Some wild fish come from polluted waters, and some farmed fish are raised in clean water and on healthy feed.

Fat and Cholesterol

Fat is an essential part of your diet. It helps your body:

- Regulate cholesterol metabolism
- Transport and absorb vitamins (A, D, E, and K)
- Keep your skin healthy
- Generate energy
- Support other vital functions in your body

Cholesterol and fat work together to build the structure of your cells and facilitate their function. But the combination can also build up in blood vessels, interfere with blood flow and cause heart disease. You need only a moderate amount of fat for your body's vital functions; your body makes the cholesterol it needs beyond what comes from food.

Avoid Saturated Fat

Fats, oils, and fat-containing foods have a combination of three types of fatty acids in varying proportions:

- Saturated
- Polyunsaturated
- Monounsaturated

Fatty acids are basic units of fat molecules, arranged as chains of carbon, hydrogen, and oxygen. The more hydrogen a fatty acid contains, the more saturated it is and the less healthy it is.

Saturated fat in food raises blood cholesterol more than cholesterol in food, but it's the combination of both—especially in excess—that increases blood cholesterol. Animal sources that are high in saturated fat are usually high in cholesterol and include meat, poultry, eggs, and dairy products. And while vegetable sources of fat contain no cholesterol, tropical oils such as palm and coconut are more saturated—and less healthy—than other vegetable oils.

Trans fats are the least healthy fats, significantly raising blood cholesterol. They are formed when food manufacturers harden oils to more solid forms, like a stick of margarine, in a process called hydrogenation. Labels now list trans fats separately, and fast-food franchises are under pressure to eliminate trans fats from their foods.

℘ Solutions

E mbracing the power of nutrition to improve your health requires you to think in new ways, break bad habits, make sacrifices, try new things, modify routines and rituals, and develop the patience and persistence to stick to your plan. You will need to make a commitment to a new style of eating for health.

Find the Right Balance

Probably the best advice for a balanced diet comes from Michael Pollan, professor of journalism at the University of California, Berkeley, and well-known author: "Eat real food, not too much, mostly plants."

The tried-and-true standard healthy diet recommendations are to eat plenty of fruits and vegetables (five to nine servings a day) and high-fiber foods (35 g of fiber daily). Substitute nuts, beans, grains, or soy foods for some meat, poultry, and dairy products. Restrict the amount of fat you eat, and only use the healthiest kinds. Limit your consumption of red meat, alcohol, salt, and smoked and nitrite-cured foods. Avoid hormones, industrial fertilizers, and pesticides in your food. When possible, buy organic foods. Limit portion size and watch total calories. You're more likely to get high-quality food, save money, and manage your weight by cooking at home.

The diet that most fully embraces these recommendations is the Mediterranean diet—consisting of plant-based, high-fiber foods, moderate fat, low calories, and small amounts of red meat. Its basic compounds are:

- *High fiber.* Eat a wide variety of fresh fruits, vegetables (with lots of tomatoes), beans, and whole grains.
- *Food preparation.* Make it sautéed, grilled, roasted, or baked. Eat few fried foods.

- *Healthy oils.* Use olive oil (canola is also good) for food preparation, dressings, sauces, and enhancement. Use butter and other saturated fats infrequently.
- *Source of protein.* Choose poultry, fish, and beans (soybeans, broad beans, kidney beans). Pinto beans and chickpeas, for instance, have a protein content of 20–34 percent as major sources of protein. Consume red meat only on occasion; limit dairy products. (For more ideas, check out Whfood.org [wh stands for world's healthiest].)
- *Fluids.* Drink six to eight glasses of water a day. Sodas are discouraged, including diet sodas with artificial sweeteners. If alcohol is part of your diet, then wine is preferable.

The success of the Mediterranean diet also depends on the healthy Mediterranean lifestyle: hard physical work, time outdoors, and hanging out with family and friends.

Eat Mostly Plants: Fruits, Vegetables, Beans, and Grains

The reason Michael Pollan strongly encourages people to eat a mostly plant-based diet is because fruit, vegetables, beans, and grains are the healthiest sources of most of the nutrients that are needed to nourish your body, regulate normal tissue function, and protect your cells against the wear and tear of everyday living. Table 17.2 describes major plant groups and the possible benefits each offers.

Get Your Essential Elements

Vitamins C, A, and E, coenzyme Q_{10}, lycopene, alpha- and beta-carotenes, flavonoids, and phenolic

SHOULD I BECOME A VEGETARIAN?

When you hear of the health benefits of a plant-based diet, you might wonder if more is better: should you become a vegetarian? Eating more produce is usually a good healthy bet, but only if it's raised with a nutrient-rich soil and clean water without unhealthy chemicals. This is particularly important for vegetarians since they eat much more produce than everyone else. Plus, you have to be extra careful to get enough protein and the full range of nutrients you need (and which are easier to get from a diet that includes animal sources of protein). (By the way, fish are animals, too.)

TABLE 17.2 Types of Vegetables to Include in Your Diet

- *Cruciferous vegetables*
  - ~**Possible benefits:** contain indols and dithiolethiones, which may block cancer-promoting substances.
  - ~**Sources:** broccoli, cauliflower, Brussels sprouts, cabbage, kale, and mustard and collard greens.
- *Umbelliferous vegetables*
  - ~**Possible benefits:** contain key vitamins and enzymes that may protect you against free radicals and other toxic substances.
  - ~**Sources:** carrots, celery, parsley, and parsnips.
- *Alliums*
  - ~**Possible benefits:** contain allicin, which may help lower cholesterol levels.
  - ~**Sources:** onion family, garlic (fresh cloves, garlic powder, or supplements).
- *Lycopersicons*
  - ~**Possible benefits:** contain high levels of a natural carotenoid called lycopene, a powerful antioxidant.
  - ~**Sources:** tomatoes, pink grapefruit, watermelon, and guava.

---

acids (such as ellagic acid) are the main plant-based antioxidants that neutralize and remove free radicals. Your body normally makes free radicals to attack any possible threat to your body (such as bacteria, viruses, and cancer cells), but they sometimes turn against your body's own cells, causing damage—including genetic (DNA) damage, which might possibly lead to the start of a cancer. Your plant-derived antioxidant SWAT team can protect you against this risk.

Vitamin D, the B vitamins, indols, dithiolethiones, allicin, selenium, and fiber promote normal cell function and may also help reduce your risk of cancer. The mineral calcium is a key building block. Table 17.3 provides you with sources of these important ingredients, found in plant and other food types.

Selecting the Best Foods

What you put in your grocery cart has a huge impact on what you eat. You want the good without the bad. Some foods are safer than others.

TABLE 17.3 Vitamins, Minerals, Supplements

- *Vitamin A,* including retinoids and carotenoids
  - ~**Possible benefits:** reduces the production of prostaglandin, fatty acids, and free radicals and may lead to lower rates of cancer and heart disease.
  - ~**Sources:** green, orange, and deep yellow vegetables, including carrots, bell peppers, green beans, squash, etc.
- *Vitamin B family,* including B_3 (niacin), B_6 (pyridoxine), B_7 (biotin), B_{12} (cobalamin), B_9 (folic acid), and folate
  - ~**Possible benefits:** the B vitamins help you grow properly, get energy from food, and manage stress. B_6 may help ease pain in the arms and legs from taxane chemotherapy. Vitamin B_{12} may boost your energy. Folic acid may help reduce anemia and the risk of birth defects and heart disease. Folate helps your body handle alcohol.
  - ~**Sources:** nuts, seeds, grains and wheat products (flour, cereals); green leafy vegetables, citrus fruits, and green tea. Animal protein is also a good source of niacin.
- *Vitamin C* (aka ascorbic acid)
  - ~**Possible benefits:** may boost the immune system, neutralize free radicals and toxins that can damage normal cell structure and function, and possibly reduce the duration of viral infection and minimize the effects of a cold.
  - ~**Sources:** fresh citrus fruits, peppers, cabbage, cranberries, and cherries. Vitamin C activity may be diminished by cooking.
- *Bioflavonoids*
  - ~**Possible benefits:** works mostly as an antioxidant to help manage allergies, infection, and inflammations. May reduce heart disease and cancer.
  - ~**Sources:** citrus, cherries, berries, grapes, radishes, rhubarb, sweet potatoes and herbs, green tea, wine (red more than white), dark chocolate.
- *Vitamin D*
  - ~**Possible benefits:** helps regulate calcium levels, important for bone and muscle strength and integrity, factors in preventing falls and fractures; may also protect against cancer.
  - ~**Sources:** dairy products, oily fish like salmon and sardines; vitamin D is activated in large part by exposure to sunshine.

- *Vitamin E*
  ~**Possible benefits:** works as an antioxidant to neutralize free radicals and reduce inflammation; may ease hot flashes.
  ~**Sources:** nuts, seeds, vegetable oils.
- *Fiber*
  ~**Possible benefits:** removes unhealthful substances from your system, regulates bowel movements, and may reduce the risk of colon cancer.
  ~**Sources:** whole-grain cereals and breads; beans, fruits, and vegetables; oat-bran; fiber products (like Metamucil, Citrucel).
- *Calcium*
  ~**Possible benefits:** helps keep bones strong.
  ~**Sources:** dairy products, tofu, and leafy green vegetables (women with advanced breast cancer may have high calcium levels and should check with their doctor before taking calcium supplements; see Chapter 12).
- *Selenium*
  ~**Possible benefits:** may reduce free radicals and inhibit the oxidation of unsaturated fats, which may reduce cancer risk.
  ~**Sources:** vegetables, cereal, seafood, dairy products, red meat, and chicken (you only need tiny amounts of selenium; supplements are unnecessary and might even be harmful).
- *Ellagic acid*
  ~**Possible benefits:** neutralizes reactive chemicals and decreases prostaglandins to limit inflammation and cell and genetic damage.
  ~**Sources:** pecans, walnuts, red grapes, red wine, raspberries, strawberries, pomegranates, and other fruits.

You want to avoid foods that contain ingredients, additives, and leftover residues of chemical treatment—pesticides, hormones, antibiotics, and preservatives—that might have a negative effect on your health over time. Here are some tips to help you make the best choices.

- Read the labels on food packages in order to figure out what's inside (and what's not).
- Pick products that are described by regulated terms and avoid products with empty claims. "USDA Organic" means produced without toxic pesticides, artificial fertilizers, synthetic hormones,

antibiotics, irradiation (to kill bacteria), genetic engineering of the seeds or plants, or any sewage or sludge (yuck, that's human waste). These organic foods generally have about two-thirds less pesticides than nonorganic foods. Terms like "natural" and "simple" sound good but have no official definition and are not regulated. Labels that say "no added hormones or pesticides" are usually meaningless because these chemicals are used during animal and crop cultivation, not added later as ingredients.

• Select food that is fresh, whole, unprocessed, grown locally, and pesticide-, herbicide-, and hormone-free. The more ingredients in food, the harder it is to track down how each was made or grown, and the more difficult it is to certify it as organic.

MANAGING THE COST OF ORGANIC FOODS

The higher cost of organic foods is a big problem for most people. To be selective with your organic purchases, look at your eating habits and preferences and save your organic purchases for:

• The foods and beverages you consume the most that are most likely to contain significant levels of pesticides (see Table 17.1)
• Dairy products
• Beef
• Food you make at home from scratch, as opposed to prepared organic meals or eating out at organic restaurants

Also keep in mind that organic products might taste different from what you might expect and they spoil faster (because they are without the preservatives and other things that extend their shelf life). So it may be best for you to purchase them in smaller quantities.

You can also save money by obtaining foods from:

• Farmers' markets, which offer local and in-season foods (requiring little or no use of pesticides, and herbicides, since the produce is delivered quickly with minimal transportation—also saving fuel). To find a farmers' market near you, go to www.localharvest.org and www.ams.usda.gov/farmersmarkets/map.htm.

- Co-ops where your family volunteers its time, to help keep costs down.
- Big store in-house organic food lines (like at Stop & Shop or Wal-mart).
- Your own garden or a community garden.

Some of these farm sources may raise chemical-free food but without official organic designation, since it takes about three years and many regulatory hurdles before full USDA organic status is obtained.

You can improve the safety of nonorganic foods by reducing any surface pollutants:

- Wash all fruits and vegetables with a produce wash solution from the grocery store. Or you can make your own wash: wipe or wash first with white vinegar, then rinse with water.
- Scrub potatoes if you plan to eat their skins.
- Peel fruits and vegetables, particularly those that are waxed (such as apples and cucumbers).
- Discard the outer leaves of heads of lettuce and cabbage.

Although peeling produce is a good option, you can end up throwing away valuable nutrients right under the skin. That's a good reason to buy organic sources of the produce you prefer to eat along with its skin, such as apples and potatoes. Another limitation: peeling and washing don't eliminate the chemicals that get absorbed inside fruits and vegetables.

Choose Food Over Supplements

Food—mostly fruits and vegetables—is the best source of these important elements, rather than pills, capsules, or powders. That's because other factors in food enhance their health-giving benefits. Plus buyer beware: the FDA does not regulate dietary supplements for their purity, content, or safety, so their manufacturers are relatively free to make promises without proof of benefits.

Cooking may reduce vitamin content in some foods, but for others like tomatoes, cooking can enhance their health value. And many people find cooking makes it easier to swallow and digest larger quantities of vegetables and fruit. Juice is not a great way to get these nutrients: you miss out on the fiber and other value from the pulp of the fruit or vegetable (plus you often consume lots more calories).

It's easier to get niacin from meat and poultry, but if you are limiting your consumption of these foods, you can get what you need from niacin-fortified flour, cereals, and breads, or a multivitamin supplement.

While it's best to get these key ingredients from fresh food, it's not always possible. You might not like fruit and vegetables, you may have limited access to the produce department, and their cost can be a real challenge. Frozen produce can serve your needs as well as fresh, if availability is an issue. But if all else fails, supplements are a good compromise. Ask your doctor about the right dose, combination, and brand of supplements for you and your situation. And beware: when it comes to vitamins, more is not necessarily better—in fact, more can be dangerous.

HEALTHY SNACKS

Steady-energy snacks can include peanut butter, cottage cheese, yogurt, nuts, beans, tofu, low-fat cheeses, chicken or vegetable broth, cooked egg whites or hard-boiled eggs, fruits, and raw vegetables. Mix 'em up—try combinations such as plain fat-free yogurt with fresh fruit, peanut butter on celery, carrots dipped in curry-flavored yogurt or cottage cheese, cucumber discs with salsa, a whipped egg mixed into hot broth, or vegetables in broth.

Play Safe with Soy

Until the controversy about the safety of soy in women with hormone receptor–positive breast cancer is resolved, it's best to play it safe. Here are a few suggestions:

- Stick to whole or lightly processed soy foods: soy milk, tofu, tempeh, soy beans (edamame).
- Avoid highly processed concentrated products in extracts, tablets, and powders, which may contain large amounts of isoflavones.

And check with your doctor before eating soy foods on a regular basis. Buy organic sources of soy to avoid concerns about exposure to the herbicides used with genetically modified crops.

Make Healthy Meat, Poultry, and Dairy Selections

While hormones may only be given to beef cattle, not to the other sources of red meat, it's recommended that you limit your consumption of red meat to once or twice a week. The most commonly used animal feeds are corn and soy—so try to select animal products that were fed healthy sources of food: grass and organic types of grains. It's also best to avoid blackening meat or poultry while grilling.

The easiest way to purchase healthy sources of these foods is to:

- Buy USDA-certified organic products.
- Look for the words *rBGH-free* or *rBST-free* on milk labels.
- Select cheese that comes from organic farms or countries that don't allow hormones to be given to dairy cows, including: Canada, Australia, New Zealand, Japan, and the countries of the European Union (e.g., Holland, France, Italy, Germany, Spain, etc.). Soon all milk sold in California must be rBGH-free or rBST-free.
- Buy meat and dairy products from small or medium local farms, which are less likely to use the large quantities of antibiotics and other chemicals used with mass production. Plus less gas is used in the transportation of the food—which is also better for the environment.
- Try to find lean, grass-fed beef and other types of red meat.
- Restrict the amount of nonorganic sources of these foods in your diet.

Best Fish Choices

You can eat cold-water fish (like salmon, haddock, and mackerel) and little fish (sardines, anchovies, herring) more than once a week. But limit your big fish (like swordfish and tuna) eating to no more than once a week, or even better, not more than once a month.

To help you figure out the best source of fish, wild or farmed, check out the nonprofit Marine Stewardship Council's website, which offers a people-healthy, environmentally friendly, location-based fish-buying guide, at www.msc.org.

Limit Your Fat Intake

Fat in your diet should be limited (but not eliminated) for a number of reasons:

- For more effective weight management (gram for gram, fat has more calories than protein and carbohydrates)
- For lower cholesterol levels and better health of your heart and blood vessels
- To potentially reduce the risk of breast cancer
- To limit your exposure to unhealthy chemicals in animal fats, including hormones, pesticides, antibiotics, and plastic residues

Try to limit your fat intake to 30 percent or less of your daily calories. Stick to healthy fats like monounsaturated, polyunsaturated, omega-3s, and omega-6s, in foods like nuts, seeds, fish, and vegetable oils (olive, canola, safflower, soybean, corn, cottonseed, and sunflower).

Saturated fats should be reduced to less than 7 percent of your total daily calories and trans fats to less than 1 percent. You also want to limit the amount of cholesterol in your diet to under 300 mg per day—or less if you already have high LDL cholesterol or blood vessel disease of the heart.

SAFE FOOD AND BEVERAGE PREPARATION AND STORAGE

The ways you cook and reheat your food and the methods of storing and carrying around your food and beverages can make a difference in their nutritional value and safety. Here are some basic recommendations:

Cooking methods
- Steam, poach, sauté, roast, grill (but not blackened), or microwave your food.
- Avoid frying.

Cooking and storage containers
- Use pans and pots made of stainless steel, ceramic, glass, or Corningware in the stove or oven. Silicone baking pans and sheets are believed to be relatively safe.

- Avoid using plastic pans or cooking bags in the regular oven, and avoid using plastic containers or wraps in the microwave oven.
- Remove restaurant take-out food from its plastic or Styrofoam container before reheating. You can also ask the restaurant if it has biodegradable containers (some are made of corn or potato starch), which are safer for you and the environment.
- Avoid the nonstick Teflon-coated surfaces, made with perfluorooctanoic acid (unhealthy for you and the environment).
- Use butcher paper, wax paper, or a paper towel (secured with a rubber band if needed) for storage. For plastic wrap, use brands without PVC (polyvinyl chloride), such as Diamant Food Wrap (without a plasticizer, which can be purchased at www.diamantfilm.com), Glad Cling Wrap, Saran with Cling Plus, or Saran Premium Wrap. Many of these options are available at www.greenfeet.com or your local supermarket. If possible, plastic wrap shouldn't come in direct contact with food.

Carrying and storing beverages

For cold drinks

- Use glass or stainless steel cups (or reuse glass jars). Try to buy beverages in glass containers (most soda cans are lined with plastic).
- If only plastic is available, check the recycling code: use 1, 2, 4, or 5 bottles when possible.
- Avoid using:
  - ~ #7 hard plastic water bottles made with bisphenol A (BPA), which can have a weak hormonal effect. With repeated use and washing, the plastic slowly breaks down and more of this chemical can leach into the drinking water.
  - ~ #6 polystyrene plastic party cups.

For hot drinks

- Use ceramic mugs or an insulated stainless steel–lined coffee cup.
- Avoid Styrofoam (polystyrene) cups (they're also really bad for the environment).
- Watch out for paper cups designed for hot or wet foods that are treated with a plastic resin (it's not usually disclosed on its label).

Pay Attention to Timing

The timing of cooking and eating can make a difference in your energy level. Cook when your energy is at its best. Prepare extra meals at one time to maximize your efficiency—like a big pot of chili or soup, trays of roasted vegetables, or an extra pan of lasagna or baked chicken. (Be sure to put away the extras rather than overeat after the cookfest—you'll be grateful for cook-free meals at the ready.) Enjoy your biggest meal when you have the most energy and the best appetite. Eat your evening meal, a lighter meal, as early as possible before you go to sleep.

❧ Moving Forward

Food is one of life's great pleasures. And some foods are especially good for you. The trick is to figure out a healthy diet that is also a pleasure to eat. Think of the improvement of your nutrition as an improvement in lifestyle that will ease the effects of growing older and the lingering effects of cancer therapy. And because increasing age is one of the greatest risk factors for breast cancer, easing the aging process on your cells also means increasing your chance of living cancer-free.

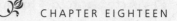

CHAPTER EIGHTEEN

Weight and Exercise: Gains and Losses

I wasn't doing too bad with my weight until I went on tamoxifen. I put on thirty pounds in no time. I managed to take off ten pounds by watching what I ate and taking the stairs instead of the elevator, but I can't seem to budge the other twenty. I feel good, so I've decided not to torture myself about those extra pounds. I think I look good enough.

While I was feeling sorry for myself, I treated myself to whatever made me happy: cheesecake, french fries, ice cream, cookies, chocolate, and more chocolate. Now I'm a fat slob and I only have myself to blame. But now that I've reached rock bottom, things can only get better, right?

I eat just what I always have—but my weight keeps growing and I can't seem to manage to get rid of what I gain. It is so frustrating.

I didn't realize how many calories were in the foods that I thought were so healthy. When I ate ten dried apricots I didn't stop to think that that was the equivalent of five whole fresh apricots. Alcohol, along with the cheese and crackers that seem to automatically go with it, can have more calories than a regular dinner. The only way I could manage my weight was to get real with the food facts. Now I have a calorie guide and measuring cups—and I always look at the nutritional information on food packaging.

✿ First Things First

A nibble here, a nibble there, and pretty soon another five pounds is sitting on your hips. Your metabolism slows as you age, decreasing by about 30 percent after menopause, and that means you use fewer calories to get through your day. If you don't cut back what you eat by a third, those unused calories are stored as fat.

If weight was a problem for you before breast cancer, it's probably a bigger problem now. At least a third of women gain weight during chemotherapy, usually an average of five to ten pounds, and for many, the tendency to gain weight continues even after chemotherapy is finished. For women taking tamoxifen or an aromatase inhibitor, the tendency to gain weight is made worse.

Causes of Weight Gain

Too many calories in, too few calories burned. Aren't you sick of hearing this? While we know it's true, it's never as simple as it seems to be. Growing older and going through breast cancer treatment appear to break all the old rules for weight—and now you're dealing with new rules written in fine print you never were informed of or agreed to. You have to eat less *and* exercise more if you want to stabilize your weight.

There are plenty of reasons for creeping or accelerated weight gain. Perhaps it's the result of the sudden arrival of menopause, or of physical inactivity, or maybe it's a consequence of "relief" eating. No matter the source, the struggle to lose those pounds is tough. Before you can solve any problem, however, you first need to understand what's causing the problem. Here is a list of forces that can pile on those pounds and relocate weight to the belly area.

Emotional issues
- *Anxiety and stress* interfere with sleep and proper function and lead to poor eating and less exercise. Chronic stress increases blood cortisol levels (a steroid that weakens muscles and shifts weight distribution to the middle).

- *Depression and feelings of hopelessness and failure* remove interest in exercise, social activities, and healthy eating and encourage bad behavior such as smoking and alcohol consumption.
- *Insomnia and fatigue* disrupt your body's healthy rhythms; sleeping, eating, and physical activity all suffer.
- *The need for comfort and pleasure* makes you seek rich foods that soothe an upset belly and gratify cravings. (Some research suggests that a taste for high-fat and high-sugar foods is common among women affected by breast cancer, because these foods create a feel-good effect by stimulating the release of endorphins.)

Treatment issues
- *Hormonal changes* can slow down your metabolism, and can occur because of:
  - ~Natural or treatment-induced menopause
  - ~Hormonal therapies such as tamoxifen or aromatase inhibitors
- *Other medications* (including steroids and pain medication) can increase your appetite and slow your metabolism.
- *Aches and pains* lead to decreased physical activity, and can result from:
  - ~Hormonal therapies
  - ~Going into menopause
  - ~Arthritis
  - ~Growing older
- *Nausea and queasiness* tend to be relieved by calorie-dense foods.

Life's other challenges
- *Unhealthy eating habits* are very hard to shake, particularly if your whole family piles high-calorie foods sky high.
- *Restaurant food* is usually rich and loaded with calories.
- *Prepared foods* are a practical solution to putting food on the table while you're feeling less than 100 percent, but they are often loaded with fat, sugar, and salt.
- *Gifts of food* tend to be rich and heavy.
- *Growing older* slows your metabolism, giving you a tendency to gain weight and making weight management an uphill battle.

• ***Stopping smoking*** causes nicotine craving and agitation, leading to increased eating.

In this chapter, you'll better understand why the pounds are piling up, and you'll find solutions to shaking off the extra weight—to help you feel better about your health and more confident about your appearance.

🌿 Challenges

FEWER CALORIES NEEDED AS YOU AGE

The facts:

• Your muscles consume the most calories of any tissue in your body.
• You lose a little bit of your muscle mass and strength every year after age thirty

The bottom line: As you grow older, your muscles get smaller, requiring fewer calories on a daily basis, even if you are just as active as you've always been. Frustrating, but it's the reality we all have to accept and live by.

Your self-image, already battered by the whole breast cancer experience, gets flogged further by weight gain. Added to that assault can be fear when you hear reports that link weight gain to an increased risk of recurrence. Losing those extra pounds can be a huge challenge, and often the energy and drive just aren't there.

Increased Breast Cancer Risk

There is significant evidence that links excess weight and a higher risk of breast cancer. Because fat cells help make estrogen, the more fat cells you have, the more estrogen there is to stimulate breast cells, including breast cancer cells, if any are present. (That's why blocking or eliminating the effects of estrogen is one of the goals of breast cancer therapy.)

Fat also collects pesticides, herbicides, hormones, and other potential unhealthy substances consumed over a lifetime, in food, beverages, personal products, water, and air (these various chemicals dissolve in fat). And some of these chemicals are accused of being carcinogenic.

BIG IN THE MIDDLE

Weight gain in the belly area is a common complaint of many women after breast cancer treatment. The main factors that put extra weight around your middle include:

- **Genetics.** Body shape is heavily influenced by the genes you inherited from your mother and father. If one or both had a potbelly, then you may develop one, too.
- **Weight gain.** Decreased metabolism, less physical activity, comfort foods, and treatment side effects all lead to weight gain, including in your belly.
- **Fat redistribution.** Age-related shifts in hormonal levels tend to park more weight in the belly area, both in front of your belly wall as well as inside your belly cavity, surrounding your intestines. Chronic stress increases your body's level of cortisol (a steroid), which also puts more weight around your middle.
- **Loss of height.** Age-related shrinkage occurs mainly along your spine: vertebral bodies and discs slowly flatten and you lose height. If the distance between your shoulders and your hips has shortened significantly, your belly tissue gets compressed and has nowhere to go but outward.

Furthermore, the location of fat cells may also impact your breast cancer risk. Studies suggest that certain female torso shapes are more at risk than others: apple-shaped women have a higher incidence of breast cancer than pear-shaped women. Maybe excess fat in the belly area is more likely to produce unhealthy amounts of hormones than fat located on the hips. In any case, there is evidence that losing weight overall and keeping it off does help lower risk.

Increased Risk of Lymphedema

Being very overweight and/or gaining a significant amount of extra weight after treatment are risk factors for lymphedema, if you've had a lymph node dissection with or without major breast surgery. That said, weight is only one of many risk factors for lymphedema, *and* it's one on the list that you can change (see Chapter 10 for more on lymphedema).

Vicious Cycles

While you're struggling to bring about a healthier you, emotional, treatment, and life issues can combine to cause continuing weight gain. It's so easy to get caught up in a whole series of interrelated destructive cycles that can run your life in the wrong direction. Here are just a few examples:

- Being heavy > less likely to exercise > more weight gain.
- Failing a diet plan > weight gain and discouragement > failing another diet plan.
- Someone's rude comment > helplessness > weight gain > another rude comment.
- Aches and pains > make you less active > weight gain > more aches and pains.

Now is a good time to break the cycles and get onto a more productive and less destructive track.

Crash Diets Do More Harm than Good

Disregard the mass of magazine cover stories and media sound bites that feature one miracle diet after another. Avoid crash diets and attempts at rapid weight loss.

If you lose weight too fast, your body goes on starvation alert. Your metabolism starts to slow down to conserve energy, defeating the very purpose of your hard efforts. The high-protein diet is another misguided notion and is also hard to maintain. It puts an unhealthy strain on your system, especially your kidneys.

Slow and steady wins the battle over the bulge and helps you stay the winner over the long haul. Every successful approach to weight loss recommends exercise and moderate consumption of nutritious foods from all the essential food groups.

Empty Calories Can Derail Healthy Eating

Empty calories—foods with high calories and no nutritional value (like soda, lemonade, and sweetened iced tea)—can destroy your diet plan from the get-go. Shortly after you load up on these foods (high in sugar

LEAVE THE ALCOHOL IN THE BOTTLE

Alcohol can destroy any weight management plan in a number of ways:

- Alcohol contains oodles of calories.
- Drink mixers add loads more calories from all the sugar they contain (whiskey sours, margaritas, etc.).
- Alcohol can make sad feelings sink lower, putting you into a total funk.
- Alcohol can diminish your self-control and allow food cravings to take over: "Let's go for the cheese and crackers with the wine!"
- Alcohol makes you sleepy and less physically active.

and carbs), a cascade of unhealthy reactions occur:

- Your blood sugar soars.
- The insulin hormone system is triggered into action.
- Your body takes the extra sugar out of your bloodstream and stores it in fat.
- Blood sugar quickly drops.

This sharp and rapid rise and fall of blood sugar makes you crave more food and lose control of your diet goals.

Weight Gain Is Even More Frustrating Now

If you're like most women, you've gained and lost weight hundreds of times before. But this time probably feels different because:

- The weight seems like it came from nowhere—it's not as if you had any pleasure putting on those extra pounds from really great food.
- The extra weight feels like more punishment from the overall breast cancer diagnosis and its treatments.
- Weight loss is harder to accomplish.

But as unkind, unfair, and bad as the extra weight gain feels, it's more important than ever to shed some pounds and get closer to a healthy weight. Sometimes it takes a major crisis, a revelation, hitting bottom, or needing to get primed for an upcoming major event (such as a reunion or wedding) for you to work up enough motivation to take charge and make the necessary changes in your life. Now is the time to put this extra weight behind you. Today and the days ahead will give you lots of new opportunities to turn things around.

❧ Solutions

Losing weight doesn't have to be an all-or-nothing or boring proposition. If you stick to a rigid diet and only one form of exercise, you're bound to find it tiresome and give up. You have to begin somewhere, go slowly in the right direction, and then build momentum. That first step is always the hardest.

You'll have the most success when you set realistic goals, combine exercise with a healthy diet (see Chapter 17), and get lots of support so you can make immediate progress, build confidence, avoid boredom, and establish the healthy habits you can sustain over time.

Get Strategic: Combined Exercise and Diet

The first step to controlling your weight is to work with your doctor, a nutritionist, and a fitness instructor to select a diet plan and exercise routine that are right for you—ones that offer you a mix of options and flexible rules. But you have to get real: 80 percent of weight management is about food; 20 percent depends on exercise. You have to put an end to overeating. Pick up a copy of Dr. David Kessler's book *The End of Overeating* for insights and ideas on cutting back.

Eating less high-calorie food and more nutritious low-calorie food is an obvious strategy. A low-fat diet that's mostly plant-based, with moderate amounts of poultry and fish and small amounts of red meat, is the healthiest way to go. Most doctors favor the Mediterranean diet. *Consumer Reports* gives a top rating to the Volumetrics Eating Plan; Weight Watchers was second, and Jenny Craig third.

Even if you're eating a very healthy diet, you won't lose weight (particularly around the belly) and keep fit without exercise. Exercise will provide you with a feeling of control, enhance your sense of well-being, and extend your life. Walking turns out to be the most sustainable form of exercise, but a mix of different forms of exercise will keep you moving and avoid the boredom. Organizing a few of your neighbors, joining

VOLUMETRICS EATING PLAN

The Volumetrics Eating Plan, created by Barbara Rolls, Ph.D., a professor of nutrition science at Pennsylvania State University, is all about feeling satisfied with fewer calories. Its basic concept is that you stop eating when you feel full. This approach has helped me and many of my patients manage their weight. Here are a few of its highlights:

- **Eat slowly to avoid overeating.** It can take twenty to thirty minutes for your stomach to tell your brain that it's full.
- **Choose low-calorie, fast-filling foods.** These will help you to feel satisfied sooner, before having to reach for all the high-calorie foods. The best choices are foods with high water and fiber content because they have the fewest calories per gram and are often the most nutritious (nonstarchy vegetables and fruit, like tomatoes, broccoli, greens, cantaloupe; whole-grain items like multigrain bread, whole-wheat pasta; low-fat sources of protein like skinless chicken breast, etc.).
- **Stack your deck.** To maximize your chance of making winning choices, fill your refrigerator with plenty of healthful foods to choose from.
- **No forbidden food.** To help minimize the tendency to crave things that are bad for you, buy only very limited amounts of calorie-dense foods (such as crackers, candy, cookies, chocolate, butter, oils). Don't deprive yourself of these foods, but eat them in very small quantities. Pick a food from a less calorie-dense group, such as grapes, instead of a more calorie-dense food, such as raisins.
- **Lots of water.** To fill you up and move food through your system, nine or more glasses of water per day are encouraged.

The good news: the Volumetrics Eating Plan is a healthy, practical, and sustainable approach to successful weight management over time.

Curves, or signing up for your local gym can all help (see more about exercise later in the chapter).

Cutting Back

You can eat a lot of things you like, even high-calorie favorites, as long as you limit the portions and understand how many calories you're actually consuming.

Restrict Portion Size

You will probably be amazed at the difference between what you consider a reasonable portion and what the label recommends. For example, a reasonable portion of chicken is 4 ounces, the size of a deck of cards. "Those labels changed my life. I don't eat a thing till I read the fat and calorie content and portion size. I'm enjoying meals more than ever, and I've lost ten pounds."

Using small or medium-sized plates will also help you avoid taking bigger portions and eating more. Weigh portions, and keep a calorie-counting book handy, along with a kitchen scale. Use measuring cups and spoons to figure the portion sizes suggested on the Nutrition Facts section of the labels on the packaged foods you buy. Also, take note of the listed calories, fat, cholesterol, sugar, salt, fiber, vitamins, and minerals. In time, you won't have to weigh and calculate everything you plan to eat.

THE MEDITERRANEAN DIET

The Mediterranean diet—consisting of high fiber, moderate fat, low calories, and small amounts of red meat—seems to win out over most others. Major features include: a diet of high fiber, lots of fruits and vegetables, and healthy sources of protein, prepared with healthy cooking techniques using olive oil (see Chapter 17, pages 346–347, for more details).

The success of the Mediterranean diet also depends on the healthy Mediterranean lifestyle: hard physical work, time outdoors, and hanging out with family and friends.

Limit Your Calories

To lose weight, you need to limit the number of calories you consume—but you need to consume enough food so you don't feel hungry. To do that, you need to know the numbers—including the number of calories in the foods you eat, the number of calories you burn off, and the number of calories to aim for. The average woman needs about 1,800 to 2,000 calories per day, but this count varies depending on your age, height, weight, and body type. It is unwise to go below a daily intake of 1,200 calories for any extended period of time.

Many people find it works best to stick to a strict number of calories for at least two weeks at the start, in order to acquire a true sense of what each food "costs." Keep in mind that all calories are not the same. For example, calories from fruit drinks (like orange juice) are more readily available to your body than the complex sugars contained inside plant fibers, like in a whole orange (minus the peel and seeds, of course), which your body only partially digests. The whole food fills you up; the complex sugars they contain keep your digestion process busy longer, muting cravings.

Limiting your calorie intake doesn't mean keeping to strict accounting forever. Once you get the drift of how calories add up, you can discard the weighing and the totaling up of exact numbers. You can average out the desired number of calories over a few days, thus allowing for an occasional splurge on one day by cutting back calories earlier the same day, the day before, or the day after. The same budgeting is required when going out to a restaurant or a friend's house for dinner.

Cut the Fat

Gram for gram, fat has more calories than protein and carbohydrates. So cutting the fat in your diet is the most effective way to limit your calories and manage your weight. As a general rule, try to limit the calories you get from fat to 30 percent or less of your total daily caloric intake.

To maximize your success, you have to pay close attention to the amount of fat in processed food. Just look at all the specialty pretzels out there—they embellish your salty crunch with a little fat to make them even more irresistible.

Remember that the leading source of fat in a woman's diet is salad dressing, followed by cheese, butter or margarine, mayonnaise, baked goods, eggs, and ground beef. These fat-cutting tips will help to keep you on track:

- Put your salad dressing on the side; dip your fork in the dressing and then spear your salad greens.
- Limit the amount of fat and oil you use for cooking, and stick with unsaturated oils (preferably olive or canola). Avoid oily foods (like carrot cake, bran muffins, cream sauces, movie theater popcorn).
- Choose beans, grains, pasta, seafood (fresh or canned in water), and skinless chicken or turkey white meat. Use cooking

techniques that require little or no fat: microwaving, broiling, and steaming (instead of deep-frying and sautéing).

• Try using applesauce or other fruit purees instead of butter when baking. Use broth instead of oil or butter to sauté your food.

• Substitute two egg whites (fat- and cholesterol-free) for one whole egg.

Single out the foods you like and familiarize yourself with low-fat ways to prepare or serve them (see Table 18.1). Once you're into the swing of the list, menu planning and calorie counting become easier. It's still a challenge to make food tasty when you're keeping fat intake low, but stick with it. Your taste will change, and you may lose your "fat tooth."

Check the bookstores for low-fat and no-fat cookbooks and for inspiration. But realize that you don't need to go to extremes to cut fats from your diet. You do need *some* fats, after all.

Eat Mindfully

Eat only when you are hungry, not when you think it's time to chow down. It takes a full twenty minutes for your body to figure out that it's had enough and to send that signal to your brain. If you're eating too fast but expecting to stop when you feel full, you're beating out the signal that will help you stop. "Think about every bite," says Sherry, a successful dieter. "Enjoy every bite you take and slow down between bites."

Schedule meals far enough apart so that you're hungry when mealtime comes around, but not so far apart that you want to consume everything in sight by the time you do get to eat. Don't eat on the run, because you'll tend to eat more than you think and you won't get the same amount of pleasure from your food.

Take Charge of Your Meals

Doing the cooking yourself, start to finish, remains the best way to manage a healthy diet. You control what comes into the house and goes onto the table and into your stomach. So while fewer and fewer people are spending time preparing meals at home these days, the healthiest plan for weight management is dining in with you as chef. It can also save you

TABLE 18.1 Tasty Low-Fat Alternatives

No, No	Yes, Yes
Apple pie with ice cream	Baked apple slices with nonfat yogurt and low-fat granola sprinkles
Sauté in butter	Sauté food in chicken or vegetable broth
Ice cream	Sorbet, ices, frozen fruit pops, or fat-free frozen yogurt
Butter	Olive oil or canola oil; unsweetened fruit preserves
Cream soups	Gazpacho, vegetable soups in broth base
Sour cream dip	Salsa
Potato chips	Thin pretzels
Donuts, iced cakes	Angel food cake
Brownies	Gingersnaps, low-fat cookies, melted chocolate thinly spread on chewy bread
Croissants	Bagels (small ones)
Salami, bologna	Turkey, lean ham
Oil-packed tuna	Water-packed tuna
French fries	Baked, roasted, or boiled potatoes
Sour cream	Yogurt or low-fat cottage cheese
Mayonnaise	Mustard
Corn chips	Air-popped popcorn
Cheese from whole milk or cream	Part-skim mozzarella, ricotta, or soy cheese
Whole eggs	Egg whites, Egg Beaters
Ham-and-cheese omelet	Vegetable and egg-white omelet
Fruit-flavored yogurt	Nonfat yogurt with sliced fresh fruit
Olives	Celery or raw vegetable strips
Whole milk	Skim milk

lots of money, making this option even more worthwhile as often as you can manage it.

It's a fact: If you cook at home, you eat less; if you eat out, you eat more.

TIPS ON DINING IN AND DINING OUT

One thing you can be sure of: restaurant food has a lot more calories and fat than you or even a trained dietitian might imagine or predict. For a restaurant to get your rave reviews and turn you into a loyal customer, the food has to taste great—and easiest way to make that happen is to use a lot of fat, sugar, and/or salt (even the tomato sauces have butter in them). So beware!

Before going out to eat, fill up on low-calorie foods (cucumbers, celery, etc.). And when you're ready to order, here are some smart choices:

- Ask what's in the dish you want to order. (Don't be embarrassed; enough people are interested in healthy eating to have made this a commonplace request.)
- Request that sauces, butter, sour cream, and salad dressing be served on the side, and the skin be taken off chicken.
- Eat no more than half of any large portion. (Ask your waiter to wrap up the other half so you can take it home for a second meal.)
- Order two appetizers and a house salad when you're with dinner guests who are enjoying a three-course meal.
- Stay away from buffet tables!

Many menus highlight healthful choices, so ordering can be less complicated and more streamlined. Even fast-food chains have joined the campaign, with lean specials and take-out literature containing nutrition facts about their popular food items.

Going to other people's homes for dinner can be very difficult. If it's a close friend, it may be worth discussing the menu ahead of time to make sure that there is a healthy option you can enjoy. Otherwise, just stick to small portions and take little bites to keep pace with everyone else. Drink lots of water.

Still, if you are cooking for a family, especially one with teenagers, you are set up for a real challenge. It can be torture to watch young people wolf down huge numbers of calories while you try to restrict yourself to an austere menu. What willpower you need! Face the problem and answer a bunch of key questions:

- Can you handle it on your own?
- Can you get your family to give up fried foods and junk foods?

- How much fat can you eliminate from the rest of your family's diet (setting them on a healthy course for their future)?
- Should you eat before the others, or at least eat something that will temper your appetite?
- Should you prepare separate dishes for yourself?

Try out different answers to these questions in order to figure out the best solutions for day-to-day meal preparation and enjoyment.

The easiest ways to take charge are to focus on your goals, design your menus, plan your grocery list, get out of the kitchen, give yourself credit for your resolve, measure your progress, and take advantage of group support.

Coping with Food Cravings

Most snacks that you reach for start off at 100 calories (there is now a whole industry that prepackages 100-calorie snacks and treats). It's wildly frustrating, budgeting calories just as you budget money. How do you satisfy your desires with the limited number of calories you can afford?

It's best to try to curb your sweet tooth. When you do use a sweetener, try complex carbohydrates such as barley, rice, and malt syrups, rather than sugar substitutes such as Sweet'N Low, NutraSweet, or Splenda. These artificial sweeteners just sustain your level of craving or desire for sweets. (Although problems have been reported with each artificial sweetener, they pose no proven health risk.)

You tend to feel better taking in protein rather than taking in foods that are high in carbohydrates. Eating protein leads to a more controlled level of blood sugar. For me, chicken broth (fat free, with some chopped veggies) or egg whites (hard-boiled eggs with yolks removed, or whites microwaved for about 90 seconds with salt and pepper in a bowl wiped or sprayed with olive oil) are good ways to satisfy hunger and carry me over to the next meal.

If the urge for food won't let up, think about how and why it's got that grip on you. Set your mind against the craving. Remind yourself that *you* are in charge of your life and your weight. And because we're not machines, allow yourself some rewards through the day or week, but plan them ahead of time so there's little chance of grabbing something you shouldn't, or worse, of bingeing.

Avoid Temptation

Concentrate on your food shopping. Never shop when you're hungry. Don't drop *anything* that isn't good for you into your shopping cart. Don't allow high-calorie foods, such as high-fat specialty ice cream or rich entrees, into your house. When you get that urge to nibble, unwholesome choices just won't be available—you'll have to settle for healthful snacks, such as:

- Lots of fresh fruits and vegetables (five to nine servings a day).
- Nonfat yogurt.
- High-fiber, low-fat snacks (like low-fat granola or Good Friends bran cereal)
- Low-fat protein sources: fish, egg whites, white-meat poultry, and lean meats.

Keep an ample supply of fruits and vegetables in your refrigerator, with plenty of cut-up raw vegetable snacks in water, crisp and ready when you are. If you need more flavor to satisfy you, toss the vegetables in a light vinaigrette (two-thirds balsamic vinegar to one-third olive oil) instead of water. Extra-tempting fruit is a smart investment; watermelon and cantaloupe go a long way. Tasty low-calorie treats are another good option. Dried fruit can be as good as candy—but here, too, the calories can quickly add up.

Keep the food *in* the kitchen and you *out* of the kitchen as much as possible; it's too easy to taste or pick up a bite of this or that. No more peanuts in the family room and pretzels in the den. Out of sight, out of your mouth. And get out of the house for exercise, yoga, work, or shopping with friends—activities where no food is served or available.

Reward Yourself

Give yourself incentives to build your resolve and motivate your weight loss:

- ***Dress up and feel sleek.*** Have a tight black catsuit or little black dress that you slip on and wear around the house to inspire you and remind you of your goals. And add a pair of jazzy shoes to finish off the look.

- *Fantasize about the "new you."* Imagine yourself as the belle of the ball, gliding down the fashion show runway, diving into the ocean with a killer bathing suit. (Fantasy is fantasy—no need to stay within reality limits!)

- *Get ready for the big event.* Let an important upcoming event inspire and drive your diet and exercise plan: a hot date, class reunion (maybe an old boyfriend or crush will be there), wedding, birthday, graduation, next summer on the beach, etc.

- *Let the skinny jeans or great outfit inspire you.* Hang up that favorite pair of jeans or bikini. Some people even buy a great outfit or a little black dress in a smaller size. Set out a series of clothes to chart your milestones.

- *Compete or work toward incentives.* Collect a pot of cash at work or with friends and let the biggest weight loser win. Or do it on your own: $5 per pound that you're able to keep off for at least a month. You can lay away a great pair of shoes until you're at your goal. Just think about something you'd really love to have or do, and let it be your incentive to lose weight. The prize, at the end, will be well deserved!

Get Support

Don't try to lose weight alone. Peer support is important. Find someone to share your pain and gains, someone you can call when food desires get overpowering, who'll shore up your resolve, who'll talk you past the desperate moments. Control leads to more control. The Weight Watchers program appears to be one of the most successful designs for long-term weight management. Group support and reinforcement along with a flexible expert diet plan are its essential ingredients: regular meetings, weigh-ins, calorie counting, kitchen-scale measurement of food, and filling yourself with large, healthy, balanced meals. The food plan is practical, healthy, and sustainable over the long term. You don't suffer food deprivation; you get to eat real food, not just powders or processed bars. Weight Watchers emphasizes behavior modification by teaching ways to alter bad eating

MAJOR OVERWEIGHT MANAGEMENT

In some cases, managing your weight may be beyond your control. Although high-calorie diets and sedentary lifestyles are responsible for most weight gain, more and more research shows that genes can be the cause of particular weight problems, such as a low metabolic rate.

There's an enormous amount of research going on about the role of genes in weight issues, as well as for weight control aids. Many people are naturally large and were not meant to be thin. It's important for each person to figure out a realistic and healthy weight to aim for, together with her doctor. However, if your weight has reached a very unhealthy level and you've had no success with weight control programs, you may be looking for more aggressive measures.

Diet pills should be used only as a last resort, after you've worked hard to lose weight through combination diet and exercise plans. The use of diet pills on a regular basis is highly controversial because of potentially life-threatening and irreversible side effects, as well as their limited long-term weight-shedding benefit. Any use of diet pills requires extreme caution, a doctor's prescription, and close medical supervision.

Diet pills should be considered only if you are 20 percent over your ideal weight with weight-related health problems, or 30 percent over your ideal weight without weight-related health problems.

Surgery to bypass the stomach or make it much narrower or smaller is an extreme measure to manage severe obesity (when you weigh 100 pounds or 100 percent more than your ideal body weight). Special bariatric surgeons must evaluate your situation to see if you're a good candidate for this procedure, measuring the potential benefits and side effects of surgery in your individual situation.

habits such as snacking, eating on the run, and consuming excessive-sized portions.

Reap the Benefits of Exercise

No matter how good you are about dieting, as already mentioned in this chapter, it's nearly impossible to lose weight and keep it off by diet alone. Couch-potato dieters seem to get only so far; they lose weight up to a point, the weight loss trails off, and then they regain what they've lost. People who exercise and diet are much more likely to continue losing weight until they hit their healthy weight; more important, they are better able to maintain that weight loss.

Exercise has importance beyond its role in weight reduction. Regular exercise can help:

- Lower risk of breast cancer—when done three or more hours per week
- Reduce your risk of heart disease
- Prevent or lessen the severity of diabetes and osteoporosis
- Enhance your sense of well-being
- Reduce body fat
- Increase muscle
- Strengthen bone
- Minimize muscle and joint discomfort
- Boost your immune system
- Lessen or overcome depression
- Cool down hot flashes
- Improve memory, sleep, and sex

That's a whole lot of dividends from something you can get for a moderate degree of effort and little or no money.

Increase Your Metabolism

Exercise builds muscle and raises your basic metabolic rate, thus increasing the number of calories burned just by breathing and being alive.

Some people's metabolic rates are slower (and actually more effi-

---

MOVIN' AND GROOVIN'

Whatever you can do to get off your rear end and keep moving will greatly build your weight management success:

- Dance lessons (ballet, ballroom, belly, whatever)
- Walk while talking with a friend, in person or on the phone (but don't use a cell phone when crossing the street)
- Walk and shop with a friend (but leave the credit cards at home)
- Walk as you listen to your favorite radio program, iTunes library, or favorite books on tape
- Walk the stairs
- Dance around your home
- Pilates
- Yoga
- Swimming
- Bicycling
- Spinning
- Aerobics

cient) than others': they need fewer calories to do the same work as people with higher metabolic rates. With age, our metabolic rate tends to decline. If people with slow metabolic rates eat what most other people do, they end up storing the calories they don't burn as fat. Increasing your metabolism through exercise allows you to burn more calories and store less, facilitating weight loss.

The most challenging and important thing is overcoming your natural inertia and getting started. Most people start off tentatively, but once you get going, you'll find it fun, or at least habit-forming.

You don't have to twist yourself out of shape or buy fancy equipment. You don't have to join a fitness club. You don't have to hire a personal trainer. To get started, you just have to take a walk, swim, climb stairs, wash your windows, or dance. Find some irresistible tapes of country and western, rock, R & B, reggae, klezmer, tango, or jazz, and improvise your own steps. Anything to get you out of your chair and moving.

Make It Part of Your Daily Routine

To make exercise a regular part of your life, integrate it into your daily routine. Plan it for a convenient time and place, no more than ten or fifteen minutes from home or work, that will allow you to keep going, season after season, year after year. And keep it interesting! Mix up various forms of exercise in your routine. Anything you can do to keep exercise social, exciting, satisfying, and regular will reinforce the pleasure of the experience, making you more inclined to keep going.

To begin with, aim for a minimum of fifteen minutes of activity,

EXERCISE: ENOUGH IS ENOUGH

Overdoing exercise is almost as bad as doing no exercise. Rest and recovery are an important part of the exercise-to-benefit equation; your body rebuilds and grows stronger in those interim rest periods.

Some experts recommend:

- Exercise only four out of seven days a week.
- Don't exercise to the point of having trouble breathing or feeling pain. (Pain is a signal that you're on the edge of injury.)
- It's better to exercise longer than harder.

The take-home message: you can injure yourself at least as much with crash exercise than with a crash diet. Start off slowly; do as much as you can at a level that's comfortable for you.

three or more times a week. Check with your doctor to work out a reasonable plan. Moderate exercise is good; vigorous exercise is better. Two hours a week is good, three hours better, four hours or more best— but any exercise is worthwhile. Thirty minutes a day is ideal, even if you break it into ten-minute segments.

Reinforcement comes from the release of those endorphins that comes with activity, plus your pride in being fit. Endorphins make you feel good—that's why runners get hooked on running.

Maintaining a Healthy Weight for the Long Term

At some point, you should weigh yourself. Many women weigh themselves once a day, but once a week is probably better. Then, if you notice an increase of a couple of pounds, you can exercise a little longer or more vigorously, or skip bread or dessert for a while.

After you've made great progress and managed to lose an impressive number of pounds, you may find you've hit a plateau—the pounds stop dropping off while you're still short of your healthy weight goal. That's how the body works; it has to protect itself from wasting away. It's also possible that as you've lost fat, you've built up heavier muscle, and that balances out the weight loss. Stick to your good habits, and the weight loss should pick up again. If the plateau hangs on too long, try to cut the calories just a bit more and rev up the exercise program, and watch for results. Or simply enjoy the success you've already achieved.

✣ Moving Forward

If you weigh more than you think you should but you've really worked on weight loss, on your own and with your physician, with limited success, don't punish yourself further. "Accept realistic weight standards and concentrate on the healthful components of your diet," suggests Dr. Kelly Brownell of Yale University. "Ease up on the concept of ideal weight." Your self-acceptance and quality of life matter as much as your place in the table of weight statistics.

Self-esteem and self-image depend on more than just weight. If you are not satisfied with your appearance, pay extra attention to what you wear. Clothes can make you feel good about yourself. Wear nice things at home just for yourself—styles that flatter your figure, colors that suit you and trim you down, not too tight, not too big. Accessories and jewelry can spice up an outfit and express your personal style. Makeup can be just as important as what you wear. Maybe it's not for everyone, but if you like to use makeup, go for it, especially if your complexion is still pale from chemotherapy. At least use a dab of lipstick to give yourself that spark of color. And add the final touch—a great pair of shoes or boots (that's why nearly all women have tons of them), but pay attention to heel height and slippery soles. You don't want a fall to end your exercise plans.

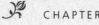

CHAPTER NINETEEN

Intimacy, Sex, and Your Love Life

I'm disfigured. And lopsided, too. I have no hair, and I've gained ten pounds. If I think my body is so repulsive, how can you say it doesn't make a difference?

I told my partner, "I miss my breast so much!" "I miss your breast, too—but I'd miss you more. It doesn't matter to me. I mean it," my partner insisted. "You're here, and that's all that counts."

My husband was there through all my meshuggaas [translation: craziness]. He stood by while I cried and screamed, and he hugged me when I let him get close enough. Our marriage is better now than it ever was before.

It takes so much work to get me aroused and, if I'm lucky, have some sort of a fleeting orgasm (if I blink, I can miss the whole thing). And all that extra work leaves me sore. So I've basically told my partner to stop trying, and sex has now become one-sided.

Sex? What sex? I've been alone for years. I'm finally working up courage to go into one of those sex shops: my doctor told me I should try a sex toy with lots of lubricants, to recondition my vagina. She makes it sound like a health prescription, but I'm still pretty embarrassed by the idea.

✄ First Things First

Sex is a vital sign of life—tied to better health, personal growth, high function, and just about every other positive aspect of ourselves. Interest in sex equals interest in living—a compelling measure of recovery after breast cancer. But penis-in-vagina is not necessarily what we mean when we talk here about sex; it's also touching, hugging, being close. Intimacy is what most people I take care of crave most—emotional intimacy along with the physical stuff. And emotional intimacy means close communication and companionship, talking and sharing about what matters most to you.

Of all the subjects you and your partner talk about, the most uncomfortable stuff is most likely your sex life and the changes that have taken place with your illness—if you talk about it at all. You may not know what needs fixing or how to fix it, but you do have a measure of what's different. Many of my patients report having less sex than before their illness. One reason is that the breast cancer experience slows your body down: it takes longer to do lots of things, including getting interested in and starting and finishing sexual intercourse.

Another big reason for having less sex is that sex may be uncomfortable or even painful for you if you've been thrown into sudden-onset menopause. Sex may be something you just want to get over in a hurry. Many women have had little or no sex from the time of diagnosis through treatment, maybe even for years.

Being single without a partner is a common reason for an absent sex life. You may be able to satisfy yourself, or you may be seeking someone to share this aspect of your life.

Bottom line: If sex was important to you before your diagnosis, losing it becomes an issue. If it wasn't a big deal to you before, it probably won't be a problem if it's gone—unless it's important to your partner. I hope what follows will help you recapture this intimate pleasure in your life.

✄ Challenges

You've just endured a program of treatment designed to beat your cancer and make it possible for you to return to a life that is meaningful, joyous, spontaneous, and significant. Are you prepared to rise to the challenge, to reclaim companionship, romance, and sexual satisfaction? The first thing to remember is that the primary sex organ is the brain, and that the best sex occurs within the context of a relationship, particularly when you're feeling self-conscious about your body and vulnerable after treatment. It's important to feel comfortable and safe with your romantic partner.

Emotional Pollution

If you harbor negative feelings about yourself or your partner, you won't have much interest in sex. Self-doubt, fear of abandonment, anger, jealousy, and resentment are just a few of the bad feelings that interfere with pleasure and destroy your ability to connect with someone in a healthy way. Despite assurances, testimonials, and sweet talk, if you see yourself as damaged goods, you assume any current or potential partner would feel as you do. Emily said, "I feel so diminished. How can it not matter to my husband? I just can't believe him when he says he doesn't care." There's a common misconception that "my experience is your experience." It isn't so, but if you are anxious and dejected, it's hard to convince you otherwise. You just cannot assume that you know how your current or future partner might feel, especially if you're feeling down and discouraged.

Your partner may be haunted by worry, anxiety, maybe even guilt, about you and about him-/herself.

> Could I have been responsible?
> Could I have been too rough, too amorous?
> Could I in some way have caused the breast cancer?
> Can I be affected by the radiation if I touch her, if I touch her breast?
> Is her cancer contagious?
> When will I be able to worry about myself for a change?
> Am I selfish because I want our old life back?

Your brain or your partner's brain may be stirring up a lot of potential problems related to the fear, pain, anger, and resentment you've been dealing with throughout treatment. It's time to drag all this baggage to the surface and get it talked out—your partner can't read your mind, and you can't read your partner's mind. If you keep these unresolved issues and feelings of discomfort submerged, you can find yourself marinating in them. Guilt, resentment, pressure, disappointment, and anger have a way of ruining any chance of recovering good feelings and sexy thoughts.

Sometimes your worst fears do come true: "Right after my diagnosis, he abandoned me emotionally, then spiritually, then physically. He just couldn't handle real life. In the end I was better off without him, though I didn't realize it at the time." Partners can leave for innumerable and often inexplicable reasons; some simply come apart under stress. But marriages or relationships that dissolve because of cancer were flawed before they were ever put to the test.

It may surprise you to learn that following a diagnosis of cancer, about as many women leave their husbands as are left by their husbands. These women decide they don't want to waste their time in an unfulfilling, unrewarding, unhappy marriage. But, in fact, flawed marriages don't have to come apart, with or without breast cancer (after all, who's perfect? What marriage is perfect?). The overall incidence of divorce does not increase substantially because of a breast cancer experience, but it could happen sooner than later.

Not uncommonly, *you* may be your biggest obstacle to a rekindled intimate life. If you're feeling depressed, sex may be the last thing you want to deal with. (You may develop an actual aversion to sex.) A sensitive partner picks up on this and holds back. But then, when you recover, your partner may continue to show no interest in sex (probably out of mistaken consideration for you), and you feel rejected and assume it's because you're no longer desirable. What a twisted circle!

If you're holding tight to the conviction that you're damaged goods and there's nothing anyone can say or do to convince you otherwise, it's time to fire that judge inside your head and get the individual therapy you need to overcome this problem.

Fear of Dependence

One woman I took care of was stunned when the end of her eleven-month treatment triggered inexplicable nastiness from her husband. It lasted a few painful weeks, then stopped as suddenly as it began. Partners may be afraid of their dependency on their sick partner, afraid of losing her, and may even withdraw affection and attention in self-defense, to prepare for life alone just in case. An unexpected, possibly shattering reaction—but not as uncommon as we'd hope.

But you may be the one who responds unpredictably instead. I had a patient who was supremely independent but upon diagnosis suddenly became overwhelmed, uncertain, and insecure. It devastated her. She had a hard time adjusting to this new frailty in herself, and her relationship with her partner went through a rough spell till she finally returned to something of her old self.

Libido Lags and Losses

Perhaps the most frustrating change in your sex life after treatment is the loss of libido—your interest, desire, and ability to enjoy sex. You may find it has become harder to get aroused, and even harder to experience orgasm. "I just don't have those urges like I did," said one woman. Another: "It takes so long to make it happen." And another: "It just doesn't happen for me anymore." This dullness of response is a consistent complaint. Loss of

MEN ≠ WOMEN, WOMEN ≠ WOMEN

Let's not forget the sexuality differences between men and women, and even between women and women. Humor is a great way to gain insight into the differences and to talk about these tough and touchy subjects with greater comfort. Have you seen *Defending the Caveman* on Broadway or DVD? "The Erogenous Zones" is a cartoon on the Internet (search on Google Images for a good laugh) that shows the distribution of men's and women's erogenous zones—where all ten zones on a man are around his penis and the ten zones on a woman are distributed between her earlobes and her knees (leaving out her feet was a big mistake).

What turns a woman on and what turns a man on tend to be very different, and each person has different preferences beyond the general rules. Knowing how to turn on your partner and exploit these differences can keep sex from becoming same-old same-old, giving it a new kick. (For plenty of partners, if same-old is working, more of the same may be just what you want.) Knowing the location of the erogenous zones gives you a good place to start and a way to suggest where he/she apply new magical manipulation to you.

desire and drive may be directly related to your lower estrogen, progesterone, or testosterone levels, induced by treatment.

Apart from the hormonal changes and their consequences, you may have lost hair, your breast is altered or gone, you've put on weight, you have no energy, you're tired, you're nauseated, and you hurt in new places. No wonder you're not feeling sexy. "I was so deep-down exhausted, I was beyond desire. I thought, 'This is gonna be permanent.' It wasn't."

In a study of breast cancer survivors by Dr. Patricia Ganz, the following factors significantly influenced the quality of their sex lives:

- Vaginal dryness
- Emotional state (for example, depression)
- Body image
- Quality of your relationship with your partner
- Partner's sexual problems

HORMONAL LIBIDO-BUSTERS

Low estrogen levels can cause painful intercourse due to:

- Shortening, narrowing, and dryness of the vagina
- Reduced fullness of the vulva and labia (outer lips around the opening to the vagina)
- Decreased size of the vaginal opening

Low estrogen and testosterone levels can cause reduced pleasure and interest in sex due to:

- Decreased desire
- Sexual numbness or reduced sensitivity
- Slow or absent arousal
- Reduced number and intensity of orgasms

Further adding to the problem, some chemotherapies may cause sores on the inside of the vagina (notably the related chemotherapies Xeloda or and 5-fluorouracil); antidepressant medications can reduce libido and cause sexual "numbness" and delayed orgasm (especially the SSRIs—Paxil, Prozac, Zoloft, Effexor). Steroids and antibiotics can cause itchy and uncomfortable yeast infections in the vagina. Pain medications (narcotics in particular), antihistamines, and antinausea medications can also reduce libido.

If treatment has sent you into early menopause, the hormonal shifts can hit you broadside. In one study of desire in women after menopause (with and without a history of breast cancer), 50 percent had a decrease in desire, 37 percent said it was unchanged, and 10 percent had an increase in desire. After Gena's breast cancer surgery, she was suddenly more interested in sex than in food, drink, or television. "I'd tell my husband I want to make love. He'd say, 'Not now, I'm tired.' I'd say, 'Now. It's therapy.' We'd laugh, and we'd make love. It was the only thing that made me feel alive. With the fear of death hanging over me, I needed that sustenance and reassurance."

Still, for most women making their way past breast cancer treatment, interest in sex is likely to be down or absent. "While men think of 101 positions, women think of 102 excuses," says sex therapist and author Dr. Sandra Leiblum, who developed a "try scale" to bring a little humor to the situation:

Age	Frequency
30–40	Try three times a week
41–50	Try weekly
51–60	Try weakly
61–70	Try
71–80	Try something else

From Dr. Sandra Leiblum's popular lecture on sexuality.

Wherever you are in your sex life, there's always a way to reclaim some of the sweetness and tenderness that can come with intimacy.

✖ Solutions

There's got to be a lot of talking to get comfortable with how things are now. It may be that you have to reassure your partner that it's okay for him or her to feel and express fear, ambivalence, and depression. That permission, the reassurance that expressing honest feelings won't destroy you, is not saying that doing so won't upset or hurt you. But it's better to get everything on the table—that's the only way you can move through and beyond it. Sharon's husband said he was no longer attracted to her after she had a bilateral mastectomy without reconstruction—but right afterward he was diagnosed with advanced prostate cancer. She later realized that his stated loss of interest in her was really an excuse for his loss of sexual potency. This gave Sharon a new sense of freedom on her own: she discovered the joy of toys and new angles on her own sexuality, while staying in the marriage.

Partners Who Are in It for the Long Haul

In spite of what you may imagine or fear, studies show that what partners of breast cancer patients care about most is that their loved one is alive. They find the loss or alteration of a loved one's breast almost meaningless in contrast. I talk to and hear from many couples, and what I've learned is that most caring partners see their lovers as having many parts to love, and as more than the sum of those parts. "My expectation was that my husband would not find me attractive after what I thought was bodily mutilation (mastectomy). I was prepared for the worst. But I was never prepared for my husband to find me the most attractive thing ever. And he was as adoring as ever. He was just so happy that I was okay. Nothing else mattered. That really surprised me. And that still surprises me."

Breast cancer has become so common that most men have someone close in their life who has suffered the disease. The mother-in-law of one of my patients had had breast cancer, and when my patient was diagnosed, her husband was calm and upbeat—he had been there before. There's no way to predict how any man will respond, but I do know, from patients of mine and others, that more men are supportive and prepared to sustain the relationship than you might imagine.

It helps the progress of treatment and recovery, and the maintenance of a sound relationship, to have your partner share in the conferences with your managing physician, so that you both get a chance to air and dispel fears when possible, and supplant myths and false information with facts.

Breast cancer is not good for relationships, but good relationships can be made stronger by sharing hardship. It's not easy, and it's only fair to appreciate that your partner can have doubts and miss and mourn the old you (just as you may be doing), but that doesn't mean the end of your intimate relationship.

Sometimes the shock of a cancer diagnosis will push partners within a troubled relationship to consider the source of their problem and seek counseling. Perhaps the excuse of this crisis will give you permission, and courage, to turn to someone who can help you help each other and stay together on new, improved terms. "I'm no longer the same person," says one survivor. "I need to be known in a new way. I don't care if he feels the same way about me. *I* don't feel the same way about me."

Romance

Are you longing for old-fashioned images that don't work anymore? You may be yearning for a little romance in your relationship, but romance can fade fast in today's daily life. By evening, when partners meet at the end of a stressful day, there's barely enough of you left to get through the basics. "Even when I go out of my way to set up a candlelit dinner, all he wants to do is blow out the candles and get into the sack."

Romance, of course, is not only candles and roses. We each have our own idea of romance. I found dance lessons with my husband surprisingly fun and intimate. For one woman it was a vasectomy. "I had to give up the pill, so John just went out and did it. What a gift!" Another survivor's husband gave up his ritual Sunday fishing to spend the day with her. Each week they have that special time together, and she sets the pace and program. Romance has reentered their lives in real, meaningful terms.

When Debbie, a thirty-five-year-old divorced single mom of a four-year-old son, was diagnosed with breast cancer, she decided to call her old college boyfriend for support. He had never married and was still carrying a torch for her. They got together the very next weekend and soon fell in love all over again. He stayed by her side through chemotherapy, hair loss, early menopause, a 25-pound weight gain, and later, the return of her period (a terrific day, as they desperately wanted children together).

Women may find it easier to talk to each other, and lesbian partners may be particularly sensitive and supportive. It is also true, however, that a woman may feel especially vulnerable and personally threatened if her partner has breast cancer, knowing this disease is one that can affect her as well.

Feeling Good About Your Body

If your self-image has been impaired by your breast cancer, you need to work at restoring a positive view of yourself: a noncritical, accepting

SINGLE: WOMEN: FINDING YOUR WAY

Much of what we've been saying has involved couples, whether men and women or women and women, but many women recovering from breast cancer are single. Some prefer to remain single, but many want to become part of a relationship, and they worry how breast cancer will affect their prospects. And they worry about how and when to tell prospective lovers about their condition.

Don't allow breast cancer to define who you are. One thing is clear: you don't need to wear a sign that reads "I've Had Breast Cancer," and you don't have to bring it up until you are ready and feel you have some stake in a relationship.

Linda Dackman was thirty-four when she had a mastectomy. She felt terribly angry, more so because she had no way at the time to find help as a single woman looking for a relationship, wanting to know when and how to tell about her mastectomy and her disease. She wrote the book *Up Front: Sex and the Post-Mastectomy Woman*, where she tells us how each time she met someone new she had to struggle with when and how to tell, and how to behave in intimate situations. In the beginning, she would blurt out her history almost immediately, frightening herself and her date. Gradually she got to a point where she was able to wait until the third or fourth meeting and discuss it without upsetting herself or her companion. And she learned to protect herself during the initial phase of a sexual encounter by wearing a silky cover-up, gradually working up to full exposure. You don't have to show all if you're not ready, not with dim lighting, bedcovers, and sexy lingerie at hand.

Renee had a really positive experience. She told Burt about her cancer history on their first date, including the fact that it was unlikely she could have children. They were married ten months later. "I worked through my fears with him—and they disappeared from my head when we had sex. Sexy lingerie helped me feel confident and attractive."

Diane met Craig at a cancer survivors support group. She was missing her right breast; he was missing his left testicle. As they joked about their situations, sparks started flying. Telling became a bonding experience; the sex came somewhat later—nothing lost despite some missing equipment.

No doubt, telling is tricky. But here are a few tips that can make it easier and better:

- Pick the time and place.
- Practice ahead; role-play with a friend.

- Assume that your date cares about you.
- Go slow.
- Don't spring your condition on your date as a surprise.
- Acknowledge that this may be different from what he/she expected.
- Don't save the "surprise" for the first time in the bedroom or when you're on vacation.

affection for who you are and how you look. "You've got to make peace with your body. After my mastectomy, I'd dress and undress in the bathroom. Then we took a second honeymoon. My husband didn't like my hiding in the bathroom. 'Come on—I love you. Two breasts are better but one is okay.'"

Are you going to great lengths not to look at the scars on your chest? Rosalie would hang a towel on her bathroom mirror so she didn't

MAKING THE CONNECTION

Finding a suitable and available companion is always a challenge, but there are enough success stories to keep up hope, take action, and make things happen. There are good single people out there looking for relationships. They may not fit your ideal fantasy, but maybe it's time to set realistic standards and look for what really counts, including character and responsibility. If he has a heart of gold, so what if he's bald and shorter than you?

Take up interesting activities that bring out interesting people. Check out bookstores with space for refreshments and socializing. Get involved in local politics; join an exercise center, a bike club, a hiking group, or an investment club; volunteer at your local hospital. Go back to school for computer programming, financial planning, or a carpentry course (you are likely to be one of relatively few women in the class). Better still, find out what activities your community center, church, or synagogue provides for single members to get together. And, of course, there are personal ads, online dating services . . . you name it. (Just be sure to meet in public places at first, until you feel confident that the person you've met virtually is worth your real time.)

In general, most couples are introduced to each other by family or friends, co-workers, classmates, or neighbors. So look to the people you know and tell them you'd really appreciate an introduction to somebody special.

have to see herself after her shower. Your reluctance to face the scars is understandable and needs to be respected, but experts on healing suggest it's important to get past this attitude. "For a very long time, I didn't really want to look straight on in the mirror. When I finally did, it wasn't that awful." But: "Frankly, why should I want to look at a mutilated part of me when I look great dressed with my prosthesis? Why do those experts need to drone on about facing reality? I have too much else to do than to worry over that kind of reality."

Fancy lingerie or nightwear may be the immediate solution to avoiding the shock of exposure. If you want that protection, go for it. Plenty of women keep their clothes on in bed. (See Chapter 6 for more on finding a prosthesis.)

Timing and Mood for Sex

I tell my patients to keep a journal of their moods through the day. When do you feel the most energized? When do you fade and get prickly? When do you think about sex? Can you detect a pattern, predict when you'd be most likely to consider a little time between the sheets? Now, can you figure out a way to schedule time with your partner that would capitalize on when you feel the sexiest? Can you arrange a lunch break together? If daylight inhibits you, close the drapes. One of my patients, even before she had breast cancer, found that cocktail-hour sex worked best for them. They both had enough energy, it didn't take too long, they took care of essentials, and she was able to get an uninterrupted night's sleep later on.

If you aren't feeling particularly attractive or sexy, your ability to become aroused may be inhibited, or you may want to avoid sex altogether or get it over with as quickly as possible. Try calling on an erotic fantasy to get you in the mood. Give this problem as much heat and attention as possible. It may be as useful to practice mental turn-ons as it is to practice physical ones.

Don't count on an exotic vacation to restart your sex life. "I can't think of a faster way to ruin a vacation," says Dr. Schover. Take the pressure off and take it slow. "Better to think in terms of mini-vacations, short breaks in your normal routine, like closing the bedroom door a couple of hours earlier than usual, with a Do Not Disturb sign hanging from the doorknob."

EASING INTO EXPOSURE

Sexy lingerie can serve as your first step to getting back into a pattern of relaxed sexual activity, but sooner or later try to come to terms with your altered appearance. Dr. Leslie Schover, author of *Sexuality and Fertility After Cancer,* suggests "mirror therapy":

- Use a full-length mirror in a private area of your home, then dress up in your favorite clothes.
- Study yourself in the mirror for fifteen minutes and pick out three things you really like about yourself.
- After that, try the same exercise in lingerie.
- Finally, taken fifteen minutes to look at yourself in the nude. Again, search out points about yourself that please you.

Focus on the positives. Try to accept your naked body, even if you never did before, to strike a truce with yourself. And little by little let your partner look at you and come to a similar point of view.

Cathy, in a new relationship, finally worked up to letting her beau see her naked chest—and he applauded. "You really did something big, letting me see you. But I told you before, it wasn't going to matter to me."

Bottom line: do what makes you comfortable, and don't force yourself into behavior that never suited you.

Take Advantage of Foreplay

Foreplay is essential for a woman to become aroused, particularly for women who find sex painful or whose libido is lagging. Some therapists suggest that couples learn to concentrate on comfort and foreplay, and delay having intercourse for some later time, thus establishing a successful pattern of foreplay—particularly genital foreplay—as part of their sexual repertoire. For some couples, incorporating movies (porn or other), erotica, and sex gadgets amplifies arousal to spice up their sex lives.

Successful arousal leads to a cascade of changes, starting with increased blood flow, and then your vagina begins a number of important jobs, starting with the production of natural lubricants. The vaginal wall relaxes, widens, and lengthens, allowing less painful and more satisfying penetration. The clitoris and nipples become erect. Your vital signs get all excited too: blood pressure, heart rate, and respiration ramp up. A woman is ready for sex after these changes occur, just as a man is ready when he has an erection. In fact, for women with severe vaginal dryness, narrowing, and shortening, they may need to have good foreplay *and* an orgasm in order to accommodate a penis during intercourse.

Lubricate and Condition

Post-treatment sex is often handicapped by conditions such as dryness and thinning of the vagina, so keeping your vagina lubricated and in condition is essential to your sex life. Begin using the lubricant during foreplay, spreading it liberally over the labia and clitoris and into the vagina, as well as on your partner's parts that will enter your vagina; you may need to add more later during intercourse. If you can't get over using your hand (or your partner's) to spread the lubricant inside your vagina, choose a product that comes with an applicator.

For some women, a combination solution works best. "It was not comfortable for me, just using over-the-counter lubrication. I tried everything, but nothing worked. So I talked to my gynecologist about estrogen—and she gave me Vagifem estrogen suppositories. It was difficult in the first ten days but in the end it was the best thing I've done. When used twice a week together with daily vaginal lubricant, the combination made a huge difference—it changed my life."

For a list of lubricants, see pages 304–305, and check out www .goodvibes.com and www.babeland .com. (You might make your choice

---

TESTOSTERONE: A LITTLE GOES A LONG WAY

If your loss of libido continues and it's a problem for you, speak to your doctor about the possibility of a hormone evaluation. Women's sex drive is somewhat dependent on the hormone testosterone (the primary hormone in men), produced in the ovaries and the adrenal glands. A little goes a long way. Adjustment of hormone levels may help restore sexual interest, but if your testosterone level is within normal range (20 to 60 ng/dL), it is unlikely that more testosterone will be of benefit.

Too much testosterone can produce acne, irritability, aggressive behavior, and male characteristics such as facial hair or a deepened voice. In addition, it's not known if testosterone replacement therapy is safe for women with a personal history of breast cancer.

based on consistency, odor, or taste.) Keep a tube in the bedroom, the bathroom, anywhere you're likely to use it. If your partner is using a condom or you're using a diaphragm, be sure to use a *water*-based lubricant; oil-based lubricants can damage condoms. Try using vaginal lubricants the same way you use moisturizing hand cream: frequently and regularly.

If intercourse continues to be painful, give it up for a while and practice with a dildo, a rubber instrument with the size, shape, and consistency of an erect penis. Don't be surprised at how realistic—veins and all—it may look. (Different sizes, shapes, and colors are available.) It will be gentler, comfortable, and perhaps fun, too. Be sure to use a lubricant with it. You can also purchase a box of small, medium, and large plastic vaginal dilators, available by special order through medical supply companies (ask your doctor or nurse). I find, however, that most women don't like this medical product because it's unnaturally hard, straight, and uncomfortable, and they end up not using it.

I often provide my patients with actual prescriptions for dildos for vaginal conditioning. It helps them overcome their embarrassment when they go to adult stores to purchase these items. (Many of these stores are aware of the use of dildos for sexual recovery after cancer treatment.)

But why stop with a dildo when you can enjoy a vibrator? High-end specialty stores, such as Babeland in New York and Seattle and Good Vibrations in San Francisco, have sex educators who can provide individual advice. Their websites, www.babeland.com and www.good vibes.com, provide a full selection and explain the various items and how to use them. Midpriced items are available through Pure Romance, on their website (www.pureromance.com) and from their in-home parties. Check out Passion Parties as well: www.passionparties.com. Shipping is done with discreet packaging. You can always pick up a Magic Wand in the small appliance section of your local pharmacy or a megastore (like Wal-mart). And if you get brave and adventurous, go with a fun friend to local, respectable adult stores in your neck of the woods.

Intercourse and Beyond

Perhaps your sexual relations have always been goal driven: you start with touching, then kissing, and finally you engage in sexual intercourse and land on orgasm. Advice from sex therapist and author Dr. Beverly

Whipple: Take the pressure off orgasm as a necessary endpoint. It may help to shift your approach to a more diverse pleasure-focused menu of activities—touching, holding, kissing, stroking, stimulation of a variety of erogenous zones, oral sex, intercourse, whatever (and wherever)—with each menu item being its own endpoint.

Sex in America tells us that people do a lot of things together. Sex isn't just penis in vagina; it's all kinds of other activities, too. For example, up to 25 percent of couples between the ages of thirty and sixty engage in oral sex on a regular basis. Maybe oral sex will allow tender parts of you to heal while providing enough gratification to keep you both content.

Now also may be the time to think about trying different positions during intercourse. Lying on your side, with your partner entering your vagina from behind, is considered the least stressful to the vagina (with the least degree of penetration compared to other positions). It also deemphasizes the breasts, a plus for some women.

Some couples enjoy the *Kama Sutra* (the age-old Indian guide to lovemaking) and how-to manuals for ideas and inspiration. Visit the adult section of a book or movie store, or go online to reputable sites dedicated to women's sexual pleasure and health.

NEW HEIGHTS

Here are a number of things sex experts recommend that you can do to heighten your orgasms:

Kegel Exercises

- Kegels strengthen the muscle in the lower vaginal area (also known as the love muscle), the muscle that contracts during orgasm. To try Kegel exercises, tense up as though you're holding back a bowel movement or stopping the flow of urine, then count to five, release, and repeat. You can practice this exercise anywhere, but we recommend that you do these while on the toilet: have legs slightly apart, then pee, squeeze, and stop; pee, squeeze, and stop; and so forth.
- Try a gadget. The Kegelcisor (www.kegelcisor.com) is a cylindrical bar-shaped stainless steel weight with rounded ends that goes inside the

vagina. You squeeze against it, following a routine, and over time, you strengthen your pelvic muscles, improve the strength of the vagina and also decrease age-related urinary incontinence.

- Check out www.kegelcompare.com. There's a whole world of related products you probably never knew about!

Zestra Botanical Oil

- Applied to the clitoris, labia, and vagina opening before sexual activity
- Increases sensitivity
- Contains borage seed oil, evening primrose oil, angelica extract, coleus extract, and vitamins C and E, plus some natural fragrances
- Use during foreplay, manual stimulation, masturbation, and intercourse
- Safe for oral sex
- Claims to work three to six minutes after application with gentle massage motions; lasts up to forty-five minutes
- Can be used with a polyurethane (not latex) condom

Eros CTD (Clitoral Therapy Device)

- A small device that applies gentle suction to the clitoris to increase blood flow, encourage engorgement, and promote arousal
- Consists of a soft plastic suction cup and tube attached to a battery-operated vacuum pump
- FDA approved and available only by your doctor's prescription (although there are plenty of knock-offs in adult stores that perform the same function, including one made by Hustler's toy product division)
- Must be used over a period of weeks in order to get any real benefit

To keep you further entertained and stimulated, check out the massagers and other toys described throughout this chapter.

Massage

If your sexual response continues to be sluggish, get your partner to give you a head-to-toe massage. Manual stimulation using a lubricant at the end of a massage can provide gratification, a welcome substitute during a period of recovery and readjustment. It also allows you to learn more about what pleases you. Tantra yoga helps many women reconnect with their inner sexual energy and boost their sexual functioning.

If your breasts were a crucial part of your sex life before your illness, you'll be experiencing new attitudes and sensations. "Believe me, you can find ways to have great sex without breasts. I was numb—so I figured, why bother?—and we had been very breast oriented before." You may want no touching, more touching, or tentative touching of the breast. Your partner may want no touching, more touching, or tentative touching. The treated breast can be sensitive after healing, painful, or numb. If your breast has been reconstructed, it will most likely have dulled sensation or none at all.

You may simply not want the area seen, much less touched. You'll have to take hold of the toucher to communicate the touching you do or don't want. You may have to learn to be more assertive than you were before all this. If you can't use words freely, you must use your hand to guide the action, especially if you don't want it going to the breast that is or was. (A few women don't want the healthy breast touched any longer because it reminds them too much of the loss of the other.) Your partner probably has only one hand free for your chest area anyway, so give some thought to how to position yourself, so that the free hand goes to the breast or area you want fondled.

I suggest that my patients do a little gentle stroking or massaging of the breast area themselves, to try to recapture sensation. If nothing else, it helps you to reacquaint yourself with that part of your body once more.

Keep your feet in play: feet are plenty sensual. We abuse them all day long—how nice to give them a little extra attention at night. You'd be amazed at how many women are thrilled by a foot massage. When your lover next wants to do something extra-special for you, ask for a foot rub.

A plain old back rub can work wonders, too. (In the good old days, any stay in the hospital guaranteed you a nightly back rub; they knew how therapeutic it was.) Massage is a wonderful relaxant and an aphrodisiac. Give it a whirl, music and body oils included.

Talk to Your Doctor or a Sex Therapist

Not all physicians and nurses are comfortable discussing sexual issues and practices. Many women with a breast cancer experience tell me their doctors don't ask them about their sex life and don't talk to them about it, either. And patients don't usually bring up discussion of their sex life with their doctors. In fact, relatively few women are asked about their sexual health during their annual gyn visit, says Lisa Martinez, R.N., founder of the Women's Sexual Health Foundation. Let me suggest you ask your doctor or nurse for help at your next visit—after all, what's the worst that can happen?

The best approach is to get help from an expert, as you did for all your breast cancer medical needs—specifically, a sex therapist. To find a sex therapist in your area, ask your doctor for a recommendation, or go to the American Association of Sexuality Educators, Counselors and Therapists website (www.aasect.org).

A support group may be more helpful than you realize: you can derive comfort and encouragement from being with other women surviving breast cancer. Women in these groups often share advice that extends to the bedroom, including ways to increase sexual pleasure that are explicit and specific for women who've had breast cancer. Advice such as this often is more accepted within the intimate confines of this kind of group.

Bottom line: if you want intimacy, if you want sex as part of your life's pleasure, with the wholehearted participation of your partner, then communication is key.

❧ Moving Forward

Cynthia was grateful for the frank and helpful information available from the hospital staff she relied on for her breast cancer therapy. "The number one issue women want help with is sexual dysfunction and happily I've learned to ask questions with absolutely no embarrassment. And I take it up with my friends who have been through similar treatment. I ask them, 'How's sex?' And they look at me, and pause, and start that opening-up process." Add various remedies, tools, toys, and tricks to good communication, and you will be much better prepared to engage in romance and intimacy in your current relationship or when the right person comes along.

CHAPTER TWENTY

A Child in Your Future: Fertility, Pregnancy, Adoption

When I got that breast cancer diagnosis, all I wanted was to get through it and be alive for my young child, but once I finished chemo I started thinking about that second child we had always wanted. I waited three years from diagnosis and it happened: I was so lucky to get pregnant again.

I waited three years from diagnosis to try to have a baby, and I did get pregnant. After my daughter was born I went on tamoxifen for four years. She is ten years old now and I'm just fine.

It took me till age forty to find the right guy and get married. Having kids was my number one priority—until I found the breast lump on our honeymoon. Our baby project was postponed for two years and by the time we got the green light, my ovaries had shut down. Now, six months later, we're looking into adoption and the surrogate option. At this point, I'd be thrilled to have a healthy baby through any source.

First Things First

Most women, from as far back as they can remember, look to the day when they can start or grow a family. They never imagine that breast cancer might swoop into their lives, screw things up, and slam them with a huge battery of issues and choices, such as: How do you protect your own life at the very moment you're thinking about starting another? Who and what come first? Is there a choice? Is it safe for you to become pregnant? Will you live long enough to raise your child? Are there close family members who will help out just in case? Does adoption make sense? Your mind floods with these kinds of questions.

Your personal circumstances may be not so settled, or you may be more than ready to go. You may not yet be in a committed relationship, you may have just married but are not quite ready to start a family, or perhaps you already have one child (or more) and want very much to have another.

If you are at a point in your life when having a baby is the biggest thing on your mind but breast cancer is also a factor, how do you decide what's possible and what you should do? You're not alone as you confront these big issues: about 25 percent of women diagnosed with breast cancer are under age fifty, and many share your strong desire. I have taken care of many women grappling with these very tough issues, and each situation is profound and unique. Yes, cancer treatment should have priority over childbearing issues—but it doesn't have to be an either/or decision. You may still have a good shot at having a baby after treatment. Other options, including adoption and surrogacy, can make you a mom, even if your body is unable to bear children.

Risk of Infertility with Cancer Treatment

While surgical removal of the ovaries and radiation directly to the ovaries causes infertility, surgery and radiation to the *breast* have no impact on your fertility. It's the medicine treatments for breast cancer, chemotherapy and hormonal therapies, that have the biggest impact on your future fertility.

Chemotherapy and Risk of Infertility

If you have just been diagnosed with breast cancer and are about to start chemotherapy, you will want to ask your medical oncologist how it will affect your future fertility. "Will chemotherapy make me infertile? Is one type of chemotherapy worse than another? Is there something I can do before chemotherapy to preserve my fertility? Will tamoxifen and other hormonal therapies interfere with my plans? What do I need to do, and how soon do I have to do it?"

Whether or not chemotherapy makes your ovaries stop working has a lot to do with your age. The younger you are, the more likely it is that your ovaries will survive treatment. The closer you are to the average age of menopause (fifty-one), the more likely it is that you will experience permanent menopause.

Even if your periods resume after chemotherapy, it's likely that your ovaries will have fewer eggs left over, resulting in fewer fertile years. Knowing this, you may feel a greater urgency to get started on the "baby project" after your periods return.

Apart from your age, your risk of infertility depends on the type and amount of chemo used. Alkylating drugs such as Cytoxan hit rapidly dividing cells the hardest—including cancer cells but also those that produce hair, sperm, and eggs. One of the original chemotherapy combinations, Cytoxan, methotrexate, and fluorouracil (CMF), produces more infertility than treatment with Cytoxan and Adriamycin in premenopausal women. Half of the women taking CMF stop menstruating. The younger the patient, the better the chance she will resume menstruating once chemo is over—as do one-half to one-quarter of women in their thirties who use this combination.

In another report of women given Cytoxan and Adriamycin chemotherapy (AC, plus or minus a few other drugs), during or immediately after treatment none of the patients younger than thirty years of age had a change in their periods. Thirty-three percent of women between thirty and thirty-nine, however, stopped menstruating; 96 percent of women between forty and forty-nine stopped menstruating; and the periods of all women fifty and over stopped completely. At some point after completion of chemotherapy, 50 percent of women under forty got their periods back, but only a few of the women over forty got theirs. Taxane chemotherapy (Taxol or Taxotere) may be gentler on the ovaries than AC. In a small group of women who went through four cycles of both AC and Taxol, the Taxol didn't increase the risk of infertility beyond AC alone.

Your doctor might suggest that you take medicine during treatment to temporarily shut down your ovaries, theoretically making them less vulnerable to damage from chemotherapy. Lupron and Zoladex are the most commonly used medicines to do this. While there is some enthusiasm for this approach, it's not clear if it actually works. And it's also not clear if it might interfere in any way with the benefits of chemo.

Ultimately, discussing all of these issues with your doctor will help you plan the best course of action and treatment for your situation.

Radiation and Risk of Infertility

Radiation to the breast doesn't cause infertility, but eggs that are rapidly dividing and ripening for your current ovulation cycle might be vulnerable to possible scatter radiation. It's unlikely for scatter radiation, however, to have any effect on the unripe, dormant eggs still enclosed within your ovaries. Eggs from future ovulations should be unaffected.

Fertility and pregnancy are delicate and complex issues, involving all of your body: ovaries, uterus, and the full cascade of substances and pro-

HOW DO YOU KNOW IF YOU ARE FERTILE AFTER TREATMENT?

Keeping your period during treatment or getting your period back after treatment is a good sign of possible future fertility, but it's not a definitive guarantee. Other factors that can affect your chance of getting pregnant include:

- The function and reserve of your whole reproductive system (ovaries, uterus, fallopian tubes, etc.)
- Your overall health
- The fertility level of the sperm
- The frequency and timing of intercourse (or sperm donation)

The time it takes for your periods to return is very variable. If they are going to return, they'll probably come back within the first six to twelve months after chemotherapy is completed. But sometimes it can take a lot longer—up to two to three years on occasion. Measuring blood hormone levels six months after chemotherapy can help figure out if your ovaries are beyond menopause and no longer functional. Blood tests usually measure follicle-stimulating hormone (FSH) and luteinizing hormone (LH), which are made in the brain and travel to the ovaries to stimulate ovulation. Once the ovaries crank out estrogen and progesterone and the eggs ripen, FSH and LH levels drop until your next ovulatory cycle. If your ovaries are beyond menopause, they don't respond to FSH and LH, but the brain keeps sending the hormones out and FSH and LH levels stay high.

If your periods do not return after treatment and both FSH and LH remain elevated six months or longer after your chemotherapy has ended, your ovaries are probably beyond menopause. But there are definitely exceptions. I have several patients who had high FSH and LH levels at six months but then—surprise—their levels eventually dropped and their periods returned one to two years later.

Your obstetrician/gynecologist might obtain other blood tests beyond FSH and LH levels to more fully assess your ovaries' ability to produce eggs, naturally or during fertility treatment, such as:

- Anti-Müllerian hormone or Müllerian inhibiting substance
- Estrogen
- Inhibin B
- Clomiphene citrate challenge test
- FSH stimulation test

Each of these tests checks out an important step in the complex dance between your hormones and your reproductive organs. By pinpointing a faulty step in the delicate process, your doctor can know better how to help you.

cesses that allow for this magical happening to take place. In this chapter, I will address many of the concerns, goals, and opportunities for motherhood after cancer, and direct you to resources as we go along.

✾ Challenges

Is It Safe to Stay Pregnant and Delay Treatment?

If you have just been diagnosed with breast cancer while pregnant, you may have to make some very big and quick decisions. Whether or not it's safe to push off treatment and keep a pregnancy depends on a number of factors:

- How far along you are in the pregnancy
- The seriousness of the breast cancer diagnosis
- The kinds of treatments required: surgery, chemotherapy, radiation, hormonal therapy, targeted therapies

The first three months of pregnancy are the most sensitive time for the baby, because that's when all of its organs are forming—including the brain. (All of the baby's organs have formed by the last three months of a normal nine-month pregnancy.)

Chemotherapy is dangerous early on during pregnancy because it interferes with organ development and can cause permanent damage to the baby. If you're in this early part of your pregnancy and your doctors are urging you to start chemotherapy immediately, it would be necessary to end the pregnancy. Chemotherapy toward the end of pregnancy, on the other hand, poses little risk to the baby. Herceptin is considered relatively safe during the middle and end of pregnancy. Antiestrogen hormonal therapy is usually withheld during the entire pregnancy (although tamoxifen and letrozole—administered differently—are sometimes given to help induce ovulation).

Surgery can usually be performed safely throughout pregnancy. Only some radiological tests can be performed during the first few months, and radiation therapy is never given at any time during pregnancy, as there can be scatter radiation that's unsafe for a growing baby.

Dealing with breast cancer treatment decisions in the middle of pregnancy—months four through six—is tricky. There are fewer clear guidelines about keeping or ending the pregnancy or delivering the baby early. If you are diagnosed during this time, you and your doctor will have to come to a decision together. You will need to weigh the nature and stage of the cancer and the need to start various treatments relative to how far along you are in your pregnancy, as well as your personal feelings and beliefs.

Weighing Prognosis and Parenthood

As you think about becoming a parent, ask your doctor to help you understand your outlook. Do things look optimistic enough to plan your future as a mother?

After much thought, you may have already decided that having a family is what's most important—knowing that your child will always be loved by you and/or your extended family, even if your survival turns out to be limited.

These decisions are extremely important and personal, and require careful consideration of a number of factors:

- Your relationship with yourself and a possible partner
- Your value system
- Your social and economic circumstances
- Your cultural and religious background
- Your support systems

Your doctor can help you by answering your questions and guiding you along the way. But ultimately, the decision to move forward and try to have a child is one only you can make—with or without a partner.

WILL TAMOXIFEN MESS UP YOUR PLANS?

You've just finished chemotherapy and your eggs are jumping up and down and ready to boogie—and then your doctor tells you he or she wants you to start tamoxifen. Taking a medication that may further mess with your hormones and one that's unsafe to take during pregnancy is probably the *last* thing you want to think about at this point. "I had a miscarriage six months prior to diagnosis. I'm thirty-eight years old now, and my periods returned five weeks ago. I'm a perfect candidate for tamoxifen, but what about babies?"

Tamoxifen will not induce early menopause unless you're already on the brink, but it does induce menopausal symptoms while you're taking it. After you stop taking tamoxifen, your body usually reverts to where it would be without the medicine. (Tamoxifen doesn't have any permanent effect on fertility.) The first question, then, to ask your doctor is "How important is it for me to take tamoxifen—and for how long?"

If the bottom line is that you would benefit from taking tamoxifen, then I suggest you take it, for at least the most important first two years. While five years of tamoxifen is supposed to be better than two, two years is better than none, and you can complete the rest later. Liz started tamoxifen and was married in the same month. "My husband would love kids, but my doctor says to stay on tamoxifen for two years; then I can come off and take about six months to a year trying to become pregnant. If it doesn't happen within that time, he says he wants me to go back on tamoxifen to finish the full five years."

You may decide to take tamoxifen for the recommended five years. Ann and her husband had been married for four years, had one child, and were about to try for another when Ann was diagnosed with breast cancer. "My husband wanted me to go the distance with the tamoxifen," Ann explained. "'I don't want you to give away any chances, even as much as we want that child,' he told me."

It's also possible that, after careful consultation with your physician, together you may decide that tamoxifen offers you only marginal benefit and you decide to forgo it.

Concern About the Safety of Pregnancy After Breast Cancer

Pregnancy produces high levels of female hormones. Estrogen in particular can stimulate the growth of breast cells—both normal and abnormal—that are already present. Although increased estrogen levels during pregnancy are unlikely to cause a new cancer to form, it's possible that you might already have cancer cells in your body that are responsive to hormones and will therefore grow faster while you're pregnant (growth will slow down once the pregnancy is over). Whether this transient period of increased growth will actually harm you has not been fully demonstrated.

It's difficult to study the safety of pregnancy, because you can't split a hundred women diagnosed with breast cancer into two equal groups (correlated by stage, age, number of prior pregnancies, hormone receptors, etc.), tell half of them to become pregnant and the other half not to, and then watch to see what happens over the years to compare outcomes. However, based on current randomized trials of young women with breast cancer that compare the results of women who become pregnant with those who don't, women who get pregnant after breast cancer therapy do better than the women who don't get pregnant. While this is good news, it needs to be interpreted with a grain of salt. Women who get pregnant after breast cancer usually are healthier and have a better outlook from the start. (It's not that the pregnancy itself makes them live longer.)

Furthermore, based on data from a number of retrospective studies that looked back over the medical records of premenopausal women with breast cancer at a particular hospital or in a small country such as Sweden, we can compare the outcomes of women who were pregnant with those of women who weren't. These studies show no apparent long-term increased risk of cancer recurrence or death in the women who became pregnant. Pregnancy didn't appear to cause new cancers; neither did it seem to cause more metastases or deaths from breast cancer. These studies also indicated that if you were diagnosed with breast cancer *during* pregnancy, the pregnancy did not affect your long-term outcome.

Therefore, even though the main concern about the safety of pregnancy after breast cancer relates to the high hormone levels during pregnancy, the results of small studies so far show that the safety of pregnancy seems to be independent of the hormone receptor status of the cancer (diagnosed prior to pregnancy).

In addition, babies born to women who have had breast cancer have no increased risk of birth defects or genetic diseases. If you have a breast cancer gene abnormality, there is a 50 percent risk of passing that gene on to your baby. That's the same risk as a woman who gets pregnant with the same genetic abnormality but without a personal history of breast cancer. Eggs obtained through in vitro fertilization (see below) can be tested for the presence of the breast cancer gene; the eggs without the gene can then be selectively utilized.

If you do become pregnant, your pregnancy is automatically considered high risk because of your history of breast cancer and because this pregnancy is extra precious. You'll need to be watched carefully throughout. If you've had treatments that could affect your heart, such as Adriamycin or Herceptin, your doctor will keep a close eye on your ticker. If you had a TRAM flap to rebuild your breast after mastectomy, your doctor needs to watch the strength of your belly wall carefully.

Cost of Fertility Treatment

In addition to the physical and emotional difficulties of fertility treatment, it can also be prohibitively expensive. How much will the fertility

AFTER TREATMENT IS OVER: HOW LONG DO YOU WAIT BEFORE YOU START TRYING?

Many doctors recommend a wait of two years to get you past the time when the risk of cancer recurrence is highest. But it's unclear when to start that countdown—from the time of diagnosis or when treatment ends. (These two points can differ by as much as a year.) Again, your risk of cancer recurrence depends on your unique situation. Also implicit in the recommended two-year waiting period is a judgment about when you should or shouldn't become a parent based on your general health and risk of recurrence.

Two years is a long time to wait when having a baby is a high priority for you and you are already in your mid-thirties or older. If your periods have returned after chemotherapy, your chances of becoming pregnant may be good, but you may have fewer fertile years ahead.

Even if you're in a terrible rush to start trying to conceive, it's advisable to wait at least six months after completion of chemotherapy and radiation before you begin trying. You need that time to recover and heal from any potential lingering side effects from treatment on your eggs, the rest of your reproductive system, and your body as a whole. After hormonal therapy is over, most doctors suggest waiting two to three months until all of the medicine is out of your system.

procedures cost? Do you have the money to pay for them? Are you able and prepared to pay for this out-of-pocket expense if your health plan won't pay? Most don't cover fertility treatment, but a few states mandate payment for this, and maybe you can negotiate ways to get part of your expenses covered.

The cost of each ovarian stimulation combined with in vitro fertilization is approximately $10,000 to $12,000 per cycle, plus a few hundred dollars a year to maintain the embryos in the freezer. The cost for natural-cycle in vitro fertilization is about $5,000 to $10,000 per cycle (you save the cost of fertility drugs). Obtaining ovarian tissue for future use costs about $12,000. Rent on the freezer is the same for all.

The cost of the donor egg process is about $20,000 to $30,000 if you're using a paid donor, or about $8,000 to $12,000 if the eggs are donated at no charge. Donated embryos are about $5,000 to $7,000 per procedure. The cost of having another woman carry the pregnancy (called a surrogate or gestational carrier) ranges from $10,000 to $100,000.

Breast-feeding

The questions don't stop once you've successfully conceived and given birth. Here's one of the first ones you'll ask: "Is it safe to breast-feed my baby?" The answer is yes. If you still have a breast, breast-feeding is possible after breast cancer.

If you had radiation to one breast, it is unlikely to produce much milk, if any. Your untreated breast can usually make enough milk to feed a baby. There won't be any harmful elements present in the milk. Under these circumstances, the milk-producing breast can get very big, and some of this asymmetry is likely to persist even after breast-feeding ends. (You'll need some special fittings to find the right bras to keep you comfortable.) If you are nursing your infant and you are advised to start chemotherapy, you should stop before you start the chemo, because the chemo gets into your breast milk.

If you are unable to breast-feed but want to capture the experience, you can try using a breast-feeding simulator—a milk reservoir that empties through a small tube positioned on your nipple. The baby sucks both the tube end and your nipple at the same time.

❧ Solutions

When I have a patient who is struggling to deal with the issues of future fertility prior to starting breast cancer treatment, I outline the issues step by step for a clear picture of what must be weighed and assessed. Here are the considerations, broken down into steps, so you can evaluate your options.

Reality Check: Assess Your Outlook

This is probably the hardest step to take because the issue is so scary to think about. Gather your strength; you can do it. Talk to your doctor about the seriousness of your cancer condition relative to the possibility of your getting pregnant after breast cancer treatment is completed. Is your prognosis relatively good, enough so that you feel encouraged to become a parent? Or is your cancer prognosis limited enough that you don't want to take added risks and responsibilities?

When you ask your doctor for a general idea of your chances of living cancer-free over the next five years, this is the range of figures you may be given:

Stage 0	95+%	(noninvasive cancer, DCIS)
Stage I	85–95%	(invasive cancer ≤ 2 cm, no nodes)
Stage II	75–85%	(invasive cancer > 2 cm to ≤ 5 cm, with or without nodes involved)
Stage III	55–65%	(invasive cancer > 5 cm, skin involved, with or without nodes involved)
Stage IV	10–20%	(metastatic spread of cancer to other parts of the body)

Of course, these numbers are just estimates, based on experience with other women. You cannot get—and you don't need—exact answers to these questions; you're not going to make any immediate, irrevocable commitments. You're just trying to get a sense of whether having a child remains a reasonable possibility for you in the future. Consider two opposite examples. One woman with noninvasive intraductal breast cancer would have an excellent prognosis. Another woman with, say, over ten lymph nodes involved or with inflammatory breast cancer would have what is considered a very aggressive cancer with an unfavorable prognosis. But I've seen exceptions to every doctor's "rule" of prognosis, so consider these as guidelines, not absolutes.

Evaluate the Safety of Becoming Pregnant

Discuss the safety of pregnancy as it relates to your particular kind of cancer. Although there is no definitive evidence that pregnancy affects your prognosis, you might have a very unusual condition that suggests an exception to this possibility. There may be circumstances that cause your doctor to say that pregnancy in your case may not be advised. For instance:

- If your cancer originated as a rapidly enlarging lump diagnosed during a previous pregnancy
- If your cancer is strongly estrogen receptor–positive
- If it was present in lymph nodes

In such a case, you would need to rethink the safety of any subsequent pregnancy for you. Fortunately, these instances are quite rare. Cynthia, diagnosed with Stage III breast cancer during her eighth month of pregnancy with her second daughter, was warned against becoming pregnant again. And so, respecting that warning, she just had a son with the help of a gestational carrier using an embryo harvested during infertility treatment years prior to her breast cancer diagnosis.

Consult with a Fertility Expert

If your doctor says your prognosis is relatively good and there is no particular reason to expect pregnancy to increase your risk for cancer recurrence, then ask a fertility specialist to explain your options for preserving your fertility. Action may need to be taken before you start treatment. There is usually a four-week break between surgery and chemotherapy, which can make it possible to use some of the technologies that harvest eggs and freeze embryos.

When selecting a fertility center for treatment, find out what experience it has taking care of women in your situation and what its pregnancy rates are. In the best programs, the pregnancy rates in general for women under forty can be as high as 50 percent, while the rates for older women may be lower than 20 percent. Those chances may be lower for women who've had chemotherapy or hormonal therapy.

You may also find the American Society of Clinical Oncology's fertility guidelines useful, available at its website: www.asco.org.

TIMING OF FERTILITY CARE

How long it takes to obtain eggs for future use depends on where you are in your cycle. The process of ovulation stimulation and egg retrieval in preparation for in vitro fertilization takes about six weeks, starting at the onset of your period. Both your medical oncologist and your fertility doc or ob-gyn need to judge how risky it might be to postpone your cancer therapy for these weeks.

How comfortable your oncologists are with postponing your treatment depends on how favorable or advanced your cancer situation is. Probably the bigger safety concern is the possible danger of the hormonal medicines used to stimulate ovulation. In general, doctors would be a lot more likely to postpone chemotherapy and/or radiation for infertility management if they felt more comfortable about the safety of the increased level of hormones flooding your body.

If you and your doctors decide that there is not enough time to pursue fertility treatment or they are concerned about its safety, you have another option: ovarian tissue freezing. Before chemotherapy is started, part or all of the ovary is removed through a small incision and then frozen. Later on, when you're ready to get pregnant after treatment, the ovary tissue is transplanted back into your body. Although still a relatively experimental procedure, there have been a significant number of success stories from centers that have developed expertise in this specialty.

You can and should hold off on chemotherapy and radiation until you gather the information you need about your risk of infertility and how to manage it. Postponing your treatment for a week or so to discuss your questions and obtain necessary information is time well spent. This short delay will not endanger your health.

You'll probably need some pull to get an immediate appointment with a fertility specialist, so ask your breast cancer doctor to please get on the phone and be persistent on your behalf. If you're facing pressure to start cancer treatment, you're entitled to special consideration, but you do have to persist and press for it.

If there is no fertility specialist in or close to your area, your regular gynecologist may have to suffice. For many fertility problems, that may be fine, but it still makes sense to do a lot of reading or to go to the Web for as much information as you can dig up. The nonprofit organization Fertile Hope (www.fertilehope.org) provides information about specific doctors and centers across the country.

In Vitro Fertilization

Getting Started

It's important to identify your source of sperm and check out the sperm's status before you pursue aggressive fertility procedures. Why go through a difficult and costly fertility procedure if the other half of the equation isn't up to the job? Make sure the "boys" are strong swimmers and present in sufficient numbers. In many fertility centers, low sperm counts can be compensated for by combining several sperm collections or directly inserting sperm into an egg to achieve fertilization. Knowing these issues ahead of time can help you make a plan and avoid going through the cost of an unsuccessful cycle.

If there is no viable sperm or no male partner in the picture, you'll have to find another source. Sperm banks offer a wide choice of donors' physical characteristics and medical, religious, and professional backgrounds. A no-strings-attached sperm bank donor will do, but most in vitro fertilization centers won't accept a designated sperm donation from a boyfriend who's not in a committed relationship with you, because of the complicated legal and ethical issues about the future rights of and to the embryos.

It's possible to use the eggs you naturally make during a regular cycle for in vitro fertilization, without using fertility drugs. This yields one or occasionally two mature eggs, and perhaps a few immature eggs

QUESTIONS TO ASK A FERTILITY SPECIALIST:

- Can I bank my embryos (fertilized eggs) now, in case I can't produce eggs later? (Most places are without the technology to freeze eggs unless they are fertilized with sperm.)
- Is ovarian stimulation (with subsequent in vitro fertilization) the only realistic option to obtaining an adequate number of eggs?
- Is natural-cycle in vitro fertilization a reasonable alternative?
- Are donated eggs an option?
- What is involved with each approach?
- How long does the process take?

And here are a couple of questions to ask yourself:

- How hard and how long are you willing to work to keep open the option of having a child?
- How much can you afford to spend at this particular time to keep open the option of having a child?

PLAN FOR YOUR EMBRYOS

Before initiating the process of in vitro fertilization, any woman (with or without breast cancer, with or without a partner) needs to consider what will happen to the frozen embryos if she and her partner divorce or if one or both partners die. Yes, this involves a whole stack of complex legal, ethical, religious, and personal issues, but you don't have to figure them out on your own. Other brave women and experienced lawyers have navigated through these issues already. Work through the issues with an experienced lawyer and incorporate your decisions into your will.

(normally produced with each month's ovulation). The advantage to using natural-cycle eggs is that it allows you to avoid the high estrogen levels produced by fertility drugs.

To bring a greater number of eggs to maturity than is normally produced in a monthly cycle, however, it's necessary to stimulate egg production. You might start with one medicine (such as Lupron) to prime your ovaries, then follow up with other medicines like Femara (letrozole) and FSH. Finally, a little HCG is used to mature the eggs. The same fertility medicines can be used to get retransplanted ovarian tissue to produce eggs.

Two medicines, letrozole and tamoxifen, that are mainly used as anticancer medicines in a low daily dose can also be used as fertility drugs in intermittent high doses. Letrozole used together with FSH produces one-third of the estrogen level usually produced by conventional fertility drugs (Pergonal, Clomid, and Metrodin). While this method of fertility treatment is still experimental, so far it appears to be safe and effective.

If you have no time to collect your own eggs or you're unable to produce your own eggs, there is still another option that can be considered after breast cancer treatment, when you're ready to start trying to get pregnant: egg donation followed by in vitro fertilization. Someone you know, or an anonymous donor, can contribute eggs, which are fertilized with your partner's or donated sperm. The resulting embryos can be used fresh, or they can be frozen and used later on.

Fertilizing the Eggs and Implanting the Embryos

The mature eggs are retrieved from the ovaries with a long suction needle under ultrasound guidance. The number of eggs obtained after ovarian stimulation depends on a bunch of things, especially your age (about ten to fifteen eggs with fertility drugs in your early thirties; about five if you're over forty). If, however, your ovaries were not functioning fully before breast cancer treatment, fertility drugs may yield only a few eggs. During a natural cycle, to increase the yield, both mature eggs and immature eggs are removed.

The mature eggs are fertilized in the laboratory with the designated sperm, as they are much easier to preserve as embryos than as eggs. The resulting embryos are frozen in liquid nitrogen and remain viable for years. The immature eggs are nourished, and when and if they mature, they, too, are fertilized and frozen.

If you have no source of sperm and don't want to use a sperm bank, and if you've decided to accept the lower odds of success

ARE FERTILITY MEDICINES SAFE?

Fertility drugs are not usually prescribed for women who have had breast cancer because they increase hormone blood levels and no one knows for sure if they're safe. (In women with no history of breast cancer, a slightly increased risk of ovarian cancer has been seen with fertility medicines.) Without studies that establish their safety, most doctors want to err on the side of caution.

Anyone with an abnormal breast cancer gene (with or without a personal history of breast cancer) is already at higher risk for developing ovarian cancer. If that's your situation, it's probably best to avoid repeated ovarian stimulation. If you're thinking of using fertility drugs for just one or a few cycles, you and your doctor will have to evaluate the nature and stage of your cancer situation and determine how safe or risky it might be for you to proceed.

with freezing of unfertilized eggs, then your eggs will be frozen right after they've been harvested.

After breast cancer treatment is over, if you're ready to get pregnant, it's time to use your stored embryos (or seek out an egg donor). If you stored unfertilized eggs, now is the time to take them out of the freezer and fertilize them to make embryos.

If your periods have not returned, estrogen and progesterone supplements will be required to put your uterus back into action. The embryos will be thawed and checked for viability, and a few embryos will be implanted into your uterus. None of the embryos may take, or one of the embryos may successfully implant and proceed to develop.

CHANCE OF PREGNANCY WITH IN VITRO FERTILIZATION

Fertility treatment using frozen embryos usually results in pregnancy rates that are about 33 percent lower than with fresh embryos. But women who are about to start breast cancer treatment don't have a choice: they must put their eggs or embryos away for later, which means freezing them. If, however, you're getting fertility treatment *after* your breast cancer treatment is over and you're still able to make eggs, eggs can be extracted and fresh embryos can be used.

After cancer, you have the same chance of getting and staying pregnant as a woman going through in vitro fertilization for any other cause of infertility. If you are in your thirties, the chance that the embryos obtained after ovarian stimulation will result in a baby range from 20 to 40 percent. If you are over forty, the chance of success is minimal: less than 10 percent. (That's why some centers have an age limit of forty.) If you are in your thirties, the chance that embryos from your natural cycle will result in a baby is less than 20 percent, because fewer embryos are available for implantation. The success rate for fertilized donor eggs runs between 25 and 50 percent. Using thawed unfertilized eggs has a 5 percent or lower pregnancy rate.

Uncommonly, more than one embryo may implant and develop, resulting in twins, triplets, or more. Usually only one or two embryos are implanted to avoid the high risks associated with a multiple pregnancy and birth.

After the embryo(s) is implanted in your uterus, the pregnancy is then sustained with supplemental hormones for about the first ten weeks, until the placenta takes over the job.

After Breast Cancer Treatment: Alternatives to Fertility Treatment

If fertility treatment did not work well or is not an option for you and you still are determined to have a child, there are other options for you after breast cancer treatment. Are you open to the idea of having a child born from another woman's egg? Are other options, such as a surrogate or adoption, acceptable to you? These answers need to come from *you*. The good news is that you have more time to find answers to these questions after breast cancer treatment is over and the status of your fertility is better known.

It's also possible that with the passage of time after treatment, your priorities might shift. Your age and situation are important factors. By the time your doctor clears you to get pregnant after treatment, you may no longer feel comfortable with the idea. In that case, you may want to arrange for someone else to carry your pregnancy (a surrogate or gestational carrier) using your frozen embryos or donor eggs. The Internet will supply you with a great deal of information (e.g., www.surromomsonline.com) as a starting place. Laws regarding surrogacy vary state by state, so be sure you are within the regulations of the state where you reside and/or where you intend to arrange for a surrogate. Because of the importance of this step and the complexities, you should consult with a lawyer who has experience in this area and who can be sure you follow all rules and have legitimate sources dealing with this pathway to a baby.

Increasingly, India has become a prime site for legal fertility procedures that include surrogacy. The lower costs of foreign medical procedures can counterweigh the stress and cost of such distant travel. They also supply egg donors to couples; the donor and the surrogate are always two different women, in order to lessen the attachment of the surrogate to the baby. While the surrogate's and donor's incentives are mainly financial, their health and exposures (alcohol, smoking, and drugs) before and during pregnancy is usually closely examined and monitored when dealing with a top-rated agency.

Adoption

Adoption being such a complex, emotional, and sometimes confusing process, it's best to seek out an adoption counselor who will work on your special needs and interests. This counselor can guide you to an adoption lawyer, an accredited agency, or an independent pathway to a child (domestic or international), take you through the home study process, and help you understand the particular psychological aspects of adoption.

Kathy and her husband found an exceptional adoption counselor who gave them a wealth of information and support: how to find the right agency, where to go inside and outside the United States, what to expect with a new child in their life, and what special legal, ethical, and psychological issues the future may hold.

Interviews with an adoption counselor are relatively inexpensive (several hundred dollars) compared with the total costs of adoption.

ADOPTION TAX CREDIT

If you qualify, you can receive up to a $10,960 federal tax credit when you adopt a child. Visit the IRS's website for more information at www.irs.gov. Given the expenses of your cancer treatment and the typical costs of a conventional adoption, this tax break is both welcome and necessary. Some employers also offer special benefits for adoption. Every bit helps, so check with your HR department (or your spouse's) to see what you qualify for.

Costs for domestic adoptions can start as low as $3,000 but can easily run up to $130,000; international adoptions range from $15,000 to $50,000. You may need to work harder to find alternative and less expensive ways to adopt a child. Just as you have had to do in finding other specialists, ask for personal recommendations from friends and physicians, then ask for credentials and references.

I tell women who are thinking of adopting to talk to people who have taken that road. You'll get a lot of personal insights, useful hints, a sense of the day-by-day details that can be so helpful—and much-needed moral support. Also, some people need that reality check to be able to trust what they're told by the professionals in the field.

As an additional resource, Adoptive Families of America (800-372-3300) is an organization designed to help anyone interested in the adoption process. One phone call, and a warm and informed organization member can set you on your way. The National Council for Adoption is a lobbying and information nonprofit organization based in Virginia (www.adoptioncouncil.org) that can also serve your needs. The information on the following pages will give you a basic overview of the different types of adoption and point you in the right direction should you choose to pursue this path to motherhood.

AGENCY ADOPTION. The traditional route to adoption is through an agency, with the advantage that the screening, the counseling, and the standards that are included in the process are for your protection as well as the child's. But it can mean a wait of up to a year (or three, or more), depending on the child you are looking for. Of course, adoption is not a matter to be rushed, but being placed on a long waiting list may be unacceptable to many women who have been through the experience of breast cancer, who come at last to the decision to adopt, and who want that child as soon as possible. "When we finally figured I was infertile and also shouldn't come off tamoxifen, and we decided that we really wanted to go for adoption, we wanted that child *now*. I'd been through so much, I wanted something good, fast."

Of primary importance for you, as a woman who has had breast cancer, is to get a strong letter from your doctor affirming your health, stating that you are free of cancer and have been for X number of years, and predicting a long and healthy future for you.

You will then go through a home study, where your background is checked (for any criminal record), you are interviewed, and your home is visited to be sure it's a child-friendly place (there is no white-glove standard). "I don't think anybody fails the study unless maybe you have a history as a child abuser." The home study can take up to two months; the search for a child can run up to a year or more.

INDEPENDENT ADOPTION. So what are the alternatives to an adoption agency? Some people choose independent adoption, through an adoption lawyer. A few people—prospective adopters as well as birth mothers—advertise on their own. And more and more people are choosing international adoption, especially if the adopting couple is older or of the same sex, or if the adoptive parent is single.

Independent adoption can be riskier than an agency adoption, however, unless all technical details are covered. Expect to do a lot more work on your own, starting with learning the details of state law that pertain to the adoption you are contemplating. (Call the state agency that handles adoption and speak with the state adoption supervisor for the information you need.) There are lawyers who specialize in adoption, whose practices handle each step along the way; legal fees may run about $2,000.

One reason adoptive parents have trouble making an independent adoption secure is that the natural father may never have agreed to give up his rights, so his signature was not on the release. You must make absolutely certain that you follow the letter of the law. If you can't get every signature (including the father's), you may be able to do a legal search. But if you get a bad feeling about the way the adoption is going, walk away.

Adoption laws vary by state. Some states allow for final adoption settlement within forty-eight hours; other states require months, almost a

year, before an adoption is considered final. Pay attention to pending leg-
islation: a lot is happening politically with adoption. New laws are always
being introduced and debated that may benefit or limit your options.

OPEN ADOPTION. With open adoption, you can meet the birth
mother, get a feel for what she's like, and get to know her background
and her history. And someday, when your child wants to know all there
is to know about his or her birth mother, you'll be able to talk about her
as a real person. Earlier and more regular contact might also be
arranged. Some adopting parents welcome this opportunity; others feel
threatened by the connection and want to know nothing about the birth
mother: "I just want to pretend she doesn't exist." Arrangements need
to be customized to each situation, with explicit legal issues spelled out
and firmly in place.

FOREIGN ADOPTION. Some people have been discouraged from
domestic adoptions because the process tends to take longer. Or they're
motivated by the terrible fear of being forced to return an adopted child
if the birth parents change their minds. (Not that this can alleviate your
pain and suffering, but there is such a thing as adoption insurance,
which reimburses you for your expenses if the birth mother changes her
mind.) In other cases, reasons for choosing a foreign adoption are more
personal. Ruth adopted two little girls (both at the same time) from
Russia; her family had come from that area many generations before,
and she was excited that her children would be connected to her family's heritage.

Kathy and her husband had been intensely involved in Chinese
therapy ever since Kathy's breast cancer diagnosis, and she was spiritually drawn to a Chinese child. Kathy arranged the adoption with their
lawyer, and they took off to China for a seven-month-old baby girl. "It
turned out to be our version of labor pains. It was hot and humid when
we arrived and we were up for another twenty-four hours straight: we
had to take two small planes and an overnight train to get to the orphan-
age that had our baby. But it was worth it. She's opened up a whole
world for us and brought in so much love."

China is a popular country to adopt from because in general there
are fewer restrictions on who can adopt, but restrictions can change

overnight. An online group at Yahoo.com, Adoption After Cancer, reports differences in how various countries handle people seeking adoption after cancer. Russia is difficult because it requires you to be cancer-free for five years. South American countries are less rigid. Each country has different guidelines, which can change at any time.

To standardize the process of international adoption, The Hague Adoption Convention has drawn up policies and protocols it hopes will eliminate any corruption in the international adoption process. To ensure smooth sailing through this process (which can be quirky and frustrating), it is advisable to work through a U.S. government–certified adoption agency.

HEALTH OF THE ADOPTED BABY

You must be cautious with any adoption, particularly regarding the health of the child and of the birth mother. The birth mother should agree to an HIV test before you get caught up in negotiations for adoption of her baby; in fact, you should have access to all her medical records, so you know as much as it's possible to know about the medical history of the child that you hope to raise. There is deep concern about babies who have been exposed to alcohol and drugs in utero, or who have suffered malnutrition, or who are developmentally delayed—conditions that for many people can add up to too much of a challenging start to parenthood. If you're prepared to consider a high-risk child, educate yourself about the demands you may be expected to address, and make a fully informed choice.

ᔉ Moving Forward

The idea of adding a child to your life can be cause for expectation and joy—as well as anxiety and fear. You may find you are more ambivalent than you expected. " When I was first diagnosed, a baby was in our future, a very real desire for us. Now, we're not sure. I know my husband is afraid of being left alone with a child. I think I've accepted that we'll skip having kids. We're older, and we like our freedom. I see my friends with their kids and I can see it's no piece of cake."

Or you may be absolutely sure of what you want to do. "Even though my husband knew my prognosis was uncertain, he wanted a child as much as I did. 'I want us to share all we can,' he said. So far, we've shared day care, carpooling, and chicken pox." With the blessing of her doctor, Ann became pregnant with the help of a sperm bank. And another woman's experience: "I'm a single mother, but with three close sisters, I felt confident about having a child knowing that if anything happened to me, she would be raised by some great other mothers."

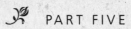

PART FIVE

Preventing and Managing Recurrence

CHAPTER TWENTY-ONE

Reducing the Risk of Breast Cancer

As an Ashkenazi Jew, I had more chance of getting breast cancer than the average woman. Sure enough, at seventy-five I had to have a mastectomy. I'm on Arimidex, it's almost five years, and I'm just counting on avoiding recurrence by working on my weight, exercising, eating healthy foods, and so on.

My sister and I have both had breast cancer and mastectomies. She has the BRCA gene but I don't, so I guess I fall into the 85 percent of women who get breast cancer from environmental factors.

I remember hearing if you wear a bra to bed, it can contribute to breast cancer. I have also heard that using too much deodorant can also contribute to breast cancer. Is this true?

Do pollutants in the atmosphere contribute to breast cancer? Are chemicals such as paraben and methylparaben, which are so often found in shampoos and body washes, contributors to breast cancer or any other kind of cancer?

❧ First Things First

Reducing the risk of breast cancer means reducing the risk of recurrence of the original breast cancer and also reducing the risk of a new cancer unrelated to the first.

Your risk of recurrence of the original cancer depends on the stage and nature of that cancer—its size, growth rate, hormone receptor levels, multiple gene profile, lymph node status, and so on. The risk of a new breast cancer in the other breast or elsewhere in the same breast is a completely different number, depending on each woman's individual risk. While the average risk is about 1 percent per year (10 percent risk over ten years), the risk is much higher for a woman with a strong family history and a known breast cancer gene abnormality: 2 to 5 percent per year (20 to 50 percent risk over ten years). In contrast, an elderly woman diagnosed with breast cancer may have a lower than average risk of 0.5 percent each year (5 percent over 10 years).

The purpose of the breast cancer treatment, including surgery, chemotherapy, and radiation, is to reduce the risk of recurrence. The higher your risk of recurrence, the more aggressive your treatment plan will be. The purpose of interventions such as prophylactic surgery or hormonal therapy is to reduce the risk of ever getting a new breast cancer, separate from the first cancer. The greater your risk of a new cancer, the more aggressive your prevention strategies will be. These two distinct goals often call for complementary strategies, since what works for treatment often works for prevention.

✣ Challenges

All breast cancers are caused by an abnormal gene that is either acquired or inherited. About 10 percent of breast cancers are due to an inherited genetic abnormality, and the rest, about 90 percent, are from an acquired genetic abnormality. Whether you inherited an abnormal breast cancer gene or acquired a gene abnormality, as long as you have at least one working gene doing its job, you can keep your breast cell growth under control and avoid breast cancer. But if this one hard-working gene stops functioning properly then an uncontrolled growth—cancer—might occur.

✿ Inherited Risk of Breast Cancer

A breast cancer gene can be passed down from your mother's side or your father's side of the family. When you're born with an inherited abnormal gene, you will then have one impaired gene from one parent and one healthy gene from your other parent. It's very rare to get an inherited abnormal gene from *both* your mother and your father, which is associated with a higher risk of developing breast cancer.

The two most common inherited types of breast cancer genes are named BRCA1 and BRCA2. Other gene abnormalities and syndromes that are associated with an increased risk of breast cancer include hereditary non-polyposis colorectal cancer (HNPCC), Cowden syndrome, Peutz-Jeghers syndrome, Li-Fraumeni syndrome, and CHEK2. In contrast, overexpression of the genes HER2 and EGFR are not inherited. These genes become abnormal during the wear and tear of living.

Most is known about BRCA1 and BRCA2. In their normal form, BRCA1 and BRCA2 are suppressor genes, whose job it is to produce a protein that suppresses uncontrolled cellular growth, preventing breast cancer. There are two copies of each of these genes in all women (and men), and as long as at least one gene is working properly, breast cell growth is normal and under control. But if both copies of this breast gene are abnormal, abnormal growth cannot be suppressed.

If your mother or father has one of these genes, there's a 50 percent risk of the gene being passed down to you. That also means a 50 percent chance of NOT getting the gene (in which case your risk of breast cancer would be similar to the average person's). But even getting the gene doesn't automatically mean you're definitely going to get breast cancer. A woman with a BRCA1 or BRCA2 abnormality has a 40–85 percent risk of breast cancer over her lifetime, depending on the type of gene, the way that particular gene behaves, the way you live your life, and the environment that surrounds you. In contrast, a man with a BRCA1 or BRCA2 abnormality has a 9 percent risk of breast cancer. *Previvor* is the term often given to a person who has a BRCA1 or BRCA2 abnormality and who has not been diagnosed with cancer.

✽ Wear and Tear from Your Environment

The environment outside your body directly affect your genes. What you bring into your body can be harmless, helpful, or harmful—for example, things that you eat, drink, and breathe.

Ongoing exposure to any harmful substances may cause trouble over time. Your genes may be able to repair or brave the damage without a problem or they may end up crippled or paralyzed. How your body weathers the damage depends on a number of factors:

- *What your cells are doing at the time of exposure to the insult.* Some cell activities are more sensitive to damage than others—for example, the process of replicating new genes in preparation for making new cells is probably the most vulnerable activity. Resting cells are least sensitive. Chemicals affect people who are actively growing and healing more than mature adults in stable health.
- *Your body's overall sensitivity to damage and ability to repair itself.*
- *Duration and dose of exposure.* Some products get into your inside environment more readily than others—for example:
  ~Bacon usually contains chemical residues (like nitrites used in the preservation of the meat as well as chemicals in the pig's food), which your body may absorb and store in your fatty tissues. In addition, bacon's high fat content means that the food moves slowly through your gastrointestinal system, giving your body more time to soak up these unhealthy ingredients.
  ~Shampoo may contain natural lavender and tea tree oil (which may have a weak estrogenlike effect) as well as a paraben preservative. But you only apply shampoo on the outside of your scalp for about a minute a few times a week, so its effects on breast health are largely negligible.

Your Risk Profile

No single factor causes cancer, and each person's risk profile is unique. If you have one or more known risk factors, your chance of getting breast cancer may be higher than for someone else who doesn't have those risk factors. If you have no risk factors, your risk of getting breast cancer is probably lower than the average person's. But even if you or someone in your family has a long list of risk factors, it still doesn't mean that you will get breast cancer once or again. And the opposite is true: women without any extra risk factors may still develop breast cancer.

Most Significant Risks

The most significant risk factors for breast cancer are beyond our control:

- *Being a woman.* Breast cancer is much more common in women than in men. Each year in the United States, about 250,000 women are diagnosed with breast cancer (invasive and noninvasive) compared to about 1,900 men.
- *Growing older.* As women grow older, their risk of breast cancer goes up.
- *Family history of breast cancer.* The impact of a family history of breast cancer depends on the type, pattern, and age at diagnosis of breast and other cancers in the family.
- *Breast cancer gene abnormality.* About 10 percent of breast cancers are due to an inherited breast cancer gene abnormality that runs in a family. Most women with a breast cancer gene abnormality also have a strong family history of breast cancer.
- *Personal history of breast cancer.* A person who has had breast cancer already is at higher risk of getting another, separate breast cancer in the future (different from recurrence, which is the return of a prior cancer).
- *Personal history of receiving radiation for Hodgkin's disease.* Having had this treatment as an adolescent or young woman raises your risk.

Minor to Moderate Risk Factors

Minor to moderate risk factors for breast cancer—which in one way or another involve stimulation by extra true hormone or hormonelike substances—are next in order of significance. Over time these extra hormones can turn on extra breast cell growth, both normal and potentially abnormal.

- *The longer you menstruate.* Starting your period at an early age (before age twelve) and stopping your period late (after age fifty-five) exposes your body to a higher level of hormones for a longer period of time.
- *No or later full-term pregnancy, no breast-feeding.* Never having had a full-term pregnancy, having your first full-term pregnancy after age 30, or never breast-feeding are all minor risk factors for breast cancer. The serial hormones of pregnancy and the lower estrogen levels during breast-feeding are protective against breast cancer. Breast-feeding enforces discipline on breast cells, making them behave, mature, and get to work making milk. With such a big job to perform, breast cells are less likely to start a cancer. (A miscarriage or abortion does not seem to make breast cancer risk go up or down.)
- *Hormone therapy after menopause.* Estrogen and progestin hormone medication taken after menopause (to relieve unpleasant symptoms such as hot flashes, low energy, and dry vagina) can lead to an increased risk of breast cancer. The longer it's taken, the higher the risk; when the hormones are discontinued, the risk eventually goes away.
- *Being overweight.* Extra fat makes extra hormones, which can lead to extra breast cell growth and a higher risk of breast cancer. Extra fat also collects chemical residues from the outside environment, and being overweight is associated with less physical activity (see Chapter 18, on weight). The impact of this risk factor depends on the amount, distribution, and duration of the excess weight.
- *Minimal physical activity.* Being physically inactive is a risk factor for breast cancer. On the flip side, if you exercise regularly, you tend to make a lot of other healthy choices, like managing your weight, eating well, not smoking, and not consuming much alcohol.
- *Alcohol.* Drinking alcohol can lead to a higher risk of breast cancer—the more alcohol consumed, the higher the risk. Beer and hard liquor seem to count a little more than wine. Alcohol may compromise your liver's ability to lower hormone levels in your blood. Also, alcohol tends to slow down your physical activity, and its high caloric content can lead to weight gain.

- *Birth control medications.* Studies based on old-fashioned pills that contained relatively higher amounts of hormones showed a small increased breast cancer risk mostly in premenopausal women that disappeared about five to ten years after the pills were stopped. Breast health risk with today's many "designer" birth control medications is not known because they have only been around for a relatively short time. That said, if you notice significant new and persistent breast enlargement and firmness soon after you go on the pill, that's probably not breast-healthy (even if you like the changes).
- *Pollutants in food, beverages, and their containers.* A tiny amount of hormonally active pollutants may be present in some foods and drinks (for example, hormones given to cows to increase their milk supply can get into their milk). Herbicide and pesticide residues on and in animal feed can get into their meat. As you ingest these pollutants over days and weeks, the tiny amounts might accumulate to potential significance. Though most of these chemicals are excreted from your body, some get stored for a long time in the body's fatty tissue.

    Chemicals with weak hormonelike activity in some plastics, such as bisphenol A and phthalates, can leak out of plastic containers and get into food or drinks. These chemicals are more likely to leak out if the plastic is older, has surface cracks, and has been washed, heated, or frozen many times. Foods and liquids that cover the container's inner surface area (sauces, soup) and have a high fat or acid content are more likely to absorb or react with the chemicals. The size of this risk depends on the amount, type, and duration of exposure to these substances.

    Public water from your town is usually considered safe, but water from a well may be unfit to drink because large amounts of farm animal waste (including antibiotic, hormone, herbicides, and pesticide residues) may go into the ground and then seep into the water supply, along with possible pollutants from local industry. Unhealthy residues from human waste (excreted natural human hormones, birth control medications, hormone replacement therapy, and other medications flushed down the drain) may find their way into a water supply. Trace amounts of these chemicals can remain in public water even after it passes through a water treatment facility. Don't assume bottled water is any better (it's usually just tap water in a bottle); it may be no safer or even less safe than your source of tap water. Furthermore, tap water is tightly regulated, whereas the purity of bottled water is largely unsupervised by objective regulators.

- *Smoking.* The chemicals in smoke can directly damage healthy tissue and increase the risk of breast cancer (in addition to many other diseases). Nicotine also narrows and hardens your blood vessels. It is thought that nicotine may make it harder for your body to get rid of potentially harmful hormones and chemicals (normally these are flushed quickly through healthy blood vessels). Smoking is also associated with other unhealthy behaviors such as drinking too much alcohol and being physically inactive.

- *Charcoal-grilled foods, red meat, high-fat foods, and fried foods.* There appears to be a connection between eating large amounts of these types of food over time and a small increase in the risk of breast cancer. There are a few possible reasons for this. Fried foods are frequently made with unhealthy fats (trans fats), and their consumption is often associated with obesity. Animal fats may contain unhealthy chemical residues. Concerns about red meat—particularly beef—have been discussed earlier in Chapter 17.

Potential Risk Factors

There are a number of products that have been accused of being possible risk factors for breast cancer, but their connection to the disease is unknown or unproven. Here are some items of concern:

- *Personal products.* All the different personal products you use to take care of your daily needs—shampoo, conditioner, makeup, lotions, and so on—contain many different ingredients, from preservatives to talc to things you can't possibly pronounce. While most of these products are used in small amounts on the outside of your body and often for just a short period of time, some of their ingredients can get absorbed into your system. There is concern about parabens, a group of widely used preservatives, because they may have very weak estrogenlike activity. Lavender and tea tree oil may stimulate breast cell growth. Talc, found in some baby powders, is unhealthy to breathe in and has been associated with an increased risk of ovarian cancer (not breast). You've also probably heard the claim that antiperspirant use—especially after shaving your underarms—increases breast cancer risk. This is based on concerns about the direct effects of its chemical ingredients (including parabens) and claims that blocking sweat traps toxins inside the body near the breast, leading to abnormal growth. While this sounds plausible and worrisome, there are no scientific studies that prove a cancer connection, and your body has many other places where it can purge its waste products.

- *Artificial sweeteners.* There is no proven connection between artificial sweeteners and breast cancer risk. But artificial sweeteners have no nutritional value and they keep you in the habit of craving sweets. Some artificial sweeteners can confuse your body's "sugar meter," leading to changes in insulin levels (the hormone that regulates blood sugar and fat energy storage). Over time, this fake-sweet habit can lead to real weight gain, which is not breast-healthy.

There are also many rumors flying around the Internet asserting that the following things can cause breast cancer: infection, tanning, wearing a bra (at all, at night, with or without an underwire), getting bumped in the breast, touching, drug use, stress, coffee, chocolate, and living near power lines. None of these is a proven risk factor.

⚘ Solutions

Keep in mind that the whole purpose of your prior and ongoing treatment for the breast cancer you've already been diagnosed with—surgery, radiation, chemotherapy, hormonal therapy, targeted therapies—was and is to get rid of the cancer and never see it again. Each of those treatments is highly effective against recurrence, and some are effective against new cancers as well (for example, hormonal therapy and prophylactic surgeries). As the scope of this book is on life after treatment, I'd like now to focus on strategies for prevention: the things you can do to reduce the risk of a new cancer, different from the first.

If you have an increased risk of breast cancer, you must make a major effort to lead a healthy life, check yourself more carefully and regularly, and work closely with your doctors for your ongoing care—everything you can do that's reasonable to reduce the risk of ever having cancer again, whether recurrence or a new cancer. While no one can promise complete cure or total prevention, there is much you can do to increase your chance of living cancer-free.

Beyond lifestyle changes that any woman can make, if your risk is high you may choose to take extra steps in prevention, early detection, and treatment:

- Follow a close and vigilant program of surveillance to monitor the health of your breasts and ovaries in order to give yourself the greatest benefit of early detection. For example, you might get a digital mammogram in January and an MRI in July in addition to twice-yearly clinical breast exams.
- Take a medication (such as hormonal therapy) to reduce your risk of developing breast cancer. For example, tamoxifen can reduce the risk of breast cancer by 40–85 percent, depending on your situation. (See Chapter 7 for more on ongoing treatment.)
- Participate in a clinical trial for new methods of detection and treatment.

Let's put aside the risks that you have no control over: being a woman, the fact that you're growing older, your family and personal history of breast cancer, whether or not you inherited a genetic abnormality, and when you started and stopped menstruating. You also can't change what you did or didn't do in the past: smoking, your weight, what you ate and drank, prior use of hormone replacement therapy or birth control pills, record of pregnancies, not breast-feeding—whatever. All of these things are history and now beyond your control. Your current goal is not to worry about these things but to focus on modifying each risk factor that you do have the power to change now and into the future.

Genetic Counseling

The main point of genetic counseling is to best determine your individual risk of breast and related cancers so you can make the best decisions for early detection and prevention. Genetic counseling starts with a detailed family cancer history consisting of cancer type, age at diagnosis, current cancer status of any blood relative, and the relationship of that person to you. Ideally, at least three generations are identified. (Most people, however, don't know much about their family beyond their grandparents.) This information is used to generate a family tree, also known as a pedigree. The pattern of your family's pedigree is then categorized in one of three ways:

- *Sporadic* means your personal or family history of breast cancer does not follow any regular pattern of inheritance. Rather, it is most consistent with breast cancer due to the wear and tear of living (acquired), with the same risk as the general public.
- *Familial* means there may be a significant family history, but that history does not follow a well-defined, specific pattern of inherited breast cancer, or, if the family history is strong but incomplete, there may be insufficient information from the pedigree to make a strong enough correlation to inheritance.
- *Hereditary* means having a pattern consistent with a breast cancer gene abnormality passing from one generation to another because of a personal or family history of one or more of the following:
  ~Premenopausal breast cancer, especially if diagnosed under age forty
  ~More than one breast cancer or gland cancer (ovary, pancreas, colon, thyroid) in one individual
  ~Multiple family members affected by breast or ovarian cancer, particularly if there are three or more on the same side of the family
  ~Ovarian cancer
  ~Male breast cancer in a blood relative
  ~Ashkenazi Jewish ancestry (Eastern European descent)
  ~A known breast cancer gene abnormality in other relatives

Genetic Testing

Testing for the presence of a gene abnormality is recommended if your family history follows a hereditary pattern. People with a familial pattern are considered at moderate risk for having a genetic abnormality. Women in the sporadic category are at low risk and are thought not to benefit from the test. Recommendations for testing also depend on special circumstances and/or your motivation to be tested.

Genetic testing can lead to clear answers—but it can also introduce new questions. Families who carry an abnormal breast cancer gene may have other factors involved in their high risk of breast cancer that are not presently understood. Families with a strong history of breast cancer may still have a genetic abnormality even if their genetic test results come back normal, because not every genetic abnormality has as yet been identified.

GENE TESTS AND PREDICTORS

Genetic testing for the various abnormalities that can occur on the BRCA1 and BRCA2 genes is best done on a blood sample (a swab of inner cheek cells or biopsy tissue is less reliable). The most common abnormalities are tested first. If they are all normal and if your personal and family history is consistent with an inherited pattern of breast cancer, then your sample can be resubmitted for full testing of both genes.

The OncoVue test estimates your genetic risk of breast cancer based on your personal and family history as well as a number of different genes in your individual genetic profile (from a swab of inner cheek cells). OncoVue then reports a breast cancer risk score that's calculated at three stages of life: premenopause, perimenopause, and postmenopause—by comparing your results to a huge database of other women.

Prophylactic Surgery

Prophylactic surgery refers to the removal of healthy tissue before cancer has a chance to form in someone at high risk for cancer. Prophylactic surgery can significantly reduce the risk of cancer of female organs. Here are some examples:

• Removal of both breasts reduces the risk of breast cancer by about 90 percent
• Removal of the ovaries and fallopian tubes reduces your risk of:

~Ovarian cancer by about 90 percent
~Breast cancer by about 60 percent if your ovaries are removed
   prior to menopause
~Fallopian tube cancers
~Peritoneal cancer (originating from the inside lining of the
   pelvis and abdomen)

The higher your risk of cancer, the greater the benefit from prophylactic surgery. Here's what a 90 percent reduction in risk from prophylactic surgery could mean:

• Breast cancer risk can drop from 80 percent to 8 percent.
• Ovarian cancer risk can fall from 50 to 5 percent.

While these reductions in risk are huge and important, you can see that prophylactic surgery is not a 100 percent guarantee. The residual risk of getting cancer still requires continued close follow-up.

Sometimes prophylactic surgery ends up discovering a hidden cancer. For example, about 5 to 10 percent of women were found to have cancer in the breasts, ovaries, or fallopian tubes at the time of prophylactic removal of these structures. While this discovery is unexpected and upsetting, this form of early detection is an important benefit of what was meant to be just prophylactic surgery. It's always better to find cancer earlier than later.

The decision to have prophylactic surgery is not an emergency, but once you have the surgery, it's irreversible. Take your time getting the information you need and discuss the option with your doctor to make the best decisions for your unique situation.

Modifying Inflexible Risk Factors

While you can't change the family you're from or the genes that they passed on to you, you can modify how these risks affect you. Prophylactic surgery is just one option. Here are other relatively inflexible risk factors that you may be able to alter:

CHOOSE THE RIGHT TYPE OF PROPHYLACTIC
SURGERY FOR YOUR SITUATION

Prophylactic Removal of the Breasts

Prophylactic removal of the breasts can reduce the high risk of a woman with a genetic abnormality down to the risk level of a woman without a genetic abnormality. Women who are most likely to pursue surgery sooner than later are those who:

- Want to do everything possible to reduce their high risk because of a strong family history or a known breast cancer gene abnormality
- Have a diagnosis of hormone receptor–negative breast cancer and are unable to count on getting any protective benefit from antiestrogen hormonal therapy
- Have lost confidence in early detection methods
- Are young and/or have young children
- Are unconvinced of any imminent cure
- Have seen family members lose their lives to breast cancer

Also, women who are about to have mastectomy for breast cancer on one side may choose prophylactic mastectomy on the other side in order to keep all reconstruction options open and obtain the best symmetrical cosmetic results (see Chapter 6).

Prophylactic Removal of Ovaries/Fallopian Tubes
(Leave Breasts Alone)

Some women who are at increased risk of breast and ovarian cancer because of a breast cancer gene abnormality may choose to have only their ovaries and fallopian tubes removed, not their breasts, because:

- Removal of the ovaries reduces the risk of both ovarian and breast cancer in premenopausal women
- Early detection of breast cancer is more reliable and accessible than early detection of ovarian cancer
- More effective ways to prevent or reduce the risk of breast cancer are available than for ovarian cancer
- Removal of your breasts has a greater negative effect on your outward self-image than removal of your ovaries

For example, a woman with a breast cancer gene abnormality and a personal history of a hormone receptor–positive breast cancer may choose hormonal medication and prophylactic removal of ovaries/fallopian tubes without prophylactic mastectomies. She is counting on both the hormonal therapy and removal of the ovaries to decrease her risk of breast cancer. (The hormone receptor status of the original cancer tends to predict the hormone receptor status of future cancers; thus it's reasonable to expect that hormonal interventions will have preventative power.) Removal of her ovaries and fallopian tubes will decrease her risk of cancers in those structures, as well as the risk of the relatively rare peritoneal cancer (originating from ovarylike cells that line the inside of your belly cavity).

Prophylactic Removal of the Breasts and Ovaries/Fallopian Tubes

A woman with a breast cancer gene abnormality and a personal history of hormone receptor–negative breast cancer would likely choose prophylactic mastectomies and no hormonal therapy, since hormonal therapy doesn't work against hormone receptor–negative breast cancer.

She would probably also choose prophylactic removal of her ovaries/fallopian tubes in order to reduce her risk of those (and peritoneal) cancers. This would offer no or minimal expected risk reduction benefit for her prior breast cancer, since it was hormone receptor–negative (but would protect against the small risk of her getting a future hormone receptor–positive breast cancer).

Start and Stop of Menstruation

As an adult woman, it's too late to modify the age when your periods started, but for young girls, weight management and athletic activity can help delay the start of menstruation. And while timing of menopause is generally beyond our control, some women at high risk of hormone receptor–positive breast cancer (because of personal history and an inherited genetic abnormality) may choose to go into menopause early to lower their risk, by removal or shutting down the ovaries with surgery or medication.

Lifestyle and Growing Older

With all of the breast cancer treatment, you've fought so hard to have a life to live. But living your life inevitably means growing older.

BREAST CANCER: NO ONE'S FAULT

I'm sorry to say that I've counseled many patients who blame themselves for their cancer. "I'm sure my breast cancer came back because I couldn't stick to that vegetarian diet and lose weight." *Not true.* Your way of life didn't cause your cancer, and simply changing your way of life isn't guaranteed to make it go away or keep it from coming back.

Getting breast cancer does *not* mean that you or anyone else did anything wrong. Sins and divorces don't lead to breast cancer. Kids who get in trouble don't increase their mother's risk of getting breast cancer. The most common risk factors for breast cancer are largely beyond your control: a personal or family history of breast cancer, being a woman, and growing older.

But a diagnosis of breast cancer is a wake-up call. It's an important opportunity to reevaluate your life, modify your risks, lead a healthy lifestyle to reduce your risk of cancer in the future, and follow a program of close surveillance to capture the benefit of early detection.

You can, however, alter the stresses and strains on your body and mind as you age. You can also heavily influence how much and what of your outside environment you bring into your inside environment. Here are some possible lifestyle changes that may help reduce your risk of breast cancer.

STOP SMOKING. The best thing of course, is never to start smoking in the first place, and the next best thing is to stop. Along with that, avoid or minimize second-hand smoke (where you breathe in other people's smoke). If a family member smokes, approach him or her with a plan that considers the health of everyone in the household. Set up some rules to create a smoke-free environment: no smoking in the house or near a doorway.

RESTRICT ALCOHOL USE. To reduce your risk of breast cancer, limit your use of alcohol to fewer than five drinks a week. Less is better. Any kind of alcohol counts, including beer, mixed drinks, hard liquor, and wine (although wine may not count quite as much). If weight is a concern and you're paying attention to good nutrition, you'll want to avoid the high number of empty calories in alcoholic beverages: one can of beer is about 120 calories, a glass of wine is 90 calories, and a 4-ounce daiquiri is about 220 calories (www.calorie-count .com). You also want to avoid overeating the high-calorie foods that often go along with drinking, including french fries, potato chips, pizza, nachos, and cheese, as well as sugary foods such as cookies and candy.

AVOID EXTRA HORMONES. Avoid bringing into your body extra hormones, such as estrogen, that might increase breast cell growth. That's why birth control medicines and the use of hormone replacement therapy following menopause are discouraged in women at elevated risk of breast cancer.

WEIGHT MANAGEMENT AND EXERCISE. Managing your weight and exercising regularly are two powerful strategies to reduce your risk of breast cancer. Much easier said than done! Taking charge in this sphere of your life requires huge willpower and persistence. To help you get to and stick with a healthy weight and exercise regimen, tap into the information available in Chapter 18 on weight management and exercise.

COOK AND EAT WELL. Follow a low-fat plant-based diet of fruit, vegetables, grains, and fiber, with relatively smaller portions of fish and poultry. Buy organic red meat and dairy products and limit your consumption of red meat to once a week. Aim for no more than 30 percent of your daily calories from fat, and use healthy oils like olive and canola. Avoid fried and blackened grilled foods. For more on making ideal nutrition decisions, see Chapter 17.

SAFE WATER. In general, the safest option is to drink filtered tap water from a glass. To find out about the safety of your tap water, check out the Environmental Working Group's website: www.ewg.org/tapwater/ yourwater. In-home charcoal water filters can help. You can also buy sterile, distilled, or purified water, but it's usually tasteless. Avoid using hard plastic water bottles that contain bisphenol A (check the recycling code—usually #7). Most bottled water is sold in #1 polyethylene bottles. You can refill them a few times with tap water and then recycle them. But it's best to use a stainless steel water bottle (look for Kleen Kanteen or other brands online). You'll make back your investment ($15 to $25) quickly by not buying bottled water and you'll also make your environment much happier.

SAFE AIR QUALITY. Clean, fresh air that's healthy to breathe is clearly important. In general, it's good to get the outside air into your house or car (unless you drive or live near oil refineries and other such chemical processing plants). Room or whole-house air filters can help if you live in a dusty or polluted region. Buy ecofriendly cleaning products and make sure to have good ventilation when using them. Avoid air fresheners. Test your home for radon and make necessary changes if high levels are detected.

HOUSEHOLD AND PERSONAL CARE PRODUCTS. There is such an enormous choice of products for every aspect of your personal care, from shampoos to suntan lotions to makeup to dishwashing liquids and floor cleaners. To help you select the safest products that perform the task and are pleasing to your senses, check out the Environmental Working Group safety reviews at www.cosmeticsdatabase.com. As detergents, soaps, and other cleaning products are always changing, it's important to check out ingredients and look for organic certification.

✿ Moving Forward

While many of these steps seem like no-brainers, some of these recommendations are based on caution rather than hard evidence of a negative effect on breast tissue in people. As a doctor, I am cautious and a true believer in the precautionary principle: better to be safe than sorry. Besides, many of the breast-healthy recommended measures are also good for the planet. So think pink, live green—and move forward with renewed resolve and bold vision to protect your health.

CHAPTER TWENTY-TWO

Recurrence: If Cancer Comes Back

Recurrence is always on my mind—sometimes it's a banging drum, other times it's background music. The slightest pain and I think it's come back.

I had my first mastectomy when I was thirty-four years old. Twenty years later, I had my second—and in a way it was an enormous relief, because I had always expected that second breast cancer. I never thought I'd reach forty, and here I am pushing sixty-five.

My lung metastases have been stable for three years now, but I keep waiting for them to go away completely—I wish. When I get my checkup every six months, I'm always a little relieved, and a little disappointed—but I'm not complaining.

Recurrence—the word is like cold fingers on my heart.

First Things First

Panic strikes when your doctor says "I think there's a problem" after your original breast cancer had come and, you thought, gone. And then if you find out a few days later that the tests show cancer, questions you're too frightened to ask stick in your throat. It's beyond unfair: double jeopardy. It's worse than the first time, most of my patients say.

When cancer comes back, it is a regrowth of the cancer you were previously diagnosed with. The newly detected cancer growth may appear at the site of the original breast cancer (local recurrence), in the lymph nodes under the arm or above the collarbone (regional recurrence), or elsewhere in your body (metastatic recurrence). In general, a new site of cancer in the other breast or in a completely different area of the same breast is considered a new, independent cancer, unrelated to the first—not a recurrence of the original cancer.

Recurrence is not a death sentence. No matter how grim your circumstances, there is *always* something that can be done to help you. Local recurrence may be curable, and metastatic disease may be put in long-term remission (sometimes never to return).

Troubling Feelings

Recurrence can bring on a flood of troubling emotions, making you feel sometimes as if you were drowning. "I just can't believe it. The first time was more frightening, the second I was angry! That first surgery was to have prevented the second!" There's a lot of anger that hovers over the crisis of recurrence: anger at your doctors for their treatments' failure to cure you, anger at yourself for not beating the disease, anger at your body for betraying you yet again.

Then comes angst over the things you did or didn't do:

Maybe I should have had the mastectomy.
Why did I stop the antiestrogen hormonal therapy when I did?
I knew I should have gone for the Adriamycin instead of the
    methotrexate.
That second opinion was right, God help me.
How could I have waited so long when I felt that lump? I was sure it
    was just scar tissue.
If I weren't so overweight . . .
I should never have used those estrogen supplements.
All that constant worrying probably made this happen.

Blame, guilt, and second-guessing are usually unfounded and get you nowhere, but it's not easy to let them go. You're trying to make sense of something that makes no sense, assign fault where there isn't any. After the shock waves settle down, it's time to go on and work with your doctor to figure out the extent and nature of the recurrence and develop a plan for treatment.

How Does the Cancer Come Back?

It's hard to make sense of recurrence, particularly if your original cancer was completely confined to the breast (with or without lymph node involvement); your blood work, CAT scans, MRIs, and bone scan were all normal; and your surgeon assured you, "I got it all." Plus, you might have had additional therapies beyond surgery, eaten all the right foods, and exercised to exhaustion. Maybe you even had mastectomy on both sides, and the idea of cancer coming back where the breasts had been seems impossible. How could this happen to you again?

Since your original diagnosis, some breast cancer cells somehow managed to escape destruction and remain undetected. But with time, they grew to a size that is now detectable by X-ray or is big enough to be felt or to cause symptoms. Mastectomy removes nearly all breast cells, but the few cells that remain behind against the skin in the front of the breast and the muscle behind could have developed into a cancer at some point along the way. That's how cancer can occur despite mastectomy.

WARNING: POWER OF SUGGESTION

If you have *not* had a recurrence but are just reading this section to keep informed, it's likely you'll shortly develop highly suspicious symptoms. This is a very natural reaction. This chapter will address the commonly felt fear of recurrence and can help you redirect your anxiety to making healthy changes in your life, particularly to reduce your risk of recurrence. (For more on reducing the risk of developing a new cancer, see Chapter 21.)

Outlook and Treatment Options Depend on the Problem

Your outlook and treatment plan depend on the extent and nature of the cancer, including:

- Type of recurrence: local, regional, and/or distant recurrence
- Nature of recurrence: the protein and genetic makeup of the cancer cells (like hormone receptors and HER2 status)
- Extent of recurrence: number of areas involved, specific organ involvement, size of recurrence
- Timing of recurrence: interval since original treatment
- Ongoing or prior cancer treatments you're currently on or have already received

As at your original diagnosis, the levels of proteins and genes, the rate of growth, and the extent and sites of spread help predict the cancer's character and behavior and will lead to the best treatment plan. "I knew I beat the odds the first time. I just figured I'd do it again."

The main purpose of this chapter is to help you understand the extent and nature of the recurrence you're up against and give you a framework for thinking things out and the willpower to carry you through the anguishing weeks between the discovery of the recurrence and the start of its treatment.

ℋ Challenges

Type and Extent of Recurrence

Breast cancer can return in one or more of these three ways:

- *Local recurrence* occurs in the breast where the original cancer started, or in the skin and underlying tissues where the breast used to be. The cancer cells that recur either weren't removed by surgery or weren't successfully eliminated by radiation or chemotherapy. After mastectomy, a cancer that recurs where the breast used to be is referred to as a *chest wall recurrence*. (When breast cancer develops in a completely separate part of the same breast or in the other breast, it is usually a new cancer, unrelated to the first. That is, it is considered not a *re*currence but another *first* occurrence.)

- *Regional recurrence* shows up in the lymph nodes next to the affected breast from cells that were presumably present but undetectable at the time of original treatment, or from cells that recurred in the breast and then later spread to lymph nodes. The nearby lymph node groups include those in the axilla (underarm), the internal mammary region (under the breastbone or sternum), and under the pectoralis muscle behind the breast (these lymph nodes are also called Rotter's nodes).
- *Metastatic recurrence* is cancer that has spread beyond the breast area and nearby lymph nodes to other parts of the body, such as the other lymph node areas, lung, liver, bones, or brain.

Cancers from other parts of the body, such as the colon or endometrium, rarely spread to the breast or to the chest wall area where the breast used to be. Metastases to the lung, liver, bones, and brain are more likely to have come from your prior breast cancer than from a new and different cancer.

Detection of Recurrence

Local Recurrence

Recurrence of breast cancer in the breast area is detected by tests or noticed because of new symptoms. It can present in different ways, depending on current anatomy and past treatments.

RECURRENCE AFTER BREAST PRESERVATION THERAPY. If you had a lumpectomy with or without breast radiation for your original breast cancer, local recurrence is suspected when you and your doctor feel or see a new, persistent, and enlarging change (a lump or a discrete area of thickening of the breast, a red rash and breast swelling) or when the breast imaging tests detect a new, worrisome abnormality in the breast, like an area of distortion, a new mass, an area of increased uptake or enhancement, or a new cluster of small calcifications (see Chapter 5, on tests).

An uncommon example of local recurrence after lumpectomy, with or without radiation, is when the whole breast swells up. The skin becomes thick and looks something like the skin of an orange, with part of the area having a reddish pink color, with or without an underlying mass; this may be an inflammatory breast cancer recurrence. This condition can sometimes be confused with breast infection, called mastitis, which is much more common, benign, and responsive to antibiotics.

RECURRENCE AFTER MASTECTOMY. If you had mastectomy for your original breast cancer, with or without reconstruction, local recurrence can also be felt or seen on the skin where the breast used to be, in the soft tissues that remain on the chest wall, or in the reconstructed breast. A new, irregular, firm to hard, pearly pink to red, fleshy, usually nontender nodule within or under the skin, with or without ulceration, is strong evidence of recurrence. The nodule is most likely to occur along the scar, but it can also occur in the general area where the breast used to be. "I have a lump on my chest now, over my mastectomy scar. I've had it for two weeks. I keep denying it, but I'm going to have it checked today." A red velvety rash with swelling of the skin can be an infection or an inflam-

FALSE ALARMS

Don't panic if you find a lump in your breast at the site of the original tumor. Within the first year of completing your cancer treatment, it is common to have a smooth, flat firmness within the area around the scar where the tumor used to be, the same area where the surgeon operated and where the radiation boost was delivered. As radiation-related swelling of the whole breast resolves, you and your doctor may find that this firmness feels relatively more prominent. This probably is normal scar tissue, but it should be evaluated further if you or your doctor is concerned.

A discrete lump in the area of the scar soon after surgery is most likely one of two things. It may be fatty tissue that disintegrated because of the effects of treatment (called fat necrosis), which can produce irregular hard lumps of various sizes that stay the same or gradually get smaller over time. The second possibility is that it is a suture granuloma along the scar, a very small (about 3 mm or ¼ inch), hard, smooth, beadlike nodule consisting of scar tissue wrapped around a little stitch your surgeon tied when sewing the area back together. This, too, does not get bigger with time.

matory type of recurrence. If the rash has areas of ulceration, it is almost certainly cancer.

Tests done to evaluate a possible recurrence in a tissue-reconstructed breast may include ultrasound, MRI, one of the uptake studies, and sometimes even a mammogram. A biopsy is done of the area of concern. After implant reconstruction, the same tests may have a role, except for mammography (since the implant blocks the view of the tissues that surround it). Chapter 5 discusses these various tests in further detail.

Regional Recurrence

After mastectomy or lumpectomy (with or without radiation), you may develop regional lymph node recurrence: a hard, persistent, and enlarging lymph node in the armpit or at the base of the neck. A large amount of lymph node involvement may cause new swelling of the arm on that side.

Regional recurrence in lymph nodes under the arm alone is uncommon. Most regional recurrences are associated with breast or chest wall recurrence, rather than being stand-alone cases. Recurrence in the axillary lymph nodes (under the arm) is more common than recurrence in the supraclavicular lymph nodes (above the collarbone), which in turn is more common than recurrence in the internal mammary lymph node chain (behind the breastbone or sternum) or infraclavicular lymph nodes (below the collarbone).

Regional recurrences can be evaluated with ultrasound, PET/CAT scans, MRIs, and biopsy.

Metastatic Recurrence

Metastatic disease may be suspected if a person develops new, persistent, and progressive symptoms in a particular part of her body, such as:

- Bone pain—most commonly back pain, but can also occur in other sites
- Cough and shortness of breath
- Headaches, changes in vision, unexplained persistent and progressive nausea, a specific area of numbness or weakness, personality change, confusion, or new seizures or falling episodes

• Belly pain
• Loss of appetite and unexplained weight loss

No one or combination of these symptoms means that the breast cancer has definitely returned, but if you have these symptoms, there is reason for concern. A careful evaluation by your doctor and nurses should be carried out.

Chapter 5 describes the tests that your doctor may order to evaluate these various symptoms, including blood work, ultrasound, a PET/CAT scan (together or separately), whole-body bone scan with or without plain bone X-rays of specific areas, or MRI.

NO BIOPSY: SPECIAL CIRCUMSTANCES

Biopsy is not usually recommended in the following situations:

• Test results clearly show spread to other parts of the body and are consistent with other signs and symptoms.
• The affected part of the body is difficult to reach safely for biopsy (such as the brain, spine, or eye).
• Biopsy would cause undue side effects, and results would not alter treatment.
• Breast cancer metastases have been established, and a new site of involvement is assumed to be caused by the same cancer.

You and your doctor will decide whether to biopsy or not, which area to biopsy, and which biopsy technique to choose.

Sometimes metastatic disease is detected on routine medical evaluation without any symptomatic clues. Regular blood work might show an elevated cancer marker (for example, the 27.29 protein), elevated liver function enzymes, or high levels of calcium or alkaline phosphatase. A routine bone scan (ordered by some oncologists) might light up in new places, indicating cancer.

Nature of the Recurrence

Your doctor will recommend a biopsy of anything that's suspicious for recurrence or a new cancer in order to rule out other, noncancer causes of the problem and establish a definitive diagnosis of recurrent breast cancer. Knowing what you are dealing with is the first step in knowing how to take care of the problem. Another type of cancer (like ovarian or colon cancer), a new strain of breast cancer (it may have become HER2-positive), or the results of new tests that were not available at your original diagnosis—any such information can shed additional light on the unique nature of your cancer recurrence and make a significant difference in your treatment.

If cancer is confirmed by a biopsy, it will then be compared with the cells from the original breast cancer. (Your prior pathology slides are stored in the pathology department's archives.) Additional studies are then done to identify the characteristics of the recurrent cancer, including hormone receptors and HER2 status. About a week after a biopsy is done, the pathology reports start rolling in. The first report will tell you the kinds of cancer cells present, their growth rate, their size, and areas of involvement; special test results on genes and proteins become available a few weeks later.

The appearance and makeup of the original and recurrent cancers are usually very similar. But sometimes the recurrent cancer appears different and has a different makeup than the original cancer. This raises the possibility that a new kind of cancer may have developed or that a distinct subset of the original cancer grew back that was different from the main cancer (described by prior tests). You can see why it's important to find out about these potential differences between episodes of cancer so that appropriate treatment can be selected.

Extent of Recurrence

Once the diagnosis of recurrence has been confirmed, you need to meet with your doctors to fully define the extent of the problem, including the number of areas involved, specific organ involvement, and size of the recurrence.

The extent of cancer in the breast and lymph nodes is determined by the size of the cancer, involvement of adjacent structures (skin in front and muscle in the back), as well as the number of lymph nodes affected.

Types of metastatic recurrences that tend to be slow growing and responsive to treatment for an extended period of time include cancer that involves the skin, lymph nodes, and eventually small lung nodules.

Aggressive forms of recurrences can involve:

- Major organs, such as the liver, brain, and a diffuse pattern in the lung
- Multiple areas—particularly if five or more different parts of the body are identified
- "Triple negative" breast cancer—meaning that the cancer is estrogen receptor–negative, progesterone receptor–negative, and HER2-negative
- Inflammatory breast cancer, involving redness and swelling of a significant part of the breast

Recurrence can happen in only one area or all over. Various tests can map out which areas are involved and track them over time.

The Timing of Recurrence

Cancer recurrence most often develops within the first five years after initial diagnosis and treatment are over. The median time for developing local and regional recurrence after initial treatment for breast cancer is three years; the median time for developing distant recurrence is two years.

But breast cancer also can come back twenty-five years or more after the original treatment, in the same place where it started or in some other part of the body. When this happens, the hibernating cancer cells have been in your body all along—they just grew very, very, very slowly.

The length of time between the original cancer and its recurrence reflects the cancer's growth rate and its response to prior treatments. The slower the regrowth rate and the better its response to initial treatments, the longer the interval until recurrence. The faster the regrowth rate and the less responsive it was to prior treatments, the shorter the interval between cancers.

Recurrence within two years of finishing treatment for your first cancer tends to be more aggressive than a recurrence that happens after two years. But no matter when recurrence occurs, there are likely new treatments developed since your first treatment that could be more effective.

Ongoing and Prior Cancer Treatments

Key to figuring out the most effective treatment strategy is knowing what did and what didn't work in the past, and how similar or different the recurrent cancer is from the first bout. In addition, some treatments can only be done once, so if you had them the first time around, you may not be able to have them again. Here are some examples of how past treatment can affect future treatment options:

Surgery

You can only have a mastectomy once; additional tissue can be removed from the breast area and reconstruction can be modified if needed. For example, if a limited-size recurrence occurs in the skin envelope that used to surround the breast, effective treatment usually involves removal of the affected skin.

You only have a limited number of lymph nodes under your arm. If you have already had a lymph node removal and then later you experience recurrence in the breast or armpit, only limited repeat lymph node dissection can be performed. To minimize associated side effects, like arm edema, this should only be done by an experienced breast surgeon.

Radiation

You can only have a full course of radiation to the whole breast area once. However, if you were to develop a recurrence in the same breast and if repeat radiation is important, then a limited amount of additional radiation may be possible. For example, if you had mastectomy for recurrence in the breast (after lumpectomy and whole breast radiation for the original breast cancer), and you later developed skin nodules, limited-dose radiation can be very helpful. And to make this limited amount of radiation go a longer way, a radiation sensitizer may be added: Xeloda (5FU chemotherapy in pill form) or hyperthermia (heat applied to the area of concern prior to delivery of radiation).

You can only receive partial breast radiation once to a particular part of the breast. But if you were to develop another breast cancer elsewhere in the same breast—and well away from the area that received the prior radiation dose—then you may be a candidate for partial breast radiation to the new area. This type of breast cancer is technically considered a new, independent cancer rather than a recurrence.

You can receive radiation to the lymph nodes next to the breast for a lymph-node-only recurrence as long as your original radiation excluded the lymph nodes.

Chemotherapy

You can only receive a limited amount of some chemotherapies because of their side effects on normal tissue (such as Adriamycin and its effect on the heart).

You would be unable to receive any chemotherapy again if you developed a serious allergy to it. For example, some people have a life-threatening allergy to Taxol.

You want to avoid taking a medication that's unlikely to help you. For example, if you were on tamoxifen when the cancer returned, it means that this medicine failed to control the cancer, so there's no reason for you to take it again.

In general, if the first set of treatments didn't work well enough to prevent recurrence, your doctors are likely to recommend a different treatment plan. But if the newly diagnosed cancer turns out to be new and distinct from the original cancer, and if the original treatments given years ago were able to stop the return of the first cancer, then your doctor may recommend repeating some elements of your original treatment plan.

❧ Solutions

Treatment for recurrence requires that you and your health care team be creative and resourceful, evaluating established and new therapies while being mindful of lessons learned from your past treatment track record. Participation in clinical trials is the best way to get access to promising new therapies.

Here are a few scenarios that can give you an idea of what treatment options your doctors might recommend.

Treatment for Local-Regional Recurrence

If the cancer returns in the breast and/or nearby lymph nodes, without spread to other parts of the body, then your treatment options are similar to any woman whose first breast cancer is:

Stage 0   (noninvasive, ductal carcinoma in situ)
Stage I   (cancer is 2 cm or smaller, no lymph node involvement)
Stage II   (cancer between 2.1 and 5 cm or there is lymph node involvement or both)
Stage III   (cancer over 5 cm, or involving skin, with or without lymph node involvement)

Your doctors will go over your treatment options, including:

• Local therapies: surgery and radiation
• Systemic therapies (to your whole system): hormonal therapy, chemotherapy, and targeted treatments

The extent and nature of the cancer in the breast and lymph nodes determine the roles of surgery, radiation, and medicines for local-regional control. The role of systemic treatments depends on the risk of cancer spreading to other parts of the body based on certain cancer characteristics such as growth rate, HER2 gene and hormone receptor status, tumor size, lymph node involvement, and combination gene tests (such as Oncotype DX). But as mentioned earlier in this chapter, your treatment options also depend on what you've had in the past. For example, a prior axillary lymph node dissection may limit your surgeon's ability to remove additional lymph nodes.

Treatment for Metastatic Recurrence

The mainstay of treatment for cancer that has spread beyond the breast and nearby lymph nodes is systemic therapy with medicines: hormonal therapy, chemotherapy, and targeted treatments. The cancer's characteristics help shape treatment recommendations. For example, treatment for a hormone receptor–positive breast cancer recurrence usually involves hormonal therapy; treatment for a HER2-positive breast cancer recurrence usually includes a medicine that targets HER2, such as Herceptin (trastuzimab).

Treatment can be as simple as switching you from tamoxifen over to an aromatase inhibitor at the time of recurrence together with a bone strengthener (e.g., Zometa) if you developed spread only to bone. Radiation to a particular site of spread is recommended if you are experiencing pain, nerve or spinal cord compromise, or weakening of a weight-bearing bone at increased risk for fracture.

A moderate approach to the treatment for metastatic breast cancer recurrence may include just one form of chemotherapy: Xeloda (taken by pill once daily, usually for several weeks each month) or low-dose weekly Taxol (delivered intravenously). This strategy can work well for someone who has a minimal amount of disease spread that occurred despite various prior hormonal therapies.

Treatment will be aggressive and more complex if the metastatic recurrence is aggressive and complex. For example, if there is cancer involving the liver, lungs, or brain, multiple chemotherapy agents will need to be used along with appropriate targeted therapies, depending on the tumor characteristics (for example, Herceptin or Tykerb if the cancer is HER2-positive). Radiation may be needed to address a specific problem such as a painful bone site, spread to the brain, or compression of the spinal cord.

Most people who have metastatic disease will require some form of ongoing therapy to get rid of the cancer, get it into remission, or keep it under control, depending on your unique situation. See Chapter 7 on ongoing therapy, stay tuned into Breastcancer.org for its section on metastatic disease and its daily updates on new treatments, and check out www.cancer.gov for available clinical trials.

You and Your Doctors

As your treatment decisions firm up, you need to select the doctors who will actually deliver the treatments and the hospital or clinic where you'll receive them. You also have to assemble your supporters and champions to help you overcome these challenges.

On top of everything else, you and your family members are probably more worried and have greater needs, demands, and expectations than you did the first time (or earlier times if you're dealing with yet another recurrence). Your relationship with your doctors becomes more critical than ever.

You probably know at least some of your doctors from before and you are probably more comfortable asking for what you need and want than you were the first time. Take the time you need, even if it means extra office visits and phone calls to go over things again—not because you forgot, but because fear and shock blurred what you heard at that first go-round. Many people get second and third opinions and consider participation in clinical trials upon a diagnosis of recurrence. All this takes time; these are not discussions that can be rushed. Too much is at stake.

New information has to be added to the picture; new perspectives and strong guidance are needed to make decisions. Support, kindness, compassion, accessibility, careful attention, and hope are all essential, even if you have to patch them together from several different members of your team. " 'We're going for cure this time, too,' said my surgeon, looking so bright and positive. I burst out: 'If you're going for cure, then so am I!' " But you also need to be realistic. "My doctor was both direct and kind: 'I'm sorry this has happened. While I can't promise any cures, we're certainly going to do everything possible to get it under control and make it go away.' " If your doctor is not as there for you as you'd like, or if you have serious misgivings about your relationship or his or her expertise, it may be time to address these issues and see if you can work them out to your satisfaction; if not, consider a change. You usually have time to make these changes; most recurrences are not emergencies.

Shifts in Support Network

You need good friends and best friends at this time, but you may find that some friends, even those who have also had breast cancer, may be unable to listen or talk with you about your news of recurrence. They may pull away—their cancer worry, their fear that it can happen to them, jumps to the surface and pushes them away from you. Now is a time when an online discussion board or a support group focused on managing recurrence can be extremely helpful, even indispensable. These are welcoming and safe places to share your concerns with others in similar situations. (See Chapter 2, on support.)

"I had two primary cancers, one in each breast; then I had the first recurrence, and then the second. I had to find someone I could talk to, who had at least as many nodes involved as I had—not five or six, but *seven*—or more. When I found her, I would call whenever I needed a support 'fix.' 'Get rid of the garbage in your life,' she'd always say. We still talk every now and then. She's been more than sixteen years 'out,' and I'm eight from that last recurrence."

Now is the time to tap into these sources of support, so you can gather your strength and confront the challenges before you.

You may be exhausted by all the tests you've been put through, and by having to gather together all those bits of information coming in from here and there—the tests, your doctors, this book—but you may also be exhausted by the uncertainty, fear and anxiety, and isolation. Stop and take a breath. I believe the sooner you and your doctors figure out what your problem is and decide on a course of action (even if your prognosis is grim and requires aggressive treatment), the sooner you can begin to renew your energy, do what needs doing, and get on with your life.

❧ Moving Forward

Many women who develop a recurrent breast cancer get a second, third, fourth, fifth, and more chance at life. One of those extra chances can stick, and you may find yourself cancer-free for an extended period of time, if not permanently. Some women are living with cancer under control with various shifting ongoing therapies, somewhat like a chronic disease (such as diabetes). Ninety-five-year-old Sadie was dealing with metastatic disease for twenty years and coping. Regardless of your path, after experiencing a recurrence, life can feel like a roller-coaster ride, with test points all along the way.

Have hope: Parallel to your efforts to fight cancer are thousands of scientists and doctors conducting research with one goal in mind: cure. Each discovery brings us closer to that shared goal. You have already benefited from this research; you are likely to benefit from the breakthroughs to come.

CHAPTER TWENTY-THREE

Endings: Comfort, Closure, and the Circle of Life

I wanted to know the worst and I wanted to know it all. I wonder if I will see my two boys graduate. Time is the thing I lack most. I try to imagine taking life easy. What if these are my last few years—or months?

I was with this woman on the West Coast also with end-stage disease who did every kind of medical thing you could think of and spent most of her last year in the hospital. I have come to accept what is happening to me: I had treatment for pain—and in between treatments, some marvelous times. What's the point of ruining what little time I have left?

Nobody ever told me how sick my grandmother was, and I never got the chance to tell her how my life was going, how good it was going to be, and to give her that last jolt of pleasure before she died. I keep hoping that somehow she knows.

First Things First

No one can accurately predict just how long you or anyone else will live, but if you have progressive metastatic breast cancer despite all available effective therapies, you may be approaching the end of your life. Despite encouraging stories of remission and amazing recovery, you inevitably think about death and want to be prepared for whatever happens. This uncertainty, in itself, is probably making you feel incredibly anxious. Your family is undoubtedly anxious as well. Knowing what to expect, getting honest answers to your questions, dealing with as few surprises as possible, and being treated with respect give you some way to hold on to a measure of control.

Before you can gather your feelings and cope with helping your children and other family members face what is happening, you need to find support for yourself and assurance that you will not be abandoned or forgotten—emotionally as well as physically—by family and doctors. If you are on your own, without someone close to you, or if you are living in an unfamiliar place without a support network, you may feel desperate and lonely and scared.

Once you recognize that you're doing all you can, as well as you can, you may be able to achieve some peace of mind, a sense of serenity you might not have expected to feel. Spiritual meaning, strength, and peace can come from becoming closer to nature, your values, and the people and places you care about. For people of faith, religion can be an enormous source of comfort and reassurance: "I know I'm part of a plan; there's a reason for what's happening to me. God doesn't make mistakes."

How you live is very important, and how you die is very important. Everyone talks about quality of life, but I feel more people need to talk about quality of death. This chapter will talk about ways to ease this final chapter of life: having precious conversations, resolving conflicts, finding answers to small and big challenges, reaching out to familiar and new sources of strength, and embracing what matters most to you.

❧ Challenges

You may have no experience handling the death of anyone close to you. Death can be terrifying to think about: a lot of what's frightening is the unknown.

Your doctor may be unable to provide an exact answer to your most compelling question: "How long will I live?" Any specific amount of time that is mentioned feels finite and frightening—an ultimatum? A self-fulfilling prophecy? Always a guess? It usually doesn't make you feel good or better. But it is important to know if you're likely to have years, months, weeks, or just days.

Certain fears may haunt you: "Will I suffer awful pain? Will I lose the ability to communicate with others? Will my wishes be respected? Will I be a burden to my family? Will I still be able to take care of myself? Will my doctor and immediate support network pull away, abandon me, leave me helpless? Will I be remembered well into the future?" These fears are real and valid, but so are the answers and the comfort your doctors and loved ones can supply.

Fears, Denial, and Avoidance

Any discussion about death is hard, especially if it means giving up your hope for a cure or remission. Many people nearing the end of their lives are prepared to endure additional rigorous treatment for the promise of a few more months of life. The desperate search for experimental or alternative treatment may represent a fierce determination to live, or it may be denial of what is so difficult to believe and accept: the end of life.

There is no generic, one-size-fits-all approach to death. Our culture's up-front presentation of a grim diagnosis is shocking to many other cultures—what we might call denial, other cultures view as a kinder, gentler approach to a terrible reality. In the old days, almost no one was told they were dying; doctors and families "protected" patients from the truth. In many cases it deprived these patients and their loved ones the opportunity to maintain control as life slipped away. And the opportunity to find closure, to say good-bye to one another, was lost forever.

Dealing with all of these intensely difficult feelings, concerns, and threats can be beyond overwhelming. Denial is a basic coping mechanism, and for many people it's the only way they can handle the situation.

I see patients who fiercely deny the seriousness of their illness, convinced that this episode is just a bad turn that will soon right itself on its own or with some newfound cure. The new reality may be just too hard to handle head-on. If they can push breast cancer out of their mind and pretend it doesn't exist, it can't hurt, and it becomes easier to protect themselves and their families. But if you are very sick, your family knows, and most want to be able to talk to you about the real issues. Going along with deep denial can force your family to experience anguish, frustration, anger, helplessness—and distance from you.

Families can also get caught up in denial, avoiding any direct talk about cancer and any discussion of death. A family member might pull me aside and ask that I not use the word *cancer*, or that I avoid anything that might "take all hope away" from their loved one. But there is hope in honesty and compassion. I tell my patients what is going on, how I can help, and how we can all work together to help them live as well as possible for as long as possible. If the most direct words are too painful at first, then we can get started with a gentler but truthful approach about "the problem," outlining the type of care that would be most helpful under the circumstances. With time, most patients gain comfort, and may ask for more about their condition as they find themselves prepared and able to handle more information. Even the most stubborn deniers may learn new ways to cope with the huge challenges of their illness, and thus enjoy a greater quality of the end of their life.

Leaving Children and Loved Ones Behind

As a parent, you want and need to know that your children will be okay and safely cared for. You may also worry how a sick husband, elderly parent, or even beloved pet will survive without you. "My kids matter most. My daughter and my two sons are my life. My husband is a great dad, but he doesn't have the same intuitive knack with my daughter as he does with my boys—and I worry about the profound loss she will suffer when I'm no longer here." The hardest departure may be that of a divorced parent who knows her children will be taken by an ex-spouse whose nurturing skills she mistrusts. What power does she have to protect them? What people can she engage to watch over them who won't inflame a potentially unstable other parent?

You want to be there for all the important moments, such as your child's wedding, especially if you know it's going to happen relatively soon: "My daughter became engaged just before I found out about the metastasis. All I can think about is how much I want to dance at her wedding." And you wonder if it's reasonable to ask your child to move up the date. "She's always dreamed of a big wedding, and they had to reserve this place a year in advance and line up this big-shot caterer and order the gown months and months ahead of time. How can I ask her to change the date? Instead, I tell her I'll be there, I'll be there. But will I?"

I am often presented with this situation, where making it to a big event becomes my patient's single focus. So I talk to her family, discuss her medical status, tell them of her driving desire, and try to work out some kind of compromise, so that some part of the event can be moved up to ensure that my patient gets to share in some of this special time before it's too late.

Difficult Feelings Erupt

Your own mix of feelings—anger, sadness, depression, anxiety, frustration, jealousy, loneliness, disappointment, exhaustion, and resignation—can move in and out like oncoming waves, sometimes at the worst times. Knowing that such feelings are normal and natural is only partly reassuring. And managing these complex feelings requires skills and insights that you may or may not have.

Don't be surprised by anger projected onto you from others. Karen lived much longer than anyone expected, and even she became exasperated that it took so long to die. Three times counselors prepared each of her four children for her death, but each time, Karen's situation turned around. By her fourth farewell, the kids were worn down by the drill. One of her teenage daughters told her to hurry up and get it over with; another daughter requested that she not die on Saturday because she had all-day plans that she didn't want to miss (again). Karen's tireless sense of humor got her through each of these challenges, and when her time finally came, she was more than ready.

Those who love you have to be angry that you are dying and leaving them. Anger and frustration swirl through the family. "I know! You're going to die! I hate you!" yelled Nancy's five-year-old daughter. Nancy let her yell and cry, then she hugged her and told her, "It's all right, it's all right. I love you." You do your best not to leave any lingering guilt generated by this anger. Children need to know it's all right for them to be angry and that their feelings can't damage you: not now, not before, not after.

Stubborn grudges can resurface. You may choose not to deal with relationships that don't work or that cause you pain and anger, even if it's a relationship with a child. Although most people see their impending death as their last chance to heal old wounds, one of my patients chose not to tell her estranged daughter that her breast cancer had become terminal. I talked to her about her decision, and I felt I had to point out how devastating it would be to her daughter—not to make my patient feel guilty but to have her consider the consequences of her decision. "If you don't say good-bye to your daughter, you'll deprive her of the final opportunity to be involved in your life and to do something meaningful for you. She'll feel terrible if she finds out you've excluded her. You may never see her again." My patient wouldn't change her mind.

You probably have high expectations of yourself and other people, and hopes that tomorrow will be a better day. You may feel blessed much of the time when people and events meet or exceed your expectations. But it's also inevitable that you may feel disappointment—in yourself, in others, and in life. If anyone lets you down, it feels awful, particularly if you are dependent upon them.

Doctors and nurses who might have been responsive and available when you were getting your care in the hospital may have nearly vanished during end-of-life care. It may just be that your in-hospital team does not perform in-home care. Or maybe their office isn't set up well enough to effectively coordinate care at a distance. Or perhaps you feel your team has lost interest in taking care of you now that all anticancer treatments have been stopped. Cruelly disappointing. But there are definitely wonderful doctors and nurses who are still there for you. That said, changing from a familiar team to an unfamiliar one can be very upsetting.

Solutions

The end of life is a process; it comes about in many steps. Sudden death—one moment you're fine, the next you're gone—is rare in breast cancer. The more you know about what to expect, the better prepared you'll be for whatever may happen, and the less frightened we hope you'll feel. Dr. David Spiegel, author of the book *Living Beyond Limits*, writes that it's best "to face the worst rather than simply to hope for the best. Facing death can intensify living. Rather than denying dying, we confront its inevitability and use that fact to help reorder life priorities, to focus on living better. Convert your anxiety to fear, and convert general fear to specific fears, to structure those fears into a series of problems that you can focus on and do something about. You do have things to do, to make your life rich and meaningful, to live more fully, to live your life right up to the end."

You and your family can be helped to develop a realistic understanding of what to expect. Support and comfort are critical every step of the way, even if you are without an immediate support network. You may, however, have to reach out in new directions and be willing to accept offers of assistance—a major shift if you've always been the caretaker.

There's no "right" way to talk about dying—except that any discussion must respect *you*. The end of life needs to honor your personal way of doing things, your values and ability to make your own decisions. The quality of your death is important, just as is the quality of your life.

Health Care Professionals

It's important for your doctor to establish permission to talk about what may trouble you (and your family) and to answer any questions you may have, such as:

- How long am I going to live?
- How will I die?
- How will you help me?
- Whom do I call?
- How can I handle the costs?

And for your family:

- How will we know the time has come?
- How will we be able to manage the last few weeks and days?

Your doctor and nurse can relieve your mind about pain management and reassure you about your connection to your family and your health care team.

Other professional caregivers may help you in significant ways. Social workers can smooth out all kinds of problems: "I couldn't make it without my social worker. She got my insurance to cover hospice and ambulance service, and she helped me figure out how to talk to my children." You may find that meeting with a psychotherapist can be the most valuable support line for you. I have known women who were able to handle a grim prognosis knowing they had a dedicated therapist available when needed.

Family and Friends

Support and comfort, the feeling of being loved by your family and friends, are essential to maintaining your spirit. You can endure the rough times and enjoy the good times much better if someone is there for you, available and attentive, engaging or quiet. Joan's partner was always there for her, but she also knew when to back off and let Joan have time alone.

On the other hand, you may choose to keep your illness private so you're not badgered by family and friends calling and asking how you feel, how you *really* feel, and how they can help. Time is precious; save it for the ones you love most, those especially dear to you, those worth the emotional energy necessary for talking, sharing, seeking comfort. To learn more about how to protect your precious energy, see Chapter 8.

Religious, Spiritual, and Philosophical Comfort

Many people turn to religion, or to a religious counselor, even if they have not been particularly observant before. Rabbi Harold Kushner (author of *When Bad Things Happen to Good People*) says, "Talk to each other, to your clergyman, to yourself. We may not be able to cure you, but we can heal you. We can share sorrow, help cherish and care for those you love, and help each other to enjoy this last part of your life." The end may be bearable when it is filled with the love of those who matter to you, with the vision they represent of a future beyond your own lifetime.

There are some people who turn to alternative sources: meditation, yoga, or philosophic dialogue. Jane and her husband went to Michael Lerner's Commonweal in Bolinas, California. "At first I thought it might be too 'California' for me, but I got past that. I wasn't looking for a cure, but for help. And I found it. I came out feeling very serene, with a core sense that it didn't matter whether I lived or died— I had *lived*. I did not have to beat this illness to continue enjoying what time I had."

Support Networks

Boosting your support network can significantly improve your quality of life. Online discussion boards or in-person support groups can be a major source of strength, relief, warmth, comfort, love, and practical advice from other people in the same situation who share similar concerns (see Chapter 2). Online communities connect you to a web of people from all over the world who are ready to zoom in to provide much-needed support, twenty-four hours a day, every day, without leaving your home or work. Women with advanced breast cancer who were part of Dr. David Spiegel's support groups were less anxious and depressed, experienced less pain, and were generally in better spirits than similar women who did not participate in support groups.

These sources of support can also help fill the gap if your family won't talk openly with you—if it's just too hard and they don't have the strength or courage to make it work. Rita had to find another source of comfort. When she and her husband were told she was dying, he burst out, "What's going to happen to *me?*"

Hospice

If you are close to the end of your life, you may find that hospice care is the most responsive and effective resource available for providing pain relief and overall support, and for respecting your final wishes.

Hospice seeks to enhance the quality of dying, to provide physical and emotional support, in a humane and professional manner. Most patients report feeling immeasurably better once they've joined hospice and have started receiving hospice services. "We had this woman come in terrible pain, and in just a little while she was back to working on her computer."

Medical, psychological, and spiritual support are all part of hospice care. Hospice also provides supportive services for your family. Care comes from hospice nurses, social workers, physical therapists, nutritionists, chaplains, and volunteers who often have personal experience with the value of hospice (see Chapter 4). The team meets regularly to review each patient's situation and each family's needs, determine whether to call for special help—a child psychologist, for instance—or request volunteer assistance for errands or social visits.

You can get help with ordinary chores like bathing, dressing, cooking, and cleaning, as well as with logistical arrangements for transportation, equipment, nursing care, blood draws, drugs for pain, and counseling—even help with financial and estate plans. Some volunteers provide their most valuable support just by sitting with you or your family, a presence that keeps you from feeling helpless and alone and helps your family cope with the demands of this difficult time.

Starting hospice requires a doctor's referral, stating that you have come to the end of treatment and you believe you have a life expectancy of six months or less. Talk with your physician about hospice care as soon as you feel you can handle it. I find that my patients very quickly get to appreciate the support and care that hospice offers, and they begin to recover some sense of well-being. Hospice has even prolonged the lives of some of the people they have cared for.

If your doctor doesn't talk to

FEAR OF HOSPICE

Hospice doesn't *make* you die. It recognizes the fact that you are near the end of your life and makes dying as easy and comfortable as possible. "We help you *live*. We don't accelerate death." Still, some people have the mistaken notion that a commitment to hospice invites a self-fulfilling prophecy, that saying anything as explicit as "six months to live" becomes a death sentence, a fact, no matter what the state of your illness or well-being. Actually, the "six months to live" estimate is prepared primarily for medical insurance purposes, qualifying you for access to all hospice benefits under most insurance plans, including Medicare.

you about hospice, you should bring it up for discussion as early as possible, to find out whether it's for you, and to receive the maximum benefits possible from this service if you elect to use it.

You may want to interview several different hospice groups—if there is more than one available to choose from—to find the one that comes closest to your spiritual beliefs, plans for end-of-life care, and other issues that matter to you; your family should participate in these interviews as well. Most important may be how all of you relate to the particular hospice nurse who will supervise your care.

The doctor who refers you to hospice usually oversees medical decisions presented by the hospice nurses. But your physician's relationship with you does change when you begin hospice care: he or she is still involved in your care, but at a greater distance. You communicate primarily by phone and seldom go to the hospital or the doctor's office. This distance can often trigger separation anxiety that adds to your stress and sense of desperation. Don't let these feelings scare you: your doctor is still just a phone call away.

Your hospice nurse in fact becomes your primary source of caregiving, communicating directly with your doctor about your condition and checking about medications, comfort management, nutrition and hydration, and so on. For example, if you are distressed or have increased pain, you call your hospice nurse, who evaluates you and gets in touch with your doctor as needed. (The hospice nurse typically has streamlined access to your physician, access you benefit from though you may be unaware of it.) Pain medication is adjusted to suit your needs, in the form of pills, patches, liquids, injections, subcutaneous pumps, or epidural catheters. Potential side effects of pain medication are also handled by your hospice nurse.

Visits from hospice workers are based on need: they can be once a week or every day. "With technology what it is today, we don't have to move the patient back and forth—to draw blood, for instance." Wherever possible, hospice service and support is provided within your own home, so that you can spend your last days in a familiar place, in peace and dignity, surrounded by people you know and love. If home is not an option, you can go to a hospice facility that serves the same purpose. Most hospice people I know consider their work a calling, not simply a job.

YOUR FAMILY'S ROLE

Your family has a crucial role to play, provided you want them involved and they are willing, able, and available. Family members are instructed in how to give medication and physical care. Your children can help in practical and meaningful ways: brushing your hair; reading you the paper; massaging your neck, hands, or feet; telling you funny stories. They want to help and they need to feel they are contributing to your well-being.

If you have no family or close friends to step in for this role, home health aides may substitute. If you cannot take care of yourself completely at home, if you need twenty-four-hour care, or if you need continuous skilled nursing care, you may qualify for some form of additional in-home care, or if necessary you can go to a hospice center, nursing facility, or hospital.

If your family has been providing continuous care and must go away, twenty-four-hour respite care is available for up to a week under the hospice benefit, and this is covered by Medicare and most other policies. Depending on your insurance policy, where you live, and how long your family is away, the care may be provided in your home or at a hospice facility. Every hospice is different and every insurance plan is different, so you'll have to investigate which benefits are available in the hospice you sign up with.

Non-Hospice Options

The whole idea of hospice may not be quite acceptable to you—but don't be too quick to seek an alternative. (So very many people are so very grateful for its care.) If you still want to keep open the possibility of additional treatment, it is possible to get something similar to hospice care a step before hospice—"oncology care" at home—but the level of care is not usually as comprehensive as what you get from hospice.

Some families don't want strangers intruding on their privacy at this difficult time in their lives; they would rather do the caregiving themselves and would rather have their physicians continue in charge until the end. One of my patients strongly objected to the religious fervor of the hospice worker she met. "I don't believe in God and I don't want these admittedly well-meaning crusaders coming into my home as

I'm dying and talking about life in the hereafter." Some hospice programs are tied to religious organizations, though most are not, but even those that are usually do not impose their personal religious beliefs on you.

Many doctors offer end-of-life care rather than referring you to hospice, and they go on seeing you regularly, arranging for home care as needed or hospitalization if required. Even after you have decided to stop treatment, your doctors can continue to help you: ready and available to explain things clearly and honestly, let you know what to expect, and guide you to the right choices.

Beyond your health care team, great comfort and support can come from your religious leader or church group, online discussion boards and in-person support groups, an individual counselor, or professional connections, neighbors, or other people in your community or spiritual center.

Final Wishes

Getting your priorities together and in order can be established with a responsible member of your family, a trusted friend, the physician you feel closest to, or a lawyer you choose to manage your affairs. A lot of people ignore the need for a will, even as they reach old age. Ignoring this chore is risky. If you care about complications in your estate or your after-death arrangements, you'd be well advised to give at least minimal thought to formal provisions for carrying out your wishes. Face it, and start talking.

Beyond your wishes for your worldly possessions, a living will and advance medical directives can give legal standing to what you want to happen concerning your care should you become unable to make those decisions yourself. For you to get the most help possible from your relationship with your doctor, the two of you should have similar approaches to your care, and your doctor should know how you feel about end-of-life issues, expressed verbally and also in writing as a living will or advance directive.

With limited time, you may feel propelled to sort through your responsibilities and obligations and then set priorities. Focus on what is fulfilling, meaningful, and pleasurable for you. You may have to make some tough decisions—where you will direct your limited energy, what

EARLY ENDINGS

Everyone wants to die with dignity, comfort, and peace. But if you are suffering and you are close to the end of your life, euthanasia (painless death, or "merciful death") may have crossed your mind. You may have even joined the Hemlock Society, a group that believes in "death with dignity," using medicine to end life sooner, to end intolerable suffering. Experiencing intense pain or fearing intense pain often drives interest in early endings, including assisted suicide, although most people who manage to procure the "final exit" medication never end up using it. But having the medicine available just in case can provide them with great peace of mind. "It would give me peace to have something available as insurance, but my preference is to die naturally." "Without my ability to choose suicide I would have killed myself long ago."

But most doctors are not comfortable with the idea of assisted suicide because it's illegal in most places. Medications used to bring on the "final exit" require a doctor's prescription, and if you ask your physician to provide the prescription, you are asking him/her to be an accomplice to an illegal action, subject to arrest and imprisonment. So while your dedication to the quality and dignity of your life and death deserves the utmost respect, it can only be honored if it doesn't incriminate the people taking care of you.

If you want your doctor to help you relieve extreme pain, agitation, uncontrollable coughing, and difficulty breathing and if you are also ready to die sooner than later, all of these goals can be accomplished by increasing doses of the medication morphine. Most doctors and nurses who take care of people at the end of life are dedicated to relieving serious symptoms and try to honor reasonable wishes. In addition to being one of the most effective pain medications, very high doses of morphine can dramatically decrease respiration and blood pressure, and can lead to death.

If controlling how you die is important to you, then you should try to find a doctor and hospice nurse who will work as partners with you to support you in your search for a peaceful and painless, dignified, *natural* death.

you must try to finish, what you will decline to do, whom you will decline to see. Getting your affairs in order is a top priority for most women; it needn't relate to whether you're dying or not.

- Reexamine your will; assign or distribute personal possessions of special sentimental value.
- Check out pension and life insurance arrangements for your beneficiaries. Discuss college plans for your children or grandchildren.
- Discuss disposition of your family home.
- Talk to your family and your physician about hospice care, advance directives and living wills, and end-of-life medical decisions such as life support and other heroic measures.
- Reassign and train others to take over your responsibilities (verbally and on paper or computer or tape recorder), such as collecting and paying bills at various times of the month, tracking expenses for medical insurance and income tax filing, scheduling routine medical and dental checkups for the children, and checkups and license registration for the car and the dog.

Asked whether two dear friends' last weeks together were spent in tears and hand-holding, Helen said, "Of course not—we had too much to do."

Elsie had planned for years to get an appraisal for what she thought might be a valuable pottery collection, but she had always been too busy to get around to it. Assembling the collection, finding an appraiser, and arranging for the disposition of the collection was a welcome distraction for her during her last weeks, and it represented some kind of meaningful closure.

Managing significant parts of your life, even as you pass on that control, gives you some measure of satisfaction, perhaps even pleasure, through this hard time.

Accepting Help Without Feeling Helpless

If you find it difficult to accept help from others, try to relax your attitude. You must allow others to come in and help you with all kinds of stuff you shouldn't be doing. There really is a middle ground in which you do some things yourself and let others do the rest for you. Don't hesitate to call on your family and close friends for help. Those who love you are suffering in their own way, feeling helpless, unable to make you better. Anything they can do for you provides some relief, some sense that they are contributing to your well-being. Kim's friends got together and delivered dinner every day for months. Maybe you need a ride to and from the doctor, or medicine from the drugstore. Asking for help is a gift from you to others, and from others to you.

"I'm letting go of things that deplete my energy." Give up the dirty work, forget dust and clutter—take that as a doctor's order, direct from me. Even if you're a cleaning fanatic, let it go. Memories last, cleanliness doesn't. Save your energy for your family and close friends.

Still, you should hold on to what is most significant to you, what defines your relationship with your family and those you care most about. A well-intentioned family member may leave you feeling useless, even invisible, if he/she's taken over planning the meals, walking the kids to the school bus, and putting them to bed. "Some people want to take over everything for you, but my sister doesn't do that. 'You can do this,' she says. I feel almost cheerful when I'm doing something that matters."

Two friends in their sixties were married to older men. One told the other, who was dying: "I always expected that someday, when we were little old ladies in tennis shoes, the two of us would travel together, on the cheap, doing what nobody but us would want to do." Friendship that had started in grade school had lasted through the births of grandchildren, but it wasn't going to last into old, old age. Instead, the one to outlive the other was asked: "Will you be godmother to my grandchildren?" With the promise from her friend came assurance that the children she loved would be watched over, that life would go on, and that memories of a grandmother would be carried into the future.

FINDING THE RIGHT WORDS AT THE RIGHT TIME

You need to connect with those you care about. Maybe there are things you've always wanted to say. " 'You have been such a generous friend all these years' are words I treasure, that *my* generous friend told me during our last visit together."

Talk, talk, talk. Don't let a day go by without connecting to those you love. Sit down together as often as you can for some kind of together time; write, phone, or email. Long distance is cheaper than it's ever been and worth every penny.

It's often hard to find the right words. Some people can manage to say the right thing at the right time; others may say nothing when they should say something. And you can be sure that someone will say the wrong thing at the worst time, whether it's something stupid in front of your children ("Have you told them yet?") or something clumsy when you're alone together ("If you're going to die, I hope I'm not around to see it").

Sometimes the wrong remark can set you off. "How can you say you know how I feel? You're not dying! You have no idea how I feel!" Most people are not confronting death, as you are, but there is still much of value they can share and offer you and your family. The quiet and thoughtful ways that friends and family show they love you can be so important.

"Tell your children how much you love them. Tell them that you want them to think about you when you are no longer here. And that when they do, they may feel sad and happy and maybe even angry because you are not there—and that all those feelings will be very normal." Kelly told her five children and the rest of her family and all of her friends, "Don't whisper my name—*talk about me* out loud!"

Preparing Your Children

How do you prepare your children for what might happen to you? Young children may be comforted believing you will be up in heaven or out among the stars; older children want more reality-grounded answers. Whatever you say, talk as much as you can with your children; let them know you are able to face this tragedy as part of life.

If your children aren't asking questions, don't assume that they don't have questions in their heads, that there aren't things they want to and need to know. They may be afraid to ask, afraid to upset you. They may not know how to put their concerns into words. Or maybe they sense your reluctance to talk about what's happening to you. It really is better if you can get some conversation going.

Of first importance, let them know that your cancer is not their fault, that they had nothing to do with your illness. Until Brenda's doctor explained to the whole family that Brenda's cancer was in no way related to any past injury, Brenda's nine-year-old son was sure the blow he'd accidentally inflicted on his mother when he was swinging his baseball bat was what caused her cancer. Younger children often believe that any bad thoughts they had about you caused your illness.

You want to establish a safe environment, open to continual dialogue. "If there is anything you want to know, ask me. Do you have any questions?" "No, unless there's anything you need to tell me." Ten-year-old Pete was afraid to know and afraid not to know. Offer a little information at a time; keep talking to each other. Remember: there is little you can tell your children that will be worse than what they may imagine.

Dana had nightmares that went on for years after her grandmother died. She was only five years old when it happened, her family gave her only partial answers to her questions, and she was too young to visit her grandmother in the hospital (because of hospital policy) before her grandmother passed away. Somehow, Dana connected remarks about her grandmother's "last struggle" with a visit she had made to the zoo, and Dana's nightmare featured her grandmother in a ferocious and deadly struggle with a huge, scary gorilla.

Children catch bits of conversation; they see you with heads together whispering, arms tight round each other, somebody crying. They usually figure out that something is very wrong, and they go right to the most dreaded conclusion. You want them to know the truth, and you want them to hear it from you. But in the beginning, don't answer more than they ask until you know what they want to know and what they can handle. Here is what some of my patients said worked best for them:

I was totally honest, but I held back details, and I never gave more than they asked for.
Go slowly; encourage their responses and reactions.
Tell them, "That is an important question. Let's talk about it.
I won't tell you anything that isn't true."
If you can't answer every question, promise that you'll ask your doctor at your next visit.

The older the child, the more you can tell. People who have studied children say even a child of three understands that death means an end, so even a child of three must be given some kind of truthful explanation. Dr. Anna Kris Wolfe, a Cambridge, Massachusetts, child analyst, says not to deprive your child of hope. You can't know *absolutely* that you're about to die, so just leave it at that: "I'm very sick. I might die, but we are all hoping I'll get better." If nothing else, being together may be somewhat less strained and difficult, and your child gets a little more time to prepare for sorrow.

The intuitive thing to do may not be the best thing to do; kids and grown-ups think differently. It's important to get advice if you have questions about a particular situation, about how to explain what has happened—and to explain how a person lives on in your memory, in rituals, traditions, stories told, jokes, and lessons learned. People have very different gifts at explaining these hard things.

Nurturing into the Future

No one can replace you, but loving people can step in and help care for your children. The network of nurturing people already present in their lives, plus those who step forward to take on necessary roles, will help see your children safely into their future. "My parents and my sisters have promised me that as long as they live, they will be there for my children, but I don't want my kids to be motherless any longer than possible. I've made it clear to my husband that I want him to remarry—the right person—as soon as he can. I've even made a few suggestions, and warned him off some less than appealing candidates who'll likely be knocking at his door."

Jenny knew she didn't have much time. With two young children, she needed to prepare them as best she could for life without her, and she needed to provide them with memories of her love for them. "My body may go, but my spirit will always be with you." Jenny and her husband debated allowing their six-year-old to come see her in the hospital because Jenny looked so weak and unnatural, but they finally decided to allow the child to visit. As the little girl was leaving, she told her mother, "I have to say good-bye because you may die, and I'll never see you again." It was in fact the last time she saw her mother; how important and precious a memory—even though upsetting—that visit would always be for her.

If you are a single or divorced parent, communicating your wishes to your ex-spouse can be challenging. You also want to be clear with members of your family or with your good friends about trying to do what they can to oversee your children's welfare. And it's worth exploring any legal

CHILDREN'S PARTICIPATION IN AFTER-DEATH RITUALS

How much should children participate in rituals after a parent's death? Dr. Wolfe says children should be part of whatever the family does to mourn and celebrate the departed. If the family will be gathering for a funeral, the child should be included. Whatever is part of the family culture will help the child with his or her grief, help make the death real, and help the child get past the very natural effort to deny what has happened.

These ceremonies are sustaining, part of the mourning process, and children need all the help they can get to do their mourning. You might say they need to learn how to do it, and the adults are there to show them the way, with the appropriate ceremonies, rituals, and memorial days, with hugging and talking and crying. Everyone who loses a loved one feels some sense of abandonment, and it helps a child to see how adults respond to this loss and then move forward. Without help learning how to mourn and to grieve, children may carry too many unresolved issues of loss into their emotional future, compromising the important relationships of their life.

How much you include a child is a very individual decision and depends very much on the age of the child. In response to the question "Should the child go along to the cemetery? Should she or he watch the coffin go into the ground?" Dr. Wolfe answers, "You don't want the child to feel left out, but I think this can be very scary for a young child, who thinks in very concrete terms of what is happening. If the child is still trying to understand what *dead* is, he or she may imagine that burial is doing further harm to the parent. It's spooky enough for adults. You have to be very careful about this.

"A lot depends on the kind of family, and the rituals that are generally observed. If there's a lot of singing and spiritual rejoicing, it might work. It's probably helpful to visit the grave later on, but watching the interment could be very frightening. Adults and children search for a place in the physical world for the person who has died, so going to visit the grave later on and talking to the departed is a good thing."

protection a creative lawyer can manage, and to formally document your wishes. At least you'll find some comfort doing all you can.

Being Remembered

You may have all kinds of ideas for preserving memories for your children but find it hard to get around to doing them. It's not an easy thing to accomplish, but perhaps it will help if you think of it as a meaningful exercise for anyone—in good health or not—who wants to leave a permanent record for later generations. Whether you live another five decades, five years, five months, or five weeks, you'll be glad you assembled this material: messages, letters, notebooks, photographs. It's a commitment to the future, no expiration date at issue.

You may want to record greetings, messages, and hopes, on paper, tape, or video, for your family to store for the future. "I'm recording favorite stories, from *Goodnight Moon* to Beverly Cleary." Jenny wrote each of her children an inspirational letter about her love for them and her hopes for their future. When Esther's grown children were told she was dying, they flew in to be with her till the end, crowding onto her bed, holding and hugging each other. Her son Gil was consumed by a need to ask questions, to benefit from her quiet, earnest wisdom: What had been most important in her life? What did she hope he and his sisters would do with their lives? What did she believe to be the goals they should pursue? Esther, who had always worked in public service, was happy to talk about her life to her children. Gil also recorded his mother's memories of the family's history. "And I wrote down her recipes for all the great stuff she cooked."

✿ Moving Forward

I hope you have lived life your way. Dying should come about your way, too. You need to manage your life through to the end, and especially at the end. Other people's ideas about illness, suffering, and dying may intrude, but don't let them get in your way. Too many people worry their whole lives about how others perceive them, how others talk about them, how others judge them, and whether what they are doing is right.

I tell my patients, "This is your time; you call the tune." Your loved ones—especially your children—are looking to you to see how you're coping, how you're managing, how you live and how you die. It's not that you're being judged; it's more that you're showing them how to face this big thing. "I want to do this right for my children, to set an example for them, an example of living."

I find it a challenge and a privilege to take care of women throughout their lifetime, and to uphold and respect their wishes to the very end. I try to do what needs to be done "their way," without violating the code of ethics I live by and the Hippocratic Oath of care I took when I became a physician. The women who are my patients have taught me many things, most especially those who have made the transition out of this life with dignity, courage, and tremendous feelings for those they love.

Kelly gave explicit instructions to her family and friends: "Bring me with you!" She arranged to have a little bit of her ashes put into silver boxes that we all bring with us to fun and interesting places: rock concerts, great restaurants, parties—whatever. She was emphatic: "I want to go, too!" So Kelly comes with me everywhere I go; she was my friend (and patient) for life, and that didn't end when her physical, mortal life ended.

TO MY CHILDREN

If I ever stop breathing,
the flowers will inhale for me.
If I ever stop writing,
the grass will dot my i's.
If I ever stop listening,
the shells on the beach will hear you.
If I ever stop talking,
the rain will sing my song.
If I ever stop loving,
the sky will embrace you.
But if I ever stop living,
then you must live on for me.

—Susan Weisgrau

Through Crisis Comes Opportunity

No one ever made me any lifetime promise, and no one comes with a guarantee. So I live with a big question over my head—but still, this is a second chance. I don't postpone what I want to do. I get pleasure in simple things, and every day is an adventure.

The journey through breast cancer does not define your life—it is a chapter in your life. Ever since my doctor came into the recovery room to tell me, "Congratulations, you're cancer-free," I've felt like the luckiest unlucky person in the world!

🌿 New Beginnings

I hope our book has helped you. Maybe you've read every word in this book; more likely, you've skipped about and read what matters most to you at the moment, and studied a few parts in depth. You've had a truly tough journey, but now is the time for healing and restoring your health.

I hope you've drawn support from the independent, courageous, and generous voices you've heard in this text: the women who've shared secrets and opened up to feelings that had been pushed out of view, remembering incidents that were painful or rewarding as they went through treatment, learning how to cope with living *well* beyond breast cancer.

"Your life is consumed with fighting cancer through the whole period of treatment. When it's all over, first you want your life back, and then you realize, 'Whoa, I have a life. I have a life. Now what's my lifestyle?' I felt like I had to prove that I was the same—or better—than I was before. I wanted to look and be the same—and for people to treat me the same as before."

✿ The Bright Side of a Bad Deal

How you move through and beyond breast cancer is unique to who you are, your circumstances, the challenges in your path, and your ability to find and create workable solutions. Your experience may seem entirely different from anyone else's—or you may know many others who've experienced much of what you have.

You may have discovered amazing new inner powers you never knew you possessed. "My marriage had gone to hell, and very soon I was a single parent raising a four-year-old. And then I got breast cancer, at thirty-three. I was scared and worried—but I found an odd kind of courage. I wrote to my college sweetheart, whom I hadn't been in touch with for twelve years. He had never married—and we got together. He stayed by me the whole way, through treatment and hair loss (the worst), and now we're married. I would never have written to him if it hadn't been for the cancer. I figured I had nothing to lose and life is so short. Anything I wanted to do, I suddenly felt I could do."

Or you learn what's important: "My husband and I fought each other on almost every issue, from how to raise our two children to what to eat for dinner. With the discovery of my cancer, we forgot all the craziness and began treating each other like human beings." "I shocked my co-workers by speaking up at staff meetings and dressing in bright colors, where before I rarely opened my mouth and always wore black."

There are mixed blessings as well. Many of my patients have told me, "I wouldn't have asked for this to happen—but my life has never been better." "Now I really know who my true friends are." "I only focus on what's most important and don't sweat the small stuff." Anger can drive positive changes in your life. "I never dreamed I could hold such anger!" Jill couldn't tell family or friends how she felt—her emotions scared even herself—so she wrote a fierce and hate-filled letter to her cancer, ending with, "I didn't choose you, and you're not going to stop me!" Then she burned it, and eased away from anger to a new sense of calm. Nancy told me "I kept a journal. I could put that anguish—my anger—on paper. I didn't have to carry it around with me." Of course, there are plenty of others who feel powerless and can manage only by denying their fears and slamming the door tight against all talk of this disease. But with time, careful thought, and sensitive attention, many of you are able to collect and focus your strength and courage and forge on.

⚘ Making a Difference

There are many opportunities to heal and make a difference by turning "Why me?" into "Why anybody?" You've had this bad thing happen; now make something good come out of it. "I got handed lemons, so I made lemonade" is a popular refrain that resonates for many of the women I care for. Amazing things have been imagined, created, and fueled by turning anger into positive action.

No doubt about it: you take care of yourself when you take care of others. Dr. David Spiegel advises, "Extract meaning from what is happening to you; use your experience to help someone else." One woman, well known in her community, went on radio and TV, telling about her diagnosis and detailing how breast cancer touches everyone's world. "Scores of women wrote and told me they went out and had their first mammogram." Another woman: "I teach breast examination using hands-on models. I show them to the men, too: 'You won't touch this? You've touched your share of breasts in your life, I'm sure.' Maybe they're embarrassed, but they laugh, and do the check along with the women. A third of breast cancers are discovered this way, and I feel I'm helping."

"One of my favorite places to be is helping other patients in the hospital where I was treated. Just walking in that door puts a smile on my face. It remains such a place of hope and healing and—surprisingly— happiness." "I used to keep quiet and to myself, but when I got cancer, I decided to break out of my shell, reach out to others, and voice my thoughts and feelings. I joined the Breastcancer.org discussion boards and made friends with women from all over the world. We've become each other's support group—and whenever possible, we find opportunities to meet offline." Others drive patients to the hospital for their daily chemotherapy or radiation treatment, or join a hospice volunteer corps. But it doesn't have to be health-related volunteerism. "I just want to make tomorrow better for someone. I work as treasurer for a homeless shelter and feeding program." "I tutor children in an inner-city school."

Participation in a clinical trial can help you and others get closer to a cure. "My mother volunteered for a clinical breast cancer prevention study. It was the way she found to handle her distress, maybe her guilt, about my getting breast cancer. She told me, 'I want to be able to tell my granddaughters how to prevent breast cancer.'"

You can really make a difference to a cause and an organization. The contribution of your time, talent, and resources is what fires the battle. For sure, it's the power of each individual involved in my organization, Breastcancer.org, that gives us the strength and compassion to help millions of people worldwide.

Direct your energy to what you care about most, to where your passion lies, and bigger things will happen. Mind the yoga blessing *namaste*, which means "honoring and uniting the divine light within us all." Amazing power can come from inside you and all of those you touch. "Helping others keeps your mind off yourself. If I don't use my experience to help others, the experience was wasted on me. I don't intend to let that happen."

❧ Redefine Your Life

D on't let breast cancer define who you are and what you do with the rest of your life. "Deciding to fight for my life made me define myself and realize for the first time why my life was valuable."

Many of you have decided to live for each moment of the day, and every day to its fullest. "Grab hold of what's bothering you about your life and shake out the good stuff."

With each year that goes by, more and more of you will get to live a longer life. Research is turning up answers that we hope and expect will lead to cures for all forms and stages of breast cancer—*and* how to prevent it. Our greatest wish is that you, your children, your grandchildren, and their families can all breathe free and no longer have anything to fear from this dreadful disease.

"My husband told me, 'You can cry for a while, but then you have to figure out how to get yourself back together.'" "My friend wanted me to sit in a rocking chair and hold his hand. I want to explore the world. I've been given this second chance—and I'm going to use it!"

Index

About the Authors

DR. MARISA C. WEISS is the president and founder of the global non-profit organization Breastcancer.org. She has a thriving practice and has had multiple appearances on *Good Morning America,* CNN's *House Call,* the CBS *Early Show,* and NBC's *Today.* She serves as a medical expert to the *Wall Street Journal, New York Times, Washington Post,* ABCNews.com, MSN.com, and numerous magazines. She has also been a guest on NPR, CNN Radio, ABC Radio, CBS Radio, and Washington Post Radio. Dr. Weiss is the founder and past president of Living Beyond Breast Cancer (LBBC), a nonprofit organization. She is also the author of *Taking Care of Your "Girls,"* the first and only book on breast health for teen and tween girls, and the book *7 Minutes: How to Get the Most from Your Doctor Visit.* She currently practices at Lankenau Hospital in the Philadelphia area, where she serves as director of Breast Radiation Oncology and director of Breast Health Outreach, and she is a member of the Marine Biological Laboratory in Woods Hole, Massachusetts. She is a mother of three children and shares her recently emptied nest with her husband, David Friedman.

ELLEN WEISS, Marisa's mother, has served as editorial consultant to LBBC and Breastcancer.org. She co-authored the first edition of *Living Beyond Breast Cancer* and is the author of *Second-Hand Super Shopper.* An elementary schoolteacher and a mother of six children, she developed her writing skills, which found full expression in this book. A breast cancer survivor herself, with a family history on her father's side, she has a personal commitment to bringing the best information in the most caring form to the many women and their families facing this disease. She lives with her husband, Leon Weiss, close to Marisa, both in the Philadelphia area and in Woods Hole, Massachusetts.

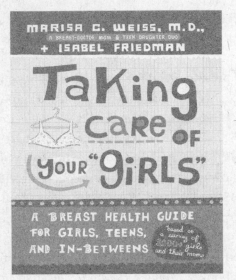